T0138336

Economic Aspects
of Health

A Conference Report
National Bureau of
Economic Research

Economic Aspects of Health

Edited by   Victor R. Fuchs

The University of Chicago Press

Chicago and London

VICTOR R. FUCHS is professor of economics at Stanford University and a research associate at the National Bureau of Economic Research. He has edited and is the author of numerous publications, including *Who Shall Live? Health, Economics, and Social Choice.*

The University of Chicago Press, Chicago 60637
The University of Chicago Press, Ltd., London

Library of Congress Cataloging in Publication Data
Main entry under title:

Economic aspects of health.

(National Bureau of Economic Research conference report)
"Papers . . . presented at the Second NBER Conference on Health Economics held at Stanford, California on July 30–31, 1980."
Includes indexes.
1. Medical economics—Congresses. 2. Health status indicators—Congresses. I. Fuchs, Victor Robert, 1924–   . II. NBER Conference on Health (2nd : 1980 : Stanford, Calif.) III. Series. [DNLM: 1. Economics, Medical—Congresses. 2. Health—Congresses. 3. Socio-economic factors—Congresses. WA 30 EL88 1980]

RA410.A2E23   362.1′042   81-15938
ISBN 0-226-26785-7   AACR2

To the memory of Walsh McDermott, M.D.

His knowledge, wisdom, and deep understanding of the multiple determinants of health benefited us all through the illumination of both policy and practice.

Contents

Acknowledgments

The Second NBER Conference on Health Economics, and the preparation of this volume, were supported by a grant from The Robert Wood Johnson Foundation to the NBER for research in health economics. This support is gratefully acknowledged. The opinions expressed herein are those of the authors and do not necessarily reflect the views of The Robert Wood Johnson Foundation.

Many people assisted in the planning and execution of the conference and in the preparation of this volume for publication. I would particularly like to express my appreciation to Alan Garber, who served as conference rapporteur and editorial assistant, to Kenneth Arrow, who was general discussant at the conference and who delivered informal remarks on health economics at the conference dinner, and to Claire Gilchrist, who did an outstanding job as conference coordinator.

Victor R. Fuchs

Introduction

Victor R. Fuchs

The papers included in this volume were presented at the Second NBER Conference on Health Economics held at Stanford, California on 30–31 July 1980. The first conference (V. Fuchs and J. Newhouse, *The Journal of Human Resources* 13, Supplement, 1978) was concerned with the economics of physician and patient behavior; i.e., it dealt with medical care markets in a traditional demand-supply framework. This second conference focused on the other principal concern of health economics— health status—as measured by mortality, morbidity, disability, and the like. Within this broad area the ten papers fall into three separate categories. Four papers report the results of empirical investigations of the determinants of health status; four are empirical studies of the consequences of ill health; and two are theoretical treatments of health in relation to public policy.

Determinants of Health

Two papers (Harris; Rosenzweig and Schultz) in the determinants category deal with fetal development and infant health; one (Fuchs) focuses on adults aged 25–64; the fourth (Taubman and Rosen) is concerned exclusively with the health of older males.

Harris pays particular attention to the relationship between prenatal care and outcome of pregnancy. He argues that previous attempts to study this question have been plagued by several significant conceptual problems. First, the relationship between the timing of prenatal medical visits and the duration of pregnancy has been poorly characterized. Although mothers with little or no care have a high proportion of preterm

Financial support from The Robert Wood Johnson Foundation and The Kaiser Family Foundation is gratefully acknowledged.

1

babies, it is possible that early termination of pregnancies from unrelated causes interrupts the course of care. In addition, the phenomena of spontaneous and induced fetal losses exert a powerful selective effect on maternal and fetal characteristics. As a result, mothers who initiate late care may have fitter infants than those who initiate early care. These differences in fitness may be difficult to observe (cf. Shepard-Zeckhauser in this volume); moreover, these unobserved maternal and infant health characteristics may affect the demand for care. It is unclear how nonexperimental, cross-section data can resolve these problems of inferring causality.

Harris's empirical work is based primarily on a sample of 6,800 black women in Massachusetts who were pregnant for at least twenty weeks during 1975–76. Using a continuous time stochastic model in which the initiation of care and the termination of pregnancy are competing risks, and controlling for other variables such as age, parity, schooling, and marital status, he finds that prenatal care appears to reduce the risk of premature birth. The relation between care and birth weight, given length of gestation, however, is much weaker.

In the last part of his paper, Harris addresses the question of the sharp decline in U.S. neonatal mortality since 1965. He shows that nearly all of the decline reflects a decrease in birth weight-specific mortality rates, not a shift in the weight distribution of births. How prenatal care might have contributed to this result is not at all clear. Harris argues that complex structural models are required to investigate this question, and presents some preliminary versions of such models. Although the conventional wisdom holds that prenatal care contributes to favorable pregnancy outcome because the physician modifies maternal behavior with respect to smoking, nutrition, and weight gain, Harris speculates that prenatal care may be serving as a proxy for a more complex set of phenomena associated with access to a wide range of social support services. Moreover, if prenatal care truly has a causal role, it may be because it permits early identification of those pregnancies which will most benefit from intensive *perinatal* care.

Rosenzweig and Schultz, like Harris, are concerned with the outcome of pregnancies, and they also devote a considerable portion of their paper to the theoretical and methodological problems that they believe have limited the usefulness of much previous research. In particular, they emphasize the necessity of jointly estimating the *demand* function for health production inputs (parental behavior) and the *production* function that relates behavior to health outcomes. Their model, which embeds a health production function in a utility-maximizing framework, distinguishes among (*a*) goods that are desired purely for their consumption value but have no effect on child health (e.g., a pretty dress); (*b*) goods that affect child health but otherwise provide no utility (e.g., medical care); and (c) goods that affect health and also directly affect utility (e.g., cigarettes). The key feature of this model is that the family does not maximize child health, but treats child health as one of many sources of utility.

One conclusion Rosenzweig and Schultz draw from their theoretical analysis is that a tax on a c-type good such as cigarettes does not unambiguously lead to better child health even if it is certain that cigarettes are harmful and that the tax will reduce the demand for cigarettes. The tax's effect on health will also depend on the relation between cigarettes, health, and other goods in the utility function. Rosenzweig and Schultz also stress that unobserved heterogeneity in the population (e.g., with respect to the health of the fetus) can bias estimates of the effects of medical care on pregnancy outcome. They propose a two-stage procedure in which the first-stage demand equations provide predicted values which can be used to obtain unbiased estimates of the production function parameters.

Along with many other authors in this volume, Rosenzweig and Schultz discuss the relation between schooling and health. They believe that greater parental schooling affects pregnancy outcome by improving parental perceptions of the true nature of the production function (leading to a different mix of inputs). They contrast this with the view that schooling improves health by raising the marginal products of a given set of inputs.

The empirical portion of the Rosenzweig-Schultz paper is based on a national probability sample of over 9,000 legitimate births in the United States during 1967, 1968, and 1969. Three measures of birth outcome are used in the analysis: birth weight, gestation period, and standardized birth weight (actual birth weight divided by predicted birth weight based on gestation).

The endogenous variables tested for potential influence on birth outcome are the number of months of elapsed pregnancy before the mother visited a medical doctor, the number of packs of cigarettes smoked by the mother while pregnant, the live birth order of the pregnancy, and the age of the mother at birth.

The exogenous variables include several related to the individual, such as schooling, income, and race, and several describing the area in which the individual resides, for example, hospital beds per capita, physicians per capita, unemployment rate of women, price of cigarettes, and availability of family planning programs.

The authors' most significant finding is that cigarette smoking by the mother has a large negative effect on birth weight, both unadjusted and adjusted for gestation. Assuming mean values for the other variables, a differential of one pack of cigarettes per day during pregnancy lowers birth weight by 279 grams, or by 8.5%. Delay in seeking prenatal care also is unfavorable to birth weight, but the effect is very small—45 grams as a result of a delay of six months. According to Rosenzweig and Schultz, the strong impact of smoking helps to explain some puzzling coefficients for other variables in the reduced-form equations. For instance, mothers with some high school education have lower weight babies than do mothers with no high school; also, residence in an SMSA (a Standard Metropolitan Statistical Area) tends to lower birth weight despite the greater availability of medical care. In both instances the authors suggest that the difference in smoking behavior is the reason.

One result which cannot be explained by smoking is the lower birth weight of babies born to black mothers. A standardized (for socioeconomic and area characteristics) differential of 185 grams is observed despite the fact that black mothers smoke much less than white mothers. After controlling for smoking, delay, age, and birth order, the black-white differential is 229 grams.

Fuchs, in his paper on time preference and health, argues that time preference (unwillingness to delay gratification) is likely to be negatively correlated with schooling, negatively correlated with investments in health (such as not smoking), and negatively correlated with health status. He believes that differences in time preference among individuals could help explain the frequently observed correlation between schooling and health, either because time preference is a determinant of investment in both, or because education changes time preference and subsequent investments in health. He assumes that capital market imperfections result in individual differences in the marginal rate of time discount, and that these differences can be measured (albeit imperfectly) by hypothetical questions.

The empirical portion of the paper reports the results of a telephone survey of five-hundred men and women aged 25–64. Time preference was measured by a series of six questions asking the respondent to choose between a sum of money now and a larger sum at a specific future time ranging from one to five years. The interest rates implicit in the questions varied from 10% to 50% per annum. Other questions dealt with family background, education, health behavior, health status, work and income variables, and expectations about inflation.

About two-thirds of the respondents gave consistent replies to the six money questions; any implied preference for a lower over a higher discount rate was defined as inconsistent. In analyses limited to the consistent replies, the implicit interest rate was found to be correlated with years of schooling (negative), cigarette smoking (positive), and health status (negative). Family background, especially religion, appears to be an important determinant of time preference.

Taubman and Rosen use a relatively new longitudinal data set (the Retirement History Study) to explore several long-standing questions regarding the relationships between health and schooling and marital status. The sample consists of approximately 10,000 white men who were aged 58–63 in 1969. Health status is defined in relative terms by the subjective evaluation of the respondent and by mortality or change in health status between 1969 and subsequent surveys in 1971 and 1973. The authors analyze the effects of the independent variables on the qualitative dependent variables by calculating cell means from frequency tables, with allowance for interactions where appropriate.

The effects of schooling on health in this sample are quite large. For instance, among married men with sixteen years or more of schooling, 47% report their health as better than average and 9% say it is worse than average. By contrast, among married men with eight years or less of schooling 28% classify themselves as in better than average health, while 25% say their health is worse than average. Holding schooling constant, divorced men appear to be in the worst health; widowers, surprisingly, evaluate their health at about the same level as that of married men.

The longitudinal aspect of the survey permits Taubman and Rosen to compare mortality rates by schooling, marital status, and initial health status. The death rate of married men is substantially lower than that of widowed, divorced, or single men at each level of schooling. This is true even after controlling for initial level of health. Many of the married men do show a worsening of health, however, suggesting that the presence of a spouse prolongs life, in part, by keeping a mate alive but in a state of ill health.

Holding marital status constant, the death rate of college graduates is about 20% lower than that of men with twelve years of schooling or less. Of those men alive throughout the four years, the better educated are more likely to report an improvement in health over time and much less likely to report a worsening. This is true either conditioned or not conditioned on level of health in 1969; the differentials are, however, smaller in the conditioned case.

More fully specified models include variables such as earnings or family income in 1968 and utilization of medical care. These variables do not significantly alter the schooling-health or marital status-health relationships. For married men, spouse's education is positively and significantly related to health, but the size of the effect is smaller than that of own education.

Consequences of Ill Health

Differences in health status can affect a wide variety of economic and quasi-economic behaviors, including the demand for medical care (considered in the paper by Manning, Newhouse, and Ware), educational attainment (Shakotko and Grossman), and labor market performance (Benham and Benham, Salkever).

It is quite obvious that health status is an important determinant of the demand for medical care. It is also obvious that errors in the measurement of health status can affect the coefficients and standard errors of all other variables not orthogonal to health status as well as bias the estimates of the effect of health status itself. The paper by Manning, Newhouse, and Ware addresses two principal problems in the measurement of health—the time of measurement and the kind of health measures used.

Most previous studies of the demand for medical care that have included a health status variable have measured health at time $t+1$ to help explain utilization during the period from t to $t+1$. Manning, Newhouse, and Ware show that such "postdiction" can cause inconsistent estimates of the effects of health status, whereas "prediction" (measurement of health status at t) is not subject to the same bias. This is true even if utilization does not affect health status; the problems with postdiction may be even more severe if it does.

One frequently used measure of health status—self-evaluation on a four-point scale of excellent, good, fair, or poor—receives some critical attention from the authors. They believe it needs to be supplemented with measures of limitation of function, psychological state, and social activity as well as counts of symptoms and chronic diseases. They also suggest that measures of attitude towards and knowledge of medical care may be useful in explaining utilization.

The empirical work is based on data for the first year of the Health Insurance Study in three sites (Seattle, Washington; Fitchburg, Massachusetts; and Franklin County, Massachusetts). The sample consists of 1,557 adults aged 18–61 who answered self-administered questionnaires at the beginning and the end of the year under study. The analysis is limited to covered outpatient expenditures, excluding those for mental health and dental care. The right-hand side variables, in addition to health status, include demographic characteristics, insurance coverage, income, and other variables relating to different aspects of the health insurance experiment.

The authors conclude that the more comprehensive measures of health status do increase explanatory power significantly; the gain in precision is at least equivalent to a 10% increase in sample size. The coefficients of some of the other independent variables are also affected, but the changes are typically not large. In the prediction-postdiction comparison, the health status coefficients are typically larger in the latter equations. This may reflect an effect of medical care on reported health problems (through greater awareness) or it may reflect the effect on utilization of exogenous variation in health status subsequent to t. Which explanation is the correct one is not resolved in this paper.

In discussions of the correlation between years of schooling and health status, numerous writers have suggested that at least part of the explanation may lie in a causal chain that runs from health to schooling rather than the reverse. Poor health in childhood, it has been hypothesized, may result in lower educational attainment. To be sure, economic theory does not unambiguously predict such an effect. It is theoretically possible that persons with poor health might seek more education as an offsetting investment.

Shakotko and Grossman investigate this question empirically with a longitudinal data set in which high school seniors were surveyed in the spring of 1972 and resurveyed in October of each year through 1976. The original sample included 21,000 seniors, but exclusion of nonwhites, students with mental or emotional handicaps, and those with missing relevant data reduced the number to 10,430 young men and women. Of these, 120 were reported by the school as having a physical disability. Compared to other students, the disabled scored somewhat lower on aptitude and achievement tests. After controlling for such differences, however, Shakotko and Grossman find no evidence that the disabled are less likely to pursue post-secondary education or more likely to leave such education sooner than the nondisabled. An analysis of earnings for those individuals in the sample who were employed full time in October 1976 provides weak evidence that the disabled have lower earnings but a higher rate of return to education.

With very few exceptions,[1] research on the economics of health has concentrated on physical health. The importance of mental illness is frequently acknowledged, but the difficulty of diagnosis, the uncertainty of the effects of therapy, the chronic character of many mental health problems, and the paucity of useful data have discouraged most economists from attempting systematic analyses. In their paper, Lee and Alexandra Benham attempt to analyze the effects of mental illness on employment and earnings, but the retrospective character of the diagnoses limits the authors' ability to infer causality. Instead, they report a series of interesting "associations" between various psychiatric disorders and labor market behavior.

Their data set consists of 434 white males born between 1910 and 1930 who, when their median age was 44, were the subjects of extensive interviews conducted by sociologist Lee Robins. Of this group, 365 had been patients at the St. Louis Municipal Psychiatric Clinic between January 1, 1924 and December 30, 1929. The other 69 "controls" had been selected on the basis of St. Louis elementary school records that showed socioeconomic characteristics similar to those of the 365 patients, but no record of school failures, school expulsions, or transfer to a correctional institution while in elementary school. Some thirty years after the referral to the clinic (or graduation from elementary school in the case of the controls) two or more psychiatrists assigned each individual to a psychiatric category on the basis of a personal interview plus information from relatives, police, schools, armed forces, credit bureaus, medical and mental hospitals, welfare agencies, and coroners. The diagnostic categories are: well, neurosis, psychosis, sociopathy, alcoholism, no diagnosis but sick, and no estimate.

Simple comparisons of mean values across diagnostic categories show that compared with the well, the mentally ill tend to have lower IQ's, less schooling, lower labor force participation, and lower earnings. They also tend to be in worse physical health and much less likely to be married with spouse present. In multiple regressions that control for schooling, marital status, IQ, and physical health, the mentally ill typically show lower earnings and lower labor force participation. The one conspicuous exception to all these findings is the neurosis category. Compared with the well group, individuals with this diagnosis have higher IQ's, more schooling, and substantially higher earnings even after controlling for IQ and schooling.

Nearly all economic investigations of the effects of ill health have concentrated on the behavior of the individuals whose health is under study. But the ill health of one person can clearly have effects on others, especially on other family members. For example, the mothers and fathers of disabled children may have different hours of work and earnings than do otherwise similar parents of healthy children. David Salkever addresses these and related situations with data from the Survey of Income and Education (SIE). This random sample of 151,170 households contains 4,000 households with children aged 3–17 with reported disabilities. Restriction of the study to white, two-parent, single-family households with no married children, no children over 18, no other relatives present, and no reported maternal health problems, reduced the number with disabled children to 2,685 families. They were compared with 3,200 families with no disabled children who were randomly selected from the larger sample.

Controlling for demographic and socioeconomic characteristics, Salkever finds that the mothers of disabled children are slightly less likely to be in the labor force. Those who do participate work significantly fewer hours than do comparable mothers of children without disabilities, and earn significantly less per hour. The effect on wages tends to increase with the age of the disabled child, suggesting a cumulative impact through differential accumulation of human capital. The effects on the fathers of disabled children are less clear cut, and frequently not statistically significant.

The presence of school work or school attendance limitations in disabled children seems to have a substantial additional effect on parental employment and earnings. These limitations, which may indicate greater disability, are associated with mothers' substantially lower employment and earnings compared to those of mothers with disabled children who have no such limitations.

Health and Public Policy

The last two papers in this volume are theoretical investigations of important aspects of health policy—the effects of population heterogeneity on policy choices (Shepard and Zeckhauser), and the properties of socially optimal health insurance plans (Bergstrom).

The central thesis of the Shepard-Zeckhauser paper is that heterogeneity among members of the population with respect to health poses a variety of important problems for analysis and policy. Heterogeneity is simply the differences among individuals in their responsiveness to different treatments. For instance, some people are more susceptible to heart attacks, some are more sensitive to pollution, some will benefit more from a new drug.

Unobserved (or latent) heterogeneity can introduce serious biases into interpretations of the effects of various health interventions. One type of bias arises in estimating efficacy for individuals (or homogeneous strata) based on observed data from a mixed population. Shepard and Zeckhauser show that failure to take account of potential heterogeneity can lead to incorrect inferences even in a randomized clinical trial. If initial application of the treatment results in the differential survival of high-risk individuals, over time the composition of the experimental group will be altered compared with that of the control group. One might then observe what appears to be diminishing effects of the treatment over time, even though there would be no diminution for a homogeneous population. The other type of bias arises in extrapolating from a known effect on an individual to the impact on a population. The authors show that the benefits of a favorable intervention will tend to be overstated in a mixed population if there is a greater reduction in mortality for high-risk individuals. This is because the intervention generally increases the proportion of high-risk people among survivors. As a result, subsequent morbidity and mortality is likely to exceed that which would be experienced in a population that did not include as large a proportion of high-risk individuals.

When heterogeneity is observable the problem becomes primarily one of incorporating both efficiency and distributional considerations into the policy analysis. Whose health should be considered in setting air pollution standards? The average person's? The health of the person at the 90th percentile of susceptibility? Is society ever justified in withholding medical care from a sick person, regardless of how low the probability is that the care will do some good? The authors discuss but do not completely resolve the ethical issues involved when cost-benefit or cost-effectiveness analyses are applied in the presence of population heterogeneity. They suggest one way out of the ethical dilemma through an "original position" approach.[2]

Bergstrom's theoretical investigation of desirable properties for health insurance yields provocative results. For instance, he shows that an optimal insurance plan would not include coverage for all treatments that are technically possible. Some care would be excluded because the cost would be too great relative to the potential benefit. Thus his model provides a theoretical rationale for ceilings on insurance coverage—a phenomenon frequently observed in private plans purchased by groups or individuals in the United States. It could also explain the explicit and implicit limits on care observed in centrally imposed, uniform national plans such as the British National Health Service.

A second discussion centers around the desirability of health insurance policies which pay a predetermined amount contingent on the insured's diagnosis rather than on the amount actually spent for care. This predetermined amount would permit the insured to buy the socially optimal amount of care for that diagnosis. Insurance plans of this type would eliminate the "moral hazard" implicit in policies which reimburse for actual expenditures and thus induce excessive care. Current insurance policies which reimburse for expenditures approximate the one discussed by Bergstrom to the extent that physicians order the socially optimal amount of care at any point in the treatment process.

The final section of the paper considers a model in which survival in impaired health is a possible outcome, along with death and full health. One striking conclusion is that a medical treatment which increased the probability of being an invalid and lowered the probability of dying without changing the probability of being healthy could be socially undesirable even if it were free. It would depend on how unpleasant and how costly it is to be an invalid.

Conclusion

Although the ten conference papers are quite diverse in their topics, data, and methodologies, three subjects appear explicitly or implicitly in many of them. They are (1) the definition and measurement of health status, (2) questions of heterogeneity and selectivity, and (3) the health-schooling relationship.

The question of how best to measure health status is given most explicit consideration by Manning, Newhouse, and Ware, but it is of considerable importance in nearly all of the papers. While Manning, Newhouse, and Ware emphasize the limitation of the "excellent-good-fair-poor" measure, Taubman and Rosen find that even a three-point subjective evaluation (better-average-worse) is a good predictor of subsequent mortality. Using the same Retirement History Study data in a study of labor market behavior, Fuchs found that self-reported health limitations by working men is an excellent predictor of future participation.[3]

Economists have typically emphasized physical measures of health status, but the Benhams' paper is a useful reminder that mental and emotional illness may have major economic consequences. The Shakotko-Grossman finding that the health status of high school seniors did not significantly affect their subsequent schooling might have been different if they could have measured mental as well as physical disability. In his paper, Fuchs experimented with alternative definitions of health status and found that conclusions regarding the relationship with schooling and time preference are altered somewhat by changes in the health measures.

In general, the papers appear to underscore two important truths about health. First, it is multi-dimensional, posing complex problems of valuation, especially when one is trying to assess the costs or benefits of some intervention that alters health status. Second, there is no one measure of health status (or even one summary measure) that is best for all purposes. The health status measure that is most useful for predicting medical care utilization may be very different from the one that is best for predicting mortality, and both may differ from the measure that is most useful for understanding labor force participation or earnings.

Questions of heterogeneity and selectivity, which are treated most fully in the paper by Shepard and Zeckhauser, appear explicitly or implicitly throughout the volume. These questions are receiving increasing emphasis in general econometric discussions.[4] The most important considerations for health economists are, first, to be aware of the potential biases that may be introduced by heterogeneity, and second, to be aware that there are some techniques for partly correcting for these biases. Finally, there is a major challenge to health economists to help policymakers think through the problems posed by observable heterogeneity. As government becomes increasingly involved in setting health and safety standards in the workplace and for a wide variety of goods and services, the need for more sophisticated cost-benefit analyses increases. For instance, it would probably be inefficient to set a safety standard for an occupation so high as to protect the most susceptible potential entrant to that occupation. But if the standard implicitly or explicitly excludes some workers, the distributional consequences need to be considered. Furthermore, economists will need to help policymakers try to achieve greater consistency across the diverse programs and regulations that impact upon health.

The third subject appearing in many of the conference volume papers is the schooling-health relationship. On the whole, there is strong confirmation of previous findings that this relationship is positive, and there is additional progress toward helping to clarify the nature of the relationship. Shakotko and Grossman's paper throws doubt on the hypothesis that the causal direction runs from health to schooling. Fuchs's emphasis on time preference suggests one mechanism through which education could affect health, as well as the possibility that both health and schooling are attributable to differences in time preference. Given the importance and robustness of the health-schooling correlation, additional research that clarifies the nature of the relationship would greatly increase understanding of the factors that determine health.

In general, the studies indicate that research on economic aspects of health has made considerable progress during the past fifteen years. Herbert Klarman's thorough review of the health economics literature through the early 1960s[5] reveals that only a small fraction of earlier research dealt with health per se. Health economists, for the most part, concentrated primarily on the demand for medical care, the supply of physician and hospital services, and problems of planning and organization of care.

In recent years economists have developed more powerful theoretical and statistical tools, have acquired more insight into health processes, and have gained access to larger and more diverse bodies of data. Many of the early attempts to estimate health production functions, for instance, relied on aggregate data for countries, states, or cities. The estimates in this volume are all based on microdata sets, in some instances very large ones. The papers reveal increasing sophistication about issues of measurement, more awareness of advances in econometric methodology, and a concern with real world health problems that augurs well for the future.

Notes

1. See, e.g., Rashi Fein, *Economics of Mental Illness* (New York: Basic Books, 1958).

2. Cf. John Rawls, *A Theory of Justice* (Cambridge: Harvard University Press, Belknap Press, 1971).

3. Victor R. Fuchs, "Self-Employment and Labor Force Participation of Older Males," *Journal of Human Resources* (Summer 1982), vol. 17, no. 3.

4. James J. Heckman, "Sample Selection Bias as a Specification Error," *Econometrica* 47 (1979): 153-161.

5. Herbert E. Klarman, *The Economics of Health* (New York: Columbia University Press, 1965).

1 Determinants of Health

1   Prenatal Medical Care and Infant Mortality

Jeffrey E. Harris, M.D.

In 1969, forty-three percent of expectant black mothers and seventy-two percent of expectant white mothers began prenatal medical care during their first trimester of pregnancy. By 1977, fifty-nine percent of black mothers and seventy seven percent of white mothers had begun prenatal care during their first trimester. Only 3% of expectant black mothers and 1% of expectant white mothers currently receive no medical attention before the onset of labor (U.S. National Center for Health Statistics 1978, Table A; 1980a, Table 20).

My main purpose in this paper is to inquire: How can we determine whether prenatal medical care has favorably influenced the outcome of pregnancy?

The role of prenatal care has been the subject of serious dispute in the obstetric and public health literature for nearly four decades. This dispute has been fomented in great part by the nonexperimental nature of the evidence. Virtually all studies of prenatal care analyze cross-section data on the uncontrolled experience of thousands of women and their pregnancies. The subjects under study are therefore self-selected. There are no randomized treatments. Possible confounding variables cannot be eliminated. Nor do the data reveal how the subjects actually made use of the medical services. This paper investigates in detail what inferences can and cannot be legitimately drawn from this type of evidence.

Jeffrey E. Harris, M.D., is at the Massachusetts Institute of Technology and the Massachusetts General Hospital. This research was supported in part by a grant from the Whitaker Health Sciences Fund. The author is currently a recipient of PHS Research Career Development Award DA-00072. Previously unpublished data presented in this paper were made available by the Office of Health Planning and Statistics, Massachusetts Department of Public Health. Valuable criticisms by W. DuMouchel, H. Farber, V. Fuchs, A. Garber, M. Grossman, J. Hausman, and D. McFadden are acknowledged. The opinions expressed in this paper are the author's sole responsibility.

Prenatal care is defined here as medical attention received from the time of conception up to, but not including, labor and delivery. The analysis of perinatal care, received during labor and delivery and in the neonatal period, is another matter.

This paper does not produce a definitive benefit-cost analysis of prenatal medical care. Nor does it pass final judgment on other determinants of pregnancy outcome. My main goal is a clear statement of the issues underlying this famous controversy. Along the way, some new methodological tools and new lines of investigation are suggested.

Prenatal Care and Infant Mortality: an Initial Examination

During 1975 76, there were 138,943 recorded live births in Massachusetts. Among live births, 1,229 infants (8.8 per 1000) died within 28 days of birth. Also reported were 1,335 fetal deaths. (In Massachusetts, reporting of fetal deaths beyond twenty weeks' gestation is legally required.)

The following analysis is based upon information encoded in the individual birth certificates and, where applicable, matched death certificates of these cases. Infant deaths beyond the neonatal period (28 days of age) were not analyzed. Similar cross-section data bases on linked birth and death records have been studied by Chase (1974, 1977), Chase et al. (1973), Cunningham et al. (1976), Gortmaker (1979), Kane (1964), Kessner et al. (1973), Kleinman et al. (1978), Lewit (1977), Mellin (1972), Morris et al. (1975), Niswander and Gordon (1972), Pakter and Nelson (1974), Russell and Burke (1975), Shah and Abbey (1971), Shwartz (1962), Shwartz and Vinyard (1965), Slesinger and Travis (1975), Susser et al. (1972), Taylor (1970), Terris and Glasser (1974), Terris and Gold (1969), Williams (1975), and others.

Figure 1.1 depicts the crude relation between the total number of prenatal visits reported during pregnancy and the probability of neonatal death among all live births. Intervals of one standard error are shown around each point estimate of the neonatal mortality rate. The point at the extreme right of the figure, corresponding to "?" on the abscissa, represents the neonatal death rate among women with an unknown number of prenatal visits. Although fetal deaths were excluded from the results shown in Figure 1.1, their inclusion does not alter the qualitative relationship displayed here.

On its face, Figure 1.1 suggests that the quantity of prenatal care, as measured by the reported number of prenatal visits, has a substantial effect on pregnancy outcome. Beyond an apparent minimum of three prenatal visits, the neonatal mortality rate rapidly declines. After approximately ten visits, however, the returns to prenatal care apparently diminish. Although the neonatal mortality rates beyond twenty visits are

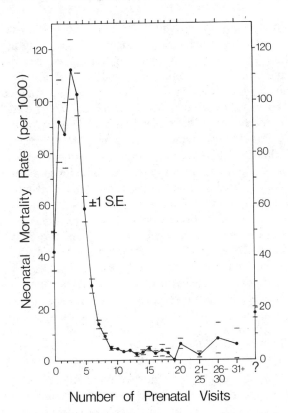

Fig. 1.1   Relation between number of prenatal visits and neonatal mortality rate per 1000 live births (Massachusetts, all races, 1975–76).

not very precise, the data suggest absolute decreasing returns to prenatal care.

In fact, not one of these conclusions is justified by the data. To see this, we must ask why some women report three prenatal visits, others report ten visits, and still others report twenty-five visits.

It is established obstetric practice in Massachusetts, and throughout the United States, for expectant mothers to follow a recommended schedule of visits—every four weeks for the first 28 weeks of pregnancy, every two weeks thereafter until the 36th week, then weekly until full term, and perhaps twice weekly if the baby is past due (U.S. National Center for Health Statistics, 1978; American College of Obstetricians and Gynecologists, 1974). The typical woman who recognizes her pregnancy at 6–8 weeks' gestation, follows the visit schedule recommended by her doctor, and delivers at 38–42 weeks will report about ten to fifteen visits. In fact, over two-thirds of the women in the sample reported a quantity of care in this range.

Those women reporting a quantity of prenatal care outside this range, however, constitute a much less homogeneous group. One important subpopulation of pregnant women, apparently concentrated among lower income and poorly educated groups, and among unmarried mothers and those of high parity, do not adhere to standard prenatal medical practice (Chase et al. 1973; Gortmaker 1979; Lewit 1977; U.S. National Center for Health Statistics 1978). These women may seek medical care only if they perceive some complication late in the course of pregnancy. Those mothers with no prenatal care may therefore represent a population with many fewer complications than those women with even one or two visits. In the range below ten prenatal visits, there is still another subpopulation of women who did follow the standard prenatal care schedule. As a result of placental insufficiency, infection, congenital anomalies, or other causes, their pregnancies—and therefore the course of prenatal care—were terminated prematurely. At the other end of the spectrum, women with previously established high risks (e.g., diabetes, rheumatic heart disease) or with increased risk detected during pregnancy (e.g., preeclampsia, intrapartum bleeding) seek care earlier and make more frequent prenatal visits. Among women with a large number of prenatal visits, however, there is also a group who were frequently monitored solely because they remained pregnant beyond their expected date of delivery.

Finally, 5.5% of live births of black women and 1.7% of live births of white women were recorded to have an unknown number of prenatal visits. Among those records with missing data on prenatal care, but with completed information on other characteristics, there was a disproportionate fraction of out-of-wedlock, higher order births, and teenage pregnancies. Since prenatal care information on live birth certificates is typically completed by hospital staff personnel and not by the mother, missing data are more likely to occur when the patient has no prior hospital record of the pregnancy (U.S. National Center for Health Statistics 1978, Technical Appendix). The unknown prenatal care category is therefore very likely to contain a disproportionate fraction of women with no prenatal care.

These facts seriously complicate the interpretation of Figure 1.1. Since early termination of pregnancy interrupts the normal course of prenatal care, the marked decline in neonatal mortality in the range of three to ten visits could mean that the extent of care is merely an indicator of fetal maturity. If the group with an unknown number of visits is composed primarily of women with no care, then the observed neonatal mortality for women who reported no care may be substantially overstated. Aside from this possible bias, the elevated neonatal mortality rate of the no care group could reflect poor socioeconomic status, illegitimacy, or other factors correlated with the demand for care. The increasing mortality rate in the range from zero to three visits, moreover, could reflect the higher complication rate among mothers who seek care only late in gestation. The possibility of increased mortality in the range beyond fifteen visits could merely reflect the higher medical risks of some mothers in that group.

Prenatal Care and the Duration of Pregnancy

To unravel these difficulties, I first examine in detail the relation between prenatal care and gestational age.

Many investigators (e.g., Eastman 1947; Oppenheimer 1961; Pakter et al. 1961) have noted that mothers with little or no prenatal care have substantially higher rates of preterm delivery. It has not gone unnoticed, however, that shortened gestation may interrupt the standard prenatal care schedule, and therefore induce a spurious correlation between prematurity and the total number of visits (Drillien 1957; Hellman 1953; Kane 1964; Shwartz 1962; Shwartz and Vinyard 1965; Terris and Glasser 1974; Terris and Gold 1969). Terris and Glasser (1974) recognized that this spurious correlation also applied to the time of initiation of care, since the interval to the first prenatal visit might just as well be truncated by early termination of pregnancy. Statistically adjusted measures of prenatal care, such as the average number of visits per week of gestation, were similarly inappropriate because the frequency of visits on the standard schedule increased later in pregnancy.

Despite repeated recognition, this paradox remains unresolved. Studies of the effect of prenatal care on other dimensions of pregnancy outcome (such as birth weight and mortality) have merely capitulated that the quantity of prenatal care and the duration of pregnancy were confounded variables. Hence, measurement of prenatal care was somehow to be adjusted for gestational age. Kane (1964), for example, excluded cases delivered prior to 38 weeks, while Chase et al. (1973, Table 3.9) excluded cases delivered prior to 36 weeks. Lewit (1977), and Russell and Burke (1975), included gestational age as an additional explanatory variable in ordinary least squares regressions of prenatal care on birth weight and infant death. (The fact that their linear specifications failed to correct for the nonlinearly increasing frequency of visits at the end of pregnancy was overlooked.) Wells et al. (1958) similarly adjusted for length of gestation in an analysis of covariance of prenatal care and perinatal death. The frequently cited Institute of Medicine study of New York City births in 1968 (Kessner et al. 1973, p. 59) constructed an a priori index of prenatal care adequacy, determined by the number of prenatal visits adjusted for gestational age. A given schedule was deemed "adequate" in this study only if the mother had private obstetrical care. The same adequacy index, exclusive of the private obstetrical care requirement, was subsequently used by Gortmaker (1979) in a multiple contingency table analysis. As in the Institute of Medicine study, this author assigned all observations with unknown care to the "inadequate" category (Gortmaker 1979, Appendix A).

None of these studies has had any bearing on the causal relation between prenatal care and the duration of pregnancy. The possibilities that prenatal attention could suppress early labor, or identify overdue mothers requiring induced labor, or screen out fetuses that are subsequently ill-fated, remain untested.

Prenatal Care and Premature Delivery as Competing Risks

At any time during gestation, a woman is subject to some instantaneous risk of termination of pregnancy. This risk of termination will depend upon the duration of pregnancy thus far, as well as other maternal and infant characteristics, including the presence of prenatal medical attention. The timing of prenatal care also represents of type of risk. That is, at any time during gestation, there is some instantaneous probability that a woman will make a prenatal visit, and in particular that a woman thus far without care will initiate prenatal care. This risk of visiting the doctor will depend in turn upon various maternal and infant characteristics.

Our problem is that the risk of visiting the doctor and the risk of termination of pregnancy are in competition. Among women who received no prenatal care, the termination of pregnancy occurred, in effect, before the initial visit could take place. Among those who did receive care, the initial visit occurred before the termination of pregnancy. In this context, we may inquire whether the initiation of prenatal care (when it does occur prior to termination of pregnancy) modifies the subsequent risk of pregnancy termination.

Let $\lambda_V(v)$ and $\lambda_T(t)$, respectively, be the instantaneous risks (or hazard rates) for making an initial visit and for termination of pregnancy. The rate $\lambda_V(v)$ is the probability that prenatal care is initiated in the short interval $(v, v+dv)$, given that no care has been received prior to time v. The rate $\lambda_T(t)$ is the probability that pregnancy will terminate in the short interval $(t, t+dt)$, given that gestation has lasted until time t. The concept underlying the hazard $\lambda_V(v)$ has been mentioned only once in the literature (Terris and Glasser 1974). The hazard $\lambda_T(t)$ is the more familiar gestational age-specific force of exit in a fetal life table (Bakketeig et al. 1978; Mellin 1962; Taylor 1970).

Consider the event that pregnancy terminates without prenatal care at time t. (Time is measured from the point of conception.) Provided that the risks of initiation of care and termination of pregnancy are initially independent, the probability of this event is

(1) $$\lambda_T(t)\exp[-\int_0^t\lambda_T(s)ds] \times \exp[-\int_0^t\lambda_V(s)ds]$$

The first expression in (1) is the probability that pregnancy terminated at time t. The second expression is the probability that prenatal care was not sought in the interval $[0,t]$. (See David and Moeschberger 1978; Lancaster 1979).

Let $\lambda_{TV}(t|v)$ be the risk of termination of pregnancy at time t, given that prenatal care was initiated at time $v\leq t$. The interdependence of hazard rates captured by this notation is a special case of the more general hypothesis that the number and timing of each prenatal visit affect the risk of termination of pregnancy. Now consider the event that care is initiated at time v and pregnancy subsequently terminates at time t. The probability of this event is

(2) $$\lambda_V(v)\exp[-\int_0^v\lambda_V(s)ds]\exp[-\int_0^v\lambda_T(s)ds]$$
$$\times \lambda_{TV}(t|v)\exp[-\int_v^t\lambda_{TV}(s|v)ds]$$

The first expression in (2) is the probability that prenatal care is initiated at time v and pregnancy did not terminate in the interval $[0,v]$. The second expression is the probability of termination of pregnancy at time t given that prenatal care was initiated at time v and that the pregnancy was intact at time v.

The hypothesis that the presence of care affects the subsequent rate of termination of pregnancy means that $\lambda_{TV}(t|v) \neq \lambda_T(t)$. When $\lambda_{TV}<\lambda_T$, prenatal care slows down the rate of termination of pregnancy; that is, it prevents prematurity. When $\lambda_{TV}>\lambda_V$, prenatal care accelerates the termination of pregnancy.

An Illustrative Test

Figure 1.2 depicts the frequency distribution of length of gestation among mothers with and without prenatal care in Massachusetts during 1975–76. The results in Figure 1.2 confirm the association between prenatal care and full term gestation: 29% of mothers with no prenatal care, as opposed to 5% of mothers with some prenatal care, had gestations less than 36 weeks' duration. (Although Massachusetts requires reporting only of pregnancies of 20 weeks' duration, a small fraction of the sample included pregnancies of shorter duration.)

To construct a statistical test of the hypothesis that prenatal care affects the duration of gestation, I need to impose some additional restrictions on the data and the model. First, I exclude cases with unknown prenatal care and unknown gestational age. (These are omitted in Figure 1.2 and constitute 4% of the entire sample.) In this illustration, the problem of

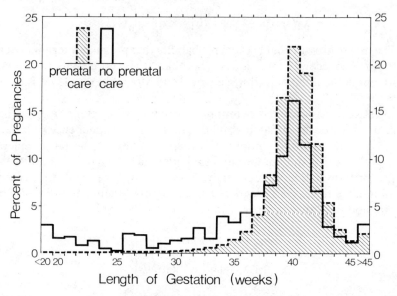

Fig. 1.2   Frequency distribution of length of gestation among women with and without prenatal care. Live births and fetal deaths (Massachusetts, all races, 1975–76).

nonrandomly missing observations is therefore not addressed. Second, I consider both live births and fetal deaths. Inclusion of fetal deaths admits the possibility that prenatal care prevents spontaneous abortion or other causes of premature delivery resulting in death during labor. Third, I examine only a subsample of 6,736 black women's pregnancies. The alternative of analyzing the pregnancies of women of all races, with indicator variables for each race, does not appear warranted at this stage. The effects of prenatal care among black mothers may differ considerably from the corresponding effects among other races.

I further restrict the model to the proportional hazards form

$$(3) \qquad \lambda_{TV}(t|v) = (1+\alpha)\lambda_T(t)$$

where $\alpha > -1$ is a constant, independent of t and v. Although the instantaneous effect of prenatal care on the rate of termination of pregnancy is assumed to be time-independent, the total effect of prenatal care on the duration of pregnancy will nevertheless depend upon the time of initiation of care.

To complete the statistical model, I need to specify how the hazards λ_T and λ_V depend upon time and other observed characteristics. Let $\underset{\sim}{X} = (X_1,...,X_K)$ be a vector of explanatory variables. I assume that λ_T and λ_V depend upon t and $\underset{\sim}{X}$ in the following way:

$$(4) \qquad \lambda_T(t|\underline{X}) = (\rho_T\omega_T)(\rho_T t)^{\omega T - 1} \prod_{k=1}^{K} (1 + \theta_{Tk}X_k)$$

$$\lambda_V(v|\underline{X}) = (\rho_V\omega_V)(\rho_V v)^{\omega V - 1} \prod_{k=1}^{K} (1 + \theta_{Vk}X_k)$$

The expressions $(\rho_T\omega_T)(\rho_T t)^{\omega T - 1}$ and $(\rho_V\omega_V)(\rho_V v)^{\omega V - 1}$ are Weibull hazard functions. The parameters ω_T and ω_V, in particular, incorporate the possibility that the rates of termination of pregnancy and initiation of prenatal care are time dependent. The hazard rate increases monotonically for $\omega > 1$, decreases monotonically for $\omega < 1$, and remains constant for $\omega = 1$. In the expressions $\prod_k(1 + \theta_{Tk}X_k)$ and $\prod_k(1 + \theta_{Vk}X_k)$, each parameter θ corresponds to the incremental effect of a given explanatory variable on one of the hazard rates. Each multiplicand $(1 + \theta X)$ represents the contribution of a specific explanatory variable to the proportional risks of termination of pregnancy and initiation of care. Under the restrictions (4), these proportional risks are assumed to be independent of gestational age. Similarly, under the restriction (3), the expression $(1 + \alpha)$ represents the contribution of prenatal care to the relative risk of termination of pregnancy.

Suppose that we have independent observations $\{t_i, \underline{X}_i: i = 1,\ldots,N\}$ on the durations of pregnancy and other explanatory variables for mothers with no prenatal care, and independent observations $\{t_j, v_j, \underline{X}_j: j = 1,\ldots,M\}$ on the durations of pregnancy, times of initiation of care and other explanatory variables among mothers with prenatal care. If the data $\{t_i, t_j, v_j\}$ are observed in continuous time, then the joint likelihood of these $N + M$ observations is

$$(5) \quad L^I = \prod_{i=1}^{N} \lambda_T(t_i|\underline{X}_i)\exp[-\Lambda_T(t_i|\underline{X}_i)]\exp[-\Lambda_V(t_i|\underline{X}_i)]$$

$$\times \prod_{j=1}^{M} \lambda_V(v_j|\underline{X}_j)\exp[-\Lambda_V(v_j|\underline{X}_j)](1+\alpha)\lambda_T(t_j|\underline{X}_j) \exp[-\Lambda_{TV}(t_j,v_j|\underline{X}_j)]$$

where $\lambda_T(t|\underline{X})$ and $\lambda_V(v|\underline{X})$ are defined in (4), and where $\Lambda_T(t|\underline{X}) = (\rho_T\omega_T)^{\omega T} \prod_k(1 + \theta_{Tk}X_k)$, and $\Lambda_V(v|\underline{X}) = (\rho_V\omega_V)^{\omega V} \prod_k(1 + \theta_{Vk}X_k)$, and $\Lambda_{TV}(t,v|\underline{X}) = (1+\alpha)\Lambda_T(t|\underline{X}) - \alpha\Lambda_T(v|\underline{X})$. This likelihood function, which I have superscripted with the numeral "I" to distinguish it from others used below, can be rewritten in the form

$$(6) \quad L^I = \prod_{i=1}^{N} \lambda_T(t_i|\underline{X}_i)\exp[-\Lambda_T(t_i|\underline{X}_i)](1+\alpha)^M\prod_{j=1}^{M} \lambda_T(t_j|\underline{X}_j)\exp[-\Lambda_{TV}(t_j,v_j|\underline{X}_j)]$$

$$\times \prod_{i=1}^{N} \exp[-\Lambda_V(t_i|\underline{X}_i)] \prod_{j=1}^{M} \lambda_T(v_j|\underline{X}_j)\exp[-\Lambda_V(v_j|\underline{X}_j)]$$

$$= L_T^I \times L_V^I$$

where L_T^I and L_V^I are multiplicatively separable in the parameters $\{\alpha, \omega_T, \rho_T, \theta_{Tk}\}$ and $\{\omega_V, \rho_V, \theta_{Vk}\}$ respectively. Hence, the maximum likelihood estimates of these two sets of parameters can be obtained separately without bias.

Table 1.1 displays the main characteristics of the subsample of black women's pregnancies. There were 82 neonatal deaths (12.3 per 1000 live births) and 43 fetal deaths. Among observations excluded from this sample because of missing information on birth weight, gestational age, initiation of prenatal care, or other explanatory variables, there were 29 additional neonatal deaths and 38 additional fetal deaths.

Table 1.2 displays the maximum likelihood estimates of the parameters of L_T^I and L_V^I in (6). The estimate of the parameter α is -0.293; that is, prenatal care reduces the risk of termination of pregnancy by 29.3%. The estimate of ω_T far exceeds 1; the risk of termination of pregnancy rises very rapidly with increasing gestational age. For the Weibull hazard function (4), the ratio of the mean gestational age of black mothers without prenatal care to the mean gestational age of black mothers with care throughout pregnancy is $(1 + \hat{\alpha})^{1/\hat{\omega}_T} = 0.978$ (approximate standard error 0.007). That is, for a 40-week pregnancy, the absence of care

Table 1.1   **Sample Characteristics of Pregnancies (6,736 Black Women, Massachusetts, 1975–76)**

Number of neonatal deaths	82	
Number of fetal deaths	43	
Percent initiated care in first trimester	74.5	
Percent initiated care in second trimester	20.9	
Percent initiated care in third trimester	3.6	
Percent with prior perinatal loss[a]	17.3	
Percent primagravida	39.7	
Percent recorded illegitimate	48.8	
Percent aged over 30 years	12.6	
Percent aged under 20 years	25.3	
Mean gestational age (weeks)	39.2	(s.d. 3.12)
Mean duration of prenatal care (weeks)[b]	28.5	(s.d. 7.90)
Mean birth weight (grams)	3123	(s.d. 619.)
Mean attained education (years)	11.6	(s.d. 0.22)
Mean annual volume of deliveries at hospital of birth (thousands)	3.1	(s.d. 2.09)

[a]Includes prior neonatal death or prior fetal death of at least 20 weeks' duration.

[b]Data on initiation of prenatal care was recorded by month of pregnancy. Calculation of weeks of care assumed that prenatal care was initiated at the midpoint of the recorded month of pregnancy.

(s.d. = standard deviation)

Table 1.2   **Maximum Likelihood Estimates of the Effect of Prenatal Care on the Rate of Termination of Pregnancy: Model I. (6,736 Black Women, Massachusetts, 1975–76.)**

		Parameter Estimates	
		L_T^I	L_V^I
Effect of prenatal care	α	−0.293	—
		(0.075)	
Weibull hazard parameters	ω	15.631	1.626
		(0.114)	(0.053)
	ρ	0.026	0.060
		(0.0001)	(0.004)
Parameters of Explanatory Variables			
Years of education	θ_1	−0.013	0.086
		(0.004)	(0.020)
Years of age over 30	θ_2	−0.003	−0.166
		(0.006)	(0.006)
Years of age under 20	θ_3	0.005	−0.076
		(0.010)	(0.008)
Illegitimacy	θ_4	−0.071	−0.260
		(0.022)	(0.017)
Prior perinatal loss	θ_5	0.091	−0.037
		(0.031)	(0.029)
Primagravida	θ_6	−0.001	0.254
		(0.028)	(0.032)
Log likelihood		−16734.3	−21371.9

Standard errors in parentheses.

reduces the mean gestational age by about 0.88 weeks (approximate standard error 0.28).

Table 1.2 also reveals statistically significant effects of attained education and prior fetal loss on the hazard of pregnancy termination. For black women with sixteen years of education, the risk of pregnancy termination is reduced by an estimated 12%, relative to black women with eight years of education (i.e., $(1 + 16\hat{\theta}_{T1}) \div (1 + 8\hat{\theta}_{T1}) = 0.88$, standard error 0.04). The interpretation of the statistically significant effect of illegitimacy (X_4) is more complicated. Since potentially confounding factors such as teenage pregnancy (X_3), first pregnancy (X_6), and reduced education (X_1) are held constant, the estimated reduced risk of early termination of pregnancy for illegitimate births may reflect the experience of relatively older black women of higher parity. I shall return to this puzzling observation later.

Table 1.2 shows that the hazard rate for the initiation of prenatal care also increases with gestational age (i.e., $\hat{\omega}_V = 1.63 > 1$.) The rate of initiation of care for black women with sixteen years of attained education is 41% greater than the rate of initiation of care for black women with eight years of attained education (i.e., $(1 + 16\hat{\theta}_{V1}) \div (1 + 8\hat{\theta}_{V1}) = 1.41$, standard error 0.06). This estimate corresponds to a 19% reduction in the mean time to initiate care (standard error 2.1%). For an expectant black mother who seeks care at 12 weeks' gestation, this represents an average reduction of 2.3 weeks in the mean time to the first visit (standard error 0.26). The combined effect of illegitimacy, advanced maternal age, and previous pregnancies is substantial. A 35-year-old multiparous woman delivering an illegitimate child has a rate of initiation of care one-tenth that of a primagravida in her 20s delivering a legitimate child (i.e., $(1 + 5\hat{\theta}_{V2}) \cdot (1 + \hat{\theta}_{V4}) \div (1 + \hat{\theta}_{V6}) = 0.1$). This corresponds to an estimated fourfold increase in the mean time to initiation of care (standard error 0.23).

These estimates were derived from a selected data base in the context of a specific parametric model. The conclusion that prenatal care reduces preterm delivery may not withstand alternative data bases, or a formulation other than the proportional hazards model of (3) and (4). It is noteworthy, however, that the estimate and standard error of the parameter α changed only minimally when I included other explanatory variables, such as type of care (private versus ward), the percentage of rental housing, the median income in the census tract corresponding to the mother's residence, or when I tried alternative specifications of the effect of maternal education and age. The results did not change substantially when fetal deaths were excluded from the sample. Although I assumed that the week of initiation of care corresponded to the midpoint of the reported month of initiation of care, the use of a more complicated likelihood function that incorporated the interval characteristics of these data also did not substantially alter the results. Finally, when I included observations with unknown care in the analysis, assuming that these women in fact received no care, the estimate of α was reduced in absolute value to -0.20.

Unobserved Characteristics and Fetal Selection

My analysis of the relation between prenatal care and the duration of pregnancy has thus far overlooked one serious problem of interpretation. Figure 1.3 depicts the relation between the month of initiation of care and the proportion of births of less than 36 weeks' gestation for white and black mothers. (Intervals of one standard error are shown for blacks. The corresponding standard errors for whites were considerably smaller, and are omitted for clarity.) Figure 1.3 shows that the increasing relation between late care and preterm delivery is interrupted during the third trimester. Since the 36th week of gestation occurs during the ninth calendar month, one can assume that this finding is not simply an artifact of the 36-week cutoff used in the figure.

In any cohort of pregnant women, the initial fetal population is likely to be extremely heterogeneous in its health characteristics. If this heterogeneity is reflected in their risks of termination of pregnancy—with the least fit infants having the highest hazard rates— then the phenomenon of fetal loss can play a powerful selective role. In comparison to the fetal population at the time of conception, those infants that have remained in utero up to the third trimester will necessarily contain a smaller fraction of ill-fated fetuses. One distinctive characteristic of mothers who initiate care in the third trimester is that their infants have remained in utero just that long. Hence, for no reason other than natural selection, late initiators of care may have infants with lower rates of pregnancy termination than earlier initiators of care. But this selection effect need not apply to mothers without care, whose infants may have been delivered at any time during gestation. These phenomena are exactly reflected in Figure 1.3.

If we could ascertain all the relevant determinants of variation in the risks of termination of pregnancy, then in principle we could fully account for this selection phenomenon. The difficulty with this solution is not merely its cost. Even if we could assemble detailed data on fetal ultrasound measurements, urinary estriol levels, maternal weight gain, and other factors for a large cross-section of women, there might still be substantial unobserved variation in fetal robustness. These unobserved characteristics would then be subject to selection. The inverse relation between late care and the duration of pregnancy might not be eliminated by conditioning on the observable characteristics.

Moreover, if the phenomenon of fetal loss selects out the least fit infants, then any factor that slows the rate of termination of pregnancy will also retard this selective process. If prenatal care, in particular, reduces the risk of termination of pregnancy, then at any given week of gestation, those mothers who had early care will tend to have a higher proportion of less fit infants. This possibility is also consistent with the data in Figure 1.3.

The problem is further complicated if the mothers under study could ascertain those health characteristics of their infants that are not revealed to the analyst in the data. Mothers who perceive their babies to be less fit, or potentially less fit, may initiate care earlier, while those with uneventful pregnancies may delay care. This hypothesis would account not only

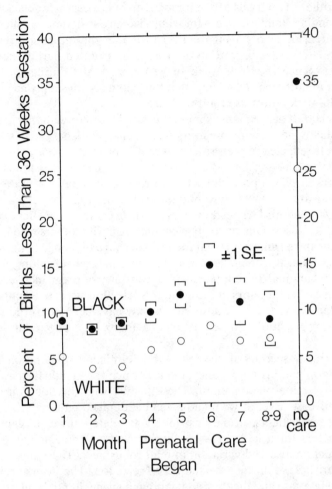

Fig. 1.3   Relation between month of initiation of prenatal care and percentage of births less than thirty-six weeks' gestation among white and black women. Live births and fetal deaths (Massachusetts, 1975–76).

for the lower proportion of preterm deliveries among late initiators of care, but also for the higher proportion of preterm deliveries among mothers who initiated care in the first month.

The data almost exclusively cover pregnancies of at least 20 weeks' duration. Hence, the cohort actually observed is likely to be more homogeneous than the original fetal cohort at the time of conception. The selective effect of fetal loss may therefore be less significant. Data from more complete fetal life table analyses (Bakketeig et al. 1978;

Mellin 1962; Taylor 1970), extending back to the weeks immediately after conception, reveal an initial period of relatively high hazard rates of pregnancy termination. As the ill-fated fetuses are progressively eliminated from the cohort, the overall hazard rate gradually falls. After approximately 20 weeks, the hazard rate then begins to rise. This increase in the hazard rate, however, does not imply that only robust infants remain in utero beyond 20 weeks. There is still likely to be substantial remaining variation in fetal characteristics up to and including the 40th week of pregnancy. Nevertheless, the censoring of early fetal deaths in our sample could bias estimates of the effect of prenatal care and other explanatory characteristics. If prenatal care prevented early fetal loss, for example, then it could extend an otherwise short pregnancy beyond the 20-week observational cutoff. On the other hand, the early medical attention could permit some women and their physicians to screen out and terminate an eventually ill-fated pregnancy before 20 weeks.

It is not at all clear how these complicated structural relationships can be identified with the available cross-section data. One possible strategy is to specify a model of the fetal selection process, and then to investigate how that model affects our inferences about the effects of prenatal care and other explanatory variables.

Let ε be a scalar index of fetal "defectiveness", whose value is restricted to be positive. Infants with low values of ε are more robust than infants with high values of ε. Although fetal defectiveness cannot be directly observed, it is assumed to affect the hazard rate for pregnancy termination. I denote this dependence by $\lambda_T(t|\underline{X},\varepsilon)$, retaining the specification that $\lambda_{TV} = (1 + \alpha)\lambda_T$. For a given cohort of pregnant women, ε initially has probability density $f(\varepsilon)$. Now let $G_{TV}(t|v,\underline{X},\varepsilon)$ be the probability that a pregnancy of defectiveness ε, with observed characteristics $\underline{X}$ and time of initiation of care v, survives at least to gestational age t. Then, by Bayes Rule, the probability density of ε among those infants with characteristics $(v,\underline{X})$ who remain in utero at least to age t is

(7)
$$f(\varepsilon|t,v,\underline{X}) = \frac{G_{TV}(t|v,\underline{X},\varepsilon)f(\varepsilon)}{\int_0^\infty G_{TV}(t|v,\underline{X},\zeta)f(\zeta)\,d\zeta}$$

A similar formula applies to mothers with no prenatal care, where G_{TV} is replaced by G_T, the corresponding probability of survival.

If λ_T is an increasing function of ε, then for a given $(v,\underline{X})$, both the mean and variance of $(\varepsilon|t,v,\underline{X})$ decline with increasing t. That is, as a result of fetal selection, those infants remaining in utero are on average less defective and more homogeneous as gestation advances.

In keeping with the proportional hazards specification, I now let $\lambda_T(t|\underline{X},\varepsilon) = \lambda_T(t|\underline{X})\varepsilon$. Moreover, I let ε have a gamma density with mean 1 and variance $1/h$. That is,

(8) $$f(\varepsilon) \propto \exp[-h\varepsilon]\varepsilon^{h-1}$$

Then for pregnancies with defectiveness ε and characteristics $(v, \underset{\sim}{X})$,

(9) $$G_{TV}(t|v, \underset{\sim}{X}, \varepsilon) = \exp[-\Lambda_{TV}(t, v|\underset{\sim}{X})\varepsilon]$$

where, in the case of mothers with no care, Λ_{TV} is replaced by Λ_T. From (7), (8), and (9), we obtain

(10) $$f(\varepsilon|t, v, \underset{\sim}{X}) \propto \exp[-(h + \Lambda_{TV}(t, v|\underset{\sim}{X}))\varepsilon]\varepsilon^{h-1}$$

where, again, in the case of mothers with no care, Λ_{TV} is replaced by Λ_T. The conditional density of ε is therefore also gamma, but with mean $h/(h + \Lambda_{TV}) < 1$ and variance $h/(h + \Lambda_{TV})^2 < 1/h$. Since Λ_{TV} is an increasing function of t, the mean and variance of ε decline with gestational age. Moreover, if $\alpha < 0$, then Λ_{TV} is an increasing function of v. That is, late care accelerates the process of selecting the least defective infants.

From (9), the probability that a woman will still be pregnant at t, given characteristics $\underset{\sim}{X}$ and initiation of care at v, is

(11) $$G_{TV}(t|v, \underset{\sim}{X}) = \int_0^\infty G_{TV}(t|v, \underset{\sim}{X}, \varepsilon)f(\varepsilon)d\varepsilon$$

$$= \left[\frac{h}{h + \Lambda_{TV}(t, v|\underset{\sim}{X})}\right]^h$$

The probability that a woman will deliver at t, given initiation of care and v and characteristics $\underset{\sim}{X}$, is therefore

(12) $$\left[-\frac{\partial}{\partial t}G_{TV}(t|v, \underset{\sim}{X})\right] \cdot G_{TV}(t|v, \underset{\sim}{X})$$

$$= (1 + \alpha)\lambda_T(t|\underset{\sim}{X})\left[\frac{h}{h + \Lambda_{TV}(t, v|\underset{\sim}{X})}\right]^{h+1}$$

Now suppose that we have independent observations $[t_i, \underset{\sim}{X_i}: i = 1, \ldots, N]$ on the durations of pregnancy and characteristics of women with no care, and independent observations $[t_j, v_j, \underset{\sim}{X_j}: j = 1, \ldots, M]$ on the durations of pregnancy, the times of initiation of care, and the characteristics of women with prenatal care. If there are no unobserved determinants of the hazard rate λ_V for initiation of care, then the joint likelihood of these observations is $L_V^{\mathrm{I}} \times L_T^{\mathrm{II}}$, where

(13) $$L_T^{\mathrm{II}} = \prod_{i=1}^N \lambda_T(t_i|\underset{\sim}{X_i})\left[\frac{h}{h + \Lambda_T(t_i|\underset{\sim}{X_i})}\right]^{h+1}(1 + \alpha)^M$$

$$\times \prod_{j=1}^M \lambda_T(t_j|\underset{\sim}{X_j})\left[\frac{h}{h + \Lambda_{TV}(t_j, v_j|\underset{\sim}{X_j})}\right]^{h+1}$$

Maximum likelihood estimates of the parameters $\{\alpha, \rho_T, \omega_T, \theta_{Tk}, 1/h\}$ in L_T^{II} are presented in Table 1.3. The estimate of the variance of ε is significantly different from zero. The maximum value of log L_T^{II} is substantially greater than the corresponding maximum value of log L_T^{II} in Table 1.2. Strictly speaking, Model I is the limiting case of Model II for $1/h \downarrow 0$. Therefore, its parameters are not properly in the interior of the parameter space of Model II. But it is sufficient to note that a null hypothesis of any arbitrarily small value of $1/h$ will be rejected in favor of Model II, and that L_T^{II} is right hand continuous at $1/h = 0$. Hence, Model II represents a substantially better fit than Model I.

The maximum likelihood estimate of α in Table 1.3 is -0.351, as compared to -0.293 in Table 1.2. That is, our previous failure to account for fetal selection in Model I resulted in a biased estimate of the effect of prenatal care. The magnitude of this bias, however, is not too large. For example, the ratio of the mean gestational age of black mothers without prenatal care to the mean gestational age of black mothers with care throughout pregnancy is $(1 + \hat{\alpha})^{1/\hat{\omega}T} = 0.977$ (standard error 0.008). (Under our proportional hazards specification, this ratio is independent of ε.) That is, for a 40-week pregnancy, the absence of care reduces the mean gestational age by about 0.94 weeks (standard error 0.32). For the parameter estimates in Model I, the corresponding reduction was 0.88 weeks (standard error 0.28).

The maximum likelihood estimate of ω_T in Table 1.3 is significantly greater than that in Table 1.2. When we ignore fetal selection, the hazard rate appears to rise more slowly because the high-ε (less robust) fetuses are being progressively eliminated from the cohort (see also Lancaster 1979). Similarly, the estimate of θ_{T5} in Table 1.3 exceeds the corresponding estimate in Table 1.2. That is, fetal selection operates more effectively on mothers with a prior history of fetal loss, and therefore failure to account for fetal selection leads to underestimates of the impact of this risk factor.

The model of equations (7) through (13) applies to the omitted regressor ε in the determination of the hazard rate λ_T. But a completely analogous argument could be applied to the determination of the hazard rate λ_V. If we assume that $\lambda_V(v|\underline{X}, \delta) = \lambda_V(v|\underline{X})\delta$, where δ is the unobserved characteristic, and if δ similarly has a gamma density at the onset of pregnancy, and if δ is distributed independently of ε, then we can derive a likelihood L_V^{II} in a manner analogous to that for L_T^{II}.

Maximum likelihood estimates of the analogous parameters for L_V^{II} are presented in the right-hand column of Table 1.3. Again, the log likelihood substantially exceeds that in Table 1.2, and the estimate of the variance of the observed regressor has a small standard error. The estimate of ω_V is similarly increased. Moreover, many of the estimates of

Table 1.3   **Maximum Likelihood Estimates of the Effect of Prenatal Care on the Rate of Termination of Pregnancy: Model II, Incorporating Unobserved Regressors (6,736 Black Women, Massachusetts, 1975–76)**

		Parameter Estimates	
		L_T^{II}	L_V^{II}
Effect of prenatal care	α	-0.351 (0.084)	—
Weibull hazard parameters	ω	18.217 (0.198)	2.094 (0.039)
	ρ	0.026 (0.0002)	0.072 (0.006)
Parameters of explanatory variables			
Years of education	θ_1	-0.012 (0.006)	0.115 (0.037)
Years of age over 30	θ_2	-0.004 (0.008)	-0.019 (0.008)
Years of age under 20	θ_3	0.012 (0.014)	-0.104 (0.008)
Illegitimacy	θ_4	-0.044 (0.032)	-0.305 (0.025)
Prior perinatal loss	θ_5	0.134 (0.048)	-0.027 (0.046)
Primagravida	θ_6	-0.028 (0.036)	0.313 (0.053)
Variance of unobserved regressor	$1/h$	0.207 (0.018)	0.427 (0.034)
Log likelihood		-16652.9	-21214.7

Standard errors in parentheses.

θ_{Vk} in Table 1.3 differ significantly from those in Table 1.2. For example, since improved education accelerates the rate of initiation of care, it will tend to eliminate high-δ mothers from the cohort, and thus reduce the average hazard rate for initiation of care. Hence, the estimates of the effect of attained education in Table 1.2 will be biased downward. This is confirmed in Table 1.3.

The most important limitation of this analysis is the assumption that the unobserved regressors ε and δ are independently distributed. This restrictive assumption does not admit the possibility that fetal and maternal health characteristics are correlated with prenatal care demand factors and in particular, that mothers' perception of the health of their pregnancy affects the rate of initiation of care. For example, the statistically significant negative estimate in Table 1.2 of the effect of illegitimacy status on the hazard rate of pregnancy termination is pulled toward zero but remains negative in Table 1.3. Among black women delivering children out of wedlock, especially those of high parity, some mothers may have very low risk pregnancies. Those who anticipate an uneventful pregnancy may also have much lower rates of initiation of care. If we do not take account of fetal selection, illegitimacy status appears to deter preterm delivery. The introduction of two independent sources of variation in the hazards λ_T and λ_V apparently eliminates some of this bias. But it does not fully incorporate the possibility that the underlying health of the pregnancy affects the demand for care.

One possible solution to this difficulty is to allow for interdependence of the omitted regressors ε and δ. In the instant case, this suggestion would require a joint distribution whose marginal densities are gamma. Although there is a class of such bivariate gamma distributions (Johnson and Kotz 1972), they do not appear to admit a correlation coefficient that can assume both positive and negative values. More important, my preliminary experiments with such bivariate densities suggested that the correlation coefficient between ε and δ and the parameter α could not be simultaneously identified. For the present competing risk model, it appears difficult if not impossible to ascertain both the effect of prenatal care on the subsequent risk of preterm delivery and the possible feedback effect of the underlying health of the pregnancy on the demand for care. A similar statistical predicament has been noted for analogous normal models with discrete endogenous variables (Schmidt 1981).

Prenatal Care and the Rate of Intrauterine Growth

I now focus on the relation between prenatal care and birth weight. Since the duration of pregnancy indirectly affects weight at birth, I concentrate on the effect of prenatal care on birth weight conditional upon gestational age.

Figure 1.4 shows the relation between gestational age and mean birth weight according to the trimester of initiation of care, among mothers of all races in Massachusetts during 1975–76. Both live births and fetal deaths are included. These data correspond to the empirical intrauterine growth curves of the obstetrical literature (Gruenwald 1966, 1974; Lubchenco 1975; Williams 1975).

Figure 1.4 appears to confirm the commonplace finding that prenatal care improves birth weight, conditional upon gestational age (Chase et al. 1973; Gortmaker 1979; Kessner et al. 1973; Lewit 1977; Russell and Burke 1975; Shah and Abbey 1971; U.S. National Center for Health

Statistics 1978). In the range from 39 to 42 weeks' gestation, mothers who initiated care in the first trimester have infants with mean birth weights 200–300 grams greater than mothers who received no care. The relation between the timing of care and birth weight follows a dose-response pattern.

The results in Figure 1.4 could merely reflect the confounding influence of such factors as education, socioeconomic status, and race, all of which could affect both the timing of care and birth weight. To eliminate this possibility, we must specify a model of the effect of care on birth weight, conditional upon these potentially confounding variables as well as upon gestational age. As in the previous sections, it is more appropriate to confine the analysis to a single race, rather than to employ an indicator variable for race in a study of the entire sample. Beyond that, however, the choice of an appropriate model is not clear.

One complicating factor is that the data of Figure 1.4 represent weight at birth among a cross-section of infants of different gestational ages, and not the intrauterine growth curve of any one infant during the course of pregnancy. If there is a systematic relation between the duration of gestation and the rate of intrauterine growth across infants, then the slopes of the empirical curves in Figure 1.4 are biased measures of the rate of intrauterine growth. Since the determinants of these variations in the risk of pregnancy termination or the rate of intrauterine growth may be difficult to observe, we must again confront the problem of fetal selection. This means that prenatal care and other explanatory factors will affect not only the intrauterine growth rate of a given infant, but also the distribution of these unobserved factors across infants. Unless we are prepared to make strong parametric assumptions, the net effect of these complicated interactions is not obvious.

In order to compare the effects of prenatal care on intrauterine growth rates with the previously discussed effects on the duration of pregnancy, I shall specify a relatively simple model. Let the rate of growth of fetal weight be a function of gestational age and other explanatory factors, including the extent of prenatal care. This function is assumed to take the form

$$(14) \qquad \frac{dw}{dt} = \Phi(t, \underset{\sim}{X}) \Psi(v) + v$$

where dw/dt is the growth rate of weight, t is gestational age, $\underset{\sim}{X}$ is a vector of explanatory variables, $\Psi(v)$ measures the proportional effect of prenatal care, and v is a stochastic error term. I further approximate $\Phi(t, \underset{\sim}{X})$ by the polynomial

$$(15) \qquad \Phi(t, \underset{\sim}{X}) = \beta_1 + 2\beta_2 t + 3\beta_3 t^2 + \sum_{k=1}^{K} \eta_k X_k$$

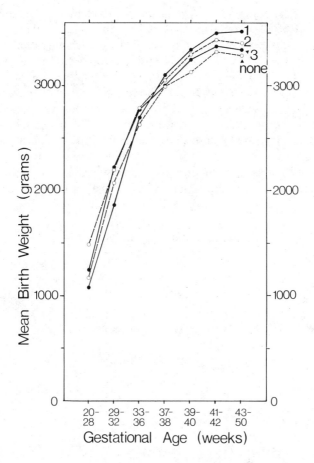

Fig. 1.4   Relation between gestational age and mean birthweight according to trimester of initiation of prenatal care. Live births and fetal deaths (Massachusetts, all races, 1975–76). Note: the gestational age intervals are of unequal duration.

In accord with the presentation of the data in Figure 1.4, I let

$$(16) \qquad \Psi(v) = \prod_{i=1}^{3} (1 + \gamma_i Y_i)$$

where $Y_i = 1$ if initiation of care occurs in trimester i, and zero otherwise. From (14), (15), and (16), and the initial condition $w(0) = 0$,

$$(17) \qquad w = (\beta_1 t + \beta_2 t^2 + \beta_3 t^3 + \sum_{k=1}^{K} \eta_k X_k t) \prod_{i=1}^{3} (1 + \gamma_i Y_i) + vt$$

In this parameterization, the parameters η_k measure the absolute contribution of each explanatory variable X_k to the rate of intrauterine growth (in grams per week), while the parameters γ_i measure the proportional effect of prenatal care. Moreover, the variance of the stochastic error vt increases with gestational age. A simple regression model of absolute birth weight with homoskedastic errors would therefore attach too much statistical weight to the high gestational age infants.

Table 1.4 presents maximum likelihood estimates of the parameters of (17) under the assumption that the error component vt is normally distributed with mean zero and variance $\sigma^2 t^2$. The estimated effects of maternal age, legitimacy status, prior perinatal loss, and parity are statistically significant. Prenatal care appears to increase the rate of intrauterine growth by about 2% in comparison to no care. But the estimated effect is statistically insignificant (at the 5% level). Moreover, there is no

Table 1.4   Effect of Trimester of Initiation of Care on Rate of Intrauterine Growth (6,736 Black Women, Massachusetts, 1975–76)

		Parameter Estimates
Gestational age (weeks)	β_1	−183.946 (7.775)
Gestational age squared (weeks²)	β_2	13.612 (0.479)
Gestational age cubed (weeks³)	β_3	−0.175 (0.007)
Years of education	η_1	0.042 (0.080)
Years of age over 30	η_2	0.533 (0.093)
Years of age under 20	η_3	−0.197 (0.147)
Illegitimacy	η_4	−2.293 (0.377)
Prior perinatal loss	η_5	−1.265 (0.463)
Primagravida	η_6	−1.208 (0.405)
Care initiated 1st trimester	γ_1	0.020 (0.020)
Care initiated 2nd trimester	γ_2	0.024 (0.020)
Care initiated 3rd trimester	γ_3	0.027 (0.024)
Variance of error term v	σ^2	187.622 (2.180)

Standard errors in parentheses.

clear dose-response relation between the onset of care and the rate of intrauterine growth.

Although the specification (17) is hardly general, a weak effect of prenatal care on birth weight was reproduced when I specified an additive effect for care rather than the multiplicative form (14), when I employed alternative measures of the quantity of care, and when I allowed for different multiplicative interactions between prenatal care and other explanatory variables.

Consider a multiparous, married black mother in her 20s, with twelve years of education, with no prior history of perinatal loss. If she received no prenatal care and delivered at 38 weeks, then from Table 1.4 her infant's birth weight is expected to be 3,063 grams. If we hold constant the duration of pregnancy, then prenatal care initiated in the first trimester adds an expected 61 grams to birth weight. However, if we calculate the total effect of initiation of care in the first trimester, inclusive of its effect on gestational age (about 1 week), then prenatal care adds an expected 169 grams to birth weight. With respect to the determination of birth weight, the contributing effect of prenatal care on the rate of intrauterine growth is considerably less than the contributing effect of prenatal care on gestational age.

The finding that prenatal care has a relatively weak effect on intrauterine growth rates among black infants is not so surprising. Although retarded fetal growth (in particular, placental insufficiency) can be detected during pregnancy, there is little in the way of treatment (Shearman et al. 1974). Although maternal cigarette smoking substantially retards intrauterine growth (Hasselmeyer et al. 1980), there is little evidence that the advice of medical practitioners has affected this practice. Only approximately 30% of current female smokers of all races quit smoking during pregnancy. Among women of all races who were last pregnant during the period 1965–75, only 35% of cigarette smokers reported receiving any physician advice about smoking (J. Harris, unpublished). Nor can I find any evidence that prenatal care has induced mothers to forego alcohol abuse. Despite all the recent advances in understanding nutrition and maternal weight gain (Niswander, Gordon et al. 1972; Habicht et al. 1974), a recent controlled trial of nutritional supplementation among black women in New York City yielded negative results (Rush et al. 1980). This study permits the striking interpretation that caloric supplementation for pregnant mothers merely ends up distributed to remaining family members (Jacobson 1980).

Prenatal Care and Infant Mortality: A Repeat Examination

Birth weight has been repeatedly found to be a critical determinant of perinatal survival (Cunningham et al. 1976; Niswander, Gordon et al. 1972; Shah and Abbey 1971; Shapiro, Schlesinger and Nesbitt 1968; U.S.

National Center for Health Statistics 1965, 1972). At any given birth weight, neonates of preterm gestational age are at greater risk than full term infants (Susser, Marolla, and Fleiss 1972). The consensus of the literature, however, is that prenatal care exerts an influence on mortality solely through its effect on birth weight. The Institute of Medicine study, for example, noted that in a linear regression with infant death as a dependent variable, the addition of a medical care "adequacy" index plus six other independent variables had no explanatory power beyond that of birth weight alone (Kessner et al. 1973, p. 63). In Gortmaker's (1979) multiple contingency table analysis, prenatal care had no consistent effect on neonatal mortality among white mothers when birth weight was included as a predetermined variable. Among black mothers, prenatal care of "intermediate" adequacy (as opposed to "adequate" or "in-adequate" care) was found to have a significant effect. Shah and Abbey (1972) similarly found birth weight to be the critical intervening variable in the determination of neonatal and post-neonatal survival. Neonatal mortality, adjusted for birth weight, they found, was lower among women who initiated care in the third trimester.

The problem with all these conclusions on the effect of prenatal care is that they do not square with a critical fact about the recent, renewed decline in infant mortality in the United States.

From 1965 to 1970, the U.S. infant mortality rate declined from 24.7 to 20.0 deaths per 1,000 live births, an absolute decrease in the mortality rate equal to that for the entire period from 1950 to 1965. By 1978, the U.S. infant mortality rate had reached an estimated 13.6 per 1,000 (U.S. National Center for Health Statistics 1977, 1979, 1980a). In contrast to the pattern of mortality decline during the first half of this century, most of the recent absolute decline in infant mortality represented an improvement in neonatal survival. At least beyond 20 weeks' gestation, a substantial decline in fetal death rates was also observed. These improvements in infant survival applied to all races.

Figure 1.5 depicts the relation between birth weight and neonatal mortality, determined from matched birth and death records for the United States in early 1950 and 1960 (U.S. National Center for Health Statistics 1972, Table D), and for Massachusetts during 1969 to 1978 (Massachusetts Department of Public Health, unpublished). From 1950 to 1960, the largest proportional decline in mortality occurred among infants weighing over 2,500 grams. This category comprised only about one-quarter of all neonatal deaths in 1960. During 1969 to 1978, by contrast, there was a substantial decrease in mortality for infants weighing between 1,000 and 2,500 grams.

The contributions of these changes in birth weight-specific mortality to the total absolute decline in neonatal mortality in Massachusetts is calculated in Figure 1.6. The height of each open bar represents the observed

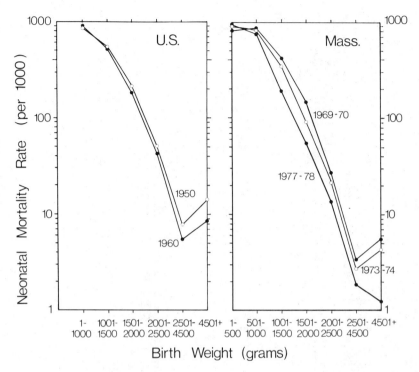

Fig. 1.5   Relation between birthweight and neonatal mortality rate per 1000 live births. United States, 1950–60; Massachusetts, 1969–78.

neonatal mortality rate among all races in Massachusetts for each year from 1969 to 1978. The height of the combined open and cross-hatched areas for the years 1970 to 1978 represents the birth weight-adjusted neonatal mortality rate. I calculated this rate by applying the birth weight-specific mortality rates for each year to the distribution of birth weights prevailing in 1969. Over 90% of the absolute decline in neonatal mortality in Massachusetts, Figure 1.6 shows, represents an improvement in birth weight-specific mortality.

There is considerable indirect evidence that the trends indicated by Figure 1.5 are representative of the entire U.S. experience (Pakter and Nelson 1974, p. 859; Kleinman et al. 1978; Chase 1977). The percentage of low birth weight and very low birth weight infants in the United States has declined somewhat during the past fifteen years. But this change is a fraction of the amount required to explain the decline in mortality if birth weight-specific mortality had remained unchanged (Lee et al. 1980).

A small fraction of the observed improvement in birth weight-specific mortality may represent favorable shifts in maternal age and parity (Mor-

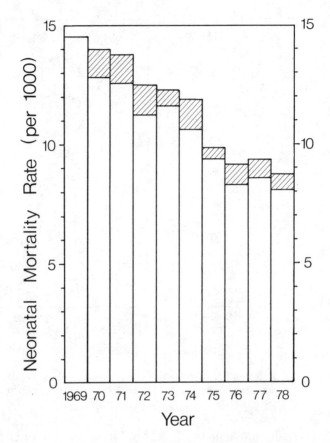

Fig. 1.6   Observed and birthweight-adjusted neonatal mortality rate per 1000 live births (Massachusetts, all races, 1969–78). Neonatal mortality rates correspond to open bars. Birthweight-adjusted neonatal mortality rates correspond to summation of open and cross-hatched bars. See text.

ris et al. 1975). Although the measurement convention for gestational age was made more precise only after 1968, there is little evidence that the joint distribution of birth weight and gestational age has changed significantly.

There are two explanations for this trend. First, we now have better medical care for the perinatal period, including labor, delivery, and early neonatal life. This improved care includes advances in neonatal intensive care, transport of high-risk mothers to regional centers, treatment of Rh-incompatibility and neonatal jaundice, and improved understanding of neonatal respiratory distress syndrome (Borkowf et al. 1979; Kitchen and Campbell 1971; T.R. Harris 1978; Stern 1976; Usher 1977).

Second, infants of a given birth weight have become healthier. This explanation frequently invokes family planning, contraception, elective abortion, genetic screening, and the elusive fact that babies are now more wanted (U.S. National Center for Health Statistics 1980*b*; Jacobowitz and Grossman 1980).

It is hardly clear what role, if any, prenatal care has played in this scenario. If the continued growth in the demand for prenatal care has had a significant impact on infant survival, then we should expect to observe a relation between prenatal care and birth weight-specific mortality in cross-section data. Moreover, if prenatal care in fact prevents early termination of pregnancy or enhances intrauterine growth rates, it is unclear why concomitant changes in the proportion of premature infants were not observed.

Table 1.5 shows the relation between birth weight and neonatal mortality according to the month of initiation of prenatal care for all races. Except for the Unknown Care category, the neonatal mortality rates for mature infants (over 2,500 grams) are indistinguishable. In the low birth weight category, those mothers who initiated care in the first month are at somewhat greater risk. The neonatal mortality rate then increases as care is delayed to the sixth month. But among those initiating care in the third trimester, the mortality rate for low birth weight infants is substantially lower.

We now see the pitfalls of a priori classifications of the amount of care based upon clinical standards (Kessner et al. 1973; Gortmaker 1979; U.S. National Center for Health Statistics 1978). Aggregation of mothers with no care and third trimester care into a single "inadequate" care category would produce a contradictory relationship between adequacy of care and birth weight-specific mortality.

The results in Table 1.5 again confront us with the problem of fetal selection. I have already suggested that the fetal population varies substantially in the rate of pregnancy termination. The sources of this variation, I further suggested, are largely unobserved. Similarly, infants of the same birth weight may vary considerably in their survival characteristics, with the sources of this heterogeneity also largely unobserved. The results in Table 1.5 suggest that those latent characteristics determining the pregnancy termination rate are correlated with those latent characteristics that determine birth weight-specific mortality.

This explanation is certainly plausible. Congenital anomalies, infection, maternal smoking, or placental insufficiency may shorten gestation and affect survival characteristics. The task of devising a structural model to test this hypothesis, however, is plagued by problems of identification.

Let μ be a latent characteristic that affects the probability of survival. An infant survives, I assume, if $\mu \leq \bar{\mu}$, where $\bar{\mu}$ may depend on various explanatory variables $\underline{X}$, including birth weight, gestational age, and the amount or timing of prenatal care. For a given cohort of pregnant

Table 1.5   Neonatal Mortality in Relation to Birth Weight and Month of Initiation of Prenatal Care (All Races, Massachusetts, 1975–76)

Month of Initiation of Care	Birth Weight ≤ 2500gm	Birth Weight > 2500gm
1st	115.4 (8.7)	1.8 (0.3)
2nd	99.0 (4.9)	1.9 (0.2)
3rd	90.8 (6.1)	2.0 (0.3)
4th	88.6 (10.4)	1.3 (0.4)
5th	94.0 (14.3)	1.2 (0.5)
6th	113.3 (22.2)	2.0 (1.0)
7th	30.5 (15.0)	2.2 (1.3)
8th or 9th	16.1 (16.0)	3.0 (2.1)
No Care	173.3 (30.9)	1.9 (1.9)
Unknown	143.3 (19.8)	5.3 (1.4)

All rates per 1,000 live births. Standard errors in parentheses.

women, if μ were distributed independently of ε, then the probability of death, conditional upon $(t, v, \underline{X})$ is

$$(18) \qquad \int^{\infty} \bar{\mu}(t, v, \underline{X}) f(\mu) \, d\mu$$

where $f(\mu)$ is the marginal density of μ. When μ has a logistic distribution, for example, equation (18) is the logistic model (Lewit 1977). When μ is normally distributed, (18) is a probit equation.

Suppose, however, that ε and μ were not independent across pregnant women. Then the distribution of μ, like ε, will change during the course of pregnancy. If ε and μ are positively correlated, then as gestation progresses, the proportion of low-ε types, and therefore the proportion of low-μ types, will increase. If $f(\mu \mid \varepsilon)$ is the conditional density of μ given ε, then the probability of death, conditional upon $(t, v, \underline{X})$ is now

$$(19) \qquad \int_0^{\infty} \int^{\infty} \bar{\mu}(t, v, \underline{X}) f(\mu \mid \varepsilon) f(\varepsilon \mid t, v, \underline{X}) \, d\mu \, d\varepsilon$$

where $f(\varepsilon \mid t, v, \underline{X})$ is defined in (7). Hence, if μ and ε are correlated, the single equation probit or logistic model (18) will lead to biased estimates of the effect of prenatal care and other explanatory variables. The structural parameters of $\bar{\mu}(t, v, \underline{X})$ cannot be estimated separately from those determining the hazard rate for pregnancy termination and therefore the density $f(\varepsilon \mid t, v, \underline{X})$.

The main problem in applying (19) to our data is that we must impose some restriction on the density $f(\mu \mid \varepsilon)$ in order to identify these structural parameters. That is, we must decide in advance how the selective process of eliminating high-ε infants affects the distribution of μ. Unfortunately, our inferences about the structural parameters are likely to be very sensitive to the type of restriction imposed.

The results of one such restriction are illustrated in Table 1.6. Both columns represent estimates of the parameters of $\bar{\mu}(t, v, \underline{X})$, which is assumed to be a linear function of gestational age, the duration of care, and other explanatory variables, including birth weight. Both neonatal and fetal deaths are included.

The left hand column of Table 1.6 (denoted Model III) corresponds to the case where μ and ε are assumed to be independently distributed (18). Specifically, I assume μ has gamma distribution with mean 1 and variance $1/h$. If we have independent observations $\{t_p, v_p, \underline{X}_p : p = 1, \ldots, P\}$ on surviving infants and $\{t_q, v_q, \underline{X}_q : q = 1, \ldots, Q\}$ on perinatal deaths, then the likelihood of these observations, conditional upon the time of initiation of care and the explanatory variables, is $L_T^{\mathrm{II}} \times L^{\mathrm{III}}$, where

$$(20) \qquad L^{\mathrm{III}} = \prod_{p=1}^{P} J(\bar{\mu}(t_p, v_p, \underline{X}_p)h; h)$$

$$\times \prod_{p=1}^{Q} [1 - J(\bar{\mu}(t_q, v_q, \underline{X}_q)h; h)]$$

where $J(x; y) = [\Gamma(y)]^{-1} \int_0^x e^{-z} z^{y-1} dz$ is the complete gamma function.

Since L^{III} does not involve any of the parameters of L_T^{II}, Table 1.6 displays only the parameters of L^{III}. The log likelihood at the bottom of this column is the maximized value of $\log L^{\mathrm{III}}$.

The right-hand column of Table 1.6 (denoted Model IV) corresponds to a special case of interdependence between ε and μ (19). Specifically, I assume that ε and μ have a degenerate one-dimensional distribution; that is, they have an identical gamma density with mean 1 and variance $1/h$. Again consider the likelihood of the observations $\{t_p, v_p, \underline{X}_p : p = 1, \ldots, P\}$ on surviving infants and $\{t_q, v_q, \underline{X}_q : q = 1, \ldots, Q\}$ on perinatal deaths. In each subset, some mothers will report prenatal care, others will not. The likelihood of these observations, conditional upon the time of initiation of care and the explanatory variables, is $L_T^{\mathrm{II}} \times L^{\mathrm{IV}}$, where

Table 1.6   Maximum Likelihood Estimates of the Effect of Prenatal Care on the Probability of Perinatal Survival (6,736 Black Women, Massachusetts, 1975–76)

	Model III Parameter Estimates	Model IV Parameter Estimates
Constant term	−0.254 (0.403)	0.379 (0.229)
Gestational age (weeks)	0.095 (0.013)	0.001 (0.007)
Duration of prenatal care (weeks)	−0.010 (0.009)	0.002 (0.002)
Birth weight (kilograms)	1.212 (0.295)	0.646 (0.032)
Annual volume of deliveries (thousands)	0.066 (0.032)	0.045 (0.018)
Years of education	−0.014 (0.023)	−0.005 (0.012)
Years of age over 30	−0.034 (0.027)	−0.013 (0.016)
Years of age under 20	−0.033 (0.034)	−0.024 (0.023)
Illegitimacy	−0.035 (0.097)	0.062 (0.064)
Prior perinatal loss	−0.224 (0.133)	−0.156 (0.077)
Primagravida	0.048 (0.151)	−0.029 (0.083)
Variance of omitted regressor μ	0.413 (0.143)	0.176 (0.015)
Log likelihood	−314.09	−17013.75

Standard errors in parentheses. Estimates of the parameters $\{\alpha, \rho_T, \omega_T, \theta_{Tk}\}$ for Model IV are not displayed.

$$(21) \qquad L^{IV} = \prod_{p=1}^{P} J(\bar{\mu}(t_p, v_p, \underset{\sim}{X}_p)[h + \Lambda_{TV}(t_p, v_p | \underset{\sim}{X}_p)]; h)$$

$$\times \prod_{q=1}^{Q} [1 - J(\bar{\mu}(t_q, v_q, \underset{\sim}{X}_q)[h + \Lambda_{TV}(t_q, v_q | \underset{\sim}{X}_q)]; h)]$$

where Λ_{TV} is replaced by Λ_T in cases where no care was obtained. The partial likelihood L^{IV} involves not only the parameters of $\bar{\mu}$, but also $\{\alpha, \rho_T, \omega_T, \theta_{TK}\}$, which appear in L_T^{II}. Unlike Model III, the parameters of L_T^{II} and L^{IV} must be estimated jointly. Since the estimates of $\{\alpha, \rho_T, \omega_T, \theta_{TK}\}$ were very close to those in Table 1.3, they are not shown in Table 1.6. The log likelihood at the bottom of the right-hand column is the maximized value of log ($L_T^{II} \times L_T^{IV}$).

For Model III, with μ independent of ε and therefore no fetal selection, birth weight and gestational age significantly affect the probability of survival. The duration of care, on the other hand, has an estimated negative effect. For Model IV, which incorporates fetal selection, the effect of prenatal care is weakly positive, whereas the influence of gestational age appears to be reduced. The latter parameter, however, captures only the direct effect of gestational age on $\bar{\mu}$, that is, the effect of increased duration of pregnancy on the survival rate of a given infant. There is also an indirect effect on Λ_{TV}, that is, the effect of increased duration of pregnancy on the distribution of latent characteristics.

From the parameter estimates in Table 1.6, I can calculate the elasticity of the perinatal mortality rate with respect to each continuous explanatory variable. For a married, multiparous black mother in her 20s, with twelve years of attained education and no prior perinatal loss, who delivers a 3,100 gram infant at 38 weeks in a hospital with 3,100 deliveries annually, I obtain the following elasticities:

	Model III		*Model IV*
Birth weight	− 7.79		− 8.72
Gestational age	− 0.75	{ direct	− 0.25
		indirect	− 0.32
Duration of care	0.52		− 0.23
Annual Volume of deliveries	− 0.42		− 0.61

In both models, birth weight has the dominant effect. Comparison of the direct and indirect elasticities for gestational age suggests that a substantial fraction of the observed effect of duration of pregnancy on mortality represents fetal selection over time. Although prenatal care has a favorable direct effect on mortality in Model IV, its elasticity is small. (The indirect effect of retarding fetal selection was negligible in this example.) Therefore, the main effect of prenatal care on perinatal mortality will still be its influence on birth weight. In this example, the complete absence of care would result in a 20% proportional increase the perinatal mortality rate, conditional upon birth weight and gestational age. Using the estimates derived in the previous section, I calculate that the absence of care, through its effect on the intrauterine growth rate and therefore birth weight, would result in a 17% proportional increase in the perinatal mortality rate. Similarly, the absence of care, through its effect on gestational age and therefore, on birth weight, would result in a 32% proportional increase in the perinatal mortality rate.

Finally, it is noteworthy that the annual volume of deliveries in the hospital of birth has a significant effect on survival. This finding supports the hypothesis that perinatal medical care, as opposed to prenatal care, has an important influence on birth weight-specific mortality.

Summary and Conclusions

Four main issues, I have demonstrated, underlie the controversy about prenatal care and pregnancy outcome.

First, the relationship between the timing of prenatal visits and the duration of pregnancy has been poorly characterized. Mothers with little or no prenatal care, it has been repeatedly observed, have a higher proportion of preterm babies. This fact suggests that prenatal care prevents premature labor. But early termination of pregnancy from any cause necessarily interrupts the course of prenatal care. In order to sort out these two confounding explanations, I devised a continuous time stochastic model in which the initiation of care and premature delivery were competing risks. Applying this model to a sample of black women's pregnancies, I found that prenatal care indeed prevented preterm delivery. The magnitude of this effect was equivalent to an approximate 1-week increase in the average duration of gestation.

Second, the risks of early termination of pregnancy vary considerably among unborn infants. These variations in risk set up a powerful selection mechanism in which less healthy fetuses are progressively eliminated from a cohort of pregnant women as gestation proceeds. As a result of this selection, those mothers who initiate care late in pregnancy necessarily have infants with characteristics quite different from those who initiate care earlier during gestation. Moreover, the underlying health characteristics subject to selection may be subtle and difficult to measure.

To investigate the potential errors of inference produced by this selection phenomenon, I included a mathematical model of fetal selection in my analysis of prenatal care and length of gestation. I showed that failure to account for fetal selection can indeed result in biased inferences about the effects of prenatal care and other prenatal risk factors. In particular, if prenatal care retards the early termination of pregnancy, then it also retards the fetal selection mechanism. Unless we incorporate the effect of prenatal care on the distribution of fetal characteristics over time, its influence on the duration of pregnancy will be understated.

Unfortunately, this solution to the problem of fetal selection requires overly restrictive assumptions about the determinants of the demand for prenatal care. There is the possibility that mothers could ascertain those fetal characteristics that are not revealed to the investigator. These latent characteristics could in turn affect the demand for medical care. When these possibilities were introduced in the analysis, it became impossible to make inferences about both the effect of prenatal care on the risk of preterm delivery and the influence of these risks on the demand for care.

Third, the frequently observed correlation between the quantity of prenatal care and birth weight lacks a convincing biological or behavioral explanation. Prenatal surveillance, to be sure, might indirectly improve birth weight by preventing early termination of pregnancy. But a mechanism for a direct effect of prenatal care on the rate of intrauterine growth is more elusive. I therefore specified a model in which the timing of care affected the rate of intrauterine growth. Applying this model to the cross-section data, I found that the influence of care on birth weight was only weakly positive and statistically insignificant. Through its effect on intrauterine growth rates, prenatal care would increase birth weight in a typical pregnancy by about 60 grams. By contrast, through its indirect effect on the duration of gestation, prenatal care would increase birth weight in a typical pregnancy by about 110 grams.

These findings are consistent with current understanding of the determinants of birth weight. In contrast to premature labor, which can be treated if not detected in advance (Chard 1974), there is no available treatment for placental insufficiency or other forms of intrauterine growth retardation (Spearman et al. 1975). Physician advice does not clearly alter maternal smoking, alcohol use, or nutrition. We cannot with certainty make any stronger inferences about the effect of prenatal care on birth weight when the underlying mechanisms of the effect remain in doubt.

Fourth, past analyses of prenatal care have not squarely confronted a critical point about the recent decline in U.S. neonatal and infant mortality; that is, the decline in mortality primarily reflects a striking improvement in the survival rates of low-birth-weight infants. By contrast, there has been comparatively little change in the proportion of low-birth-weight infants or the fraction of preterm deliveries. If the recent growth in prenatal care had a significant impact on infant survival, then we should expect to observe a relation between prenatal care and birth weight-specific mortality in cross-section data. Moreover, if prenatal care in fact affects birth weight, it is unclear why concomitant changes in the rate of prematurity were not observed.

I examined the relation between birth weight-specific mortality and the timing of prenatal care, and confirmed the frequently cited, contradictory observation that mothers who initiate care late during pregnancy have infants with considerably lower birth weight-specific mortality. This finding is consistent with the effects of fetal selection. If the fetal population varies in its risks of early termination of pregnancy, then among those mothers remaining pregnant into the third trimester, there will be a smaller proportion of high-risk infants. If the risk of premature delivery is correlated with fetal survival characteristics, then the fetal selection mechanism will also affect the distribution of these survival characteristics.

I formulated a specific model of the relation between fetal selection and fetal survival characteristics. Applying this model to the subsample of black women's pregnancies, I found that prenatal care had a weakly positive effect on birth weight-specific perinatal mortality. Unfortunately, this conclusion is contingent upon my specifying a particular mechanism of sorting unobserved characteristics. In the case where these latent regressors affect the demand for prenatal care or other fetal health characteristics, even stronger restrictions are required to identify the statistical parameters. The effect of prenatal care on fetal health, the distribution of fetal health characteristics, and the feedback effect of these characteristics on the demand for prenatal care cannot jointly be identified from cross-section data of vital records.

My analysis of the prenatal care controversy has side-stepped a number of additional difficulties. No attempt was made here to evaluate the quality, as opposed to the quantity, of prenatal care. Although I distinguished formally between prenatal care and perinatal care, the potential interaction of these factors has not been considered. Thus it is possible that prenatal care serves primarily to facilitate certain treatments in the perinatal period. This possibility is consistent with the finding that black women with prenatal care have lower risks of preterm delivery. Moreover, many of the results of this paper were derived from a sample of black women's pregnancies. Since medical intervention may vary in its influence on the health of different races, the quantitative estimates cannot be applied generally at this time. Finally, my analysis made only passing reference to the problem of nonrandomly missing observations. It ought to be recognized that those vital records with omitted entries for prenatal care and other data may be the most critical ones.

Would a detailed longitudinal study of the natural histories of many pregnancies overcome all these problems? So long as the expectant mothers choose when and if to seek prenatal care, such a study cannot overcome the problem of fetal selection. Nor can it eliminate the competition between early care and early fetal loss. Perhaps nothing short of a controlled, randomized trial will do. Even in that case, we cannot merely wait until an experimental subject recognizes her pregnancy and then assign her to a particular prenatal regimen. Instead, we would need to assign large cohorts of women to alternative experimental treatments prior to the onset of pregnancy. Moreover, independent ascertainment of the onset of pregnancy would be required. Such an experiment is surely difficult to perform.

Perhaps the most feasible approach is to design clinical studies that are more narrowly focused on certain types of prenatal intervention. They may not resolve the value of the millions of routine visits women make to their obstetricians. But we could at least learn something about prenatal diet, weight gain, vitamin supplementation, exercise, ultrasound studies, and other aspects of medical care.

References

American College of Obstetricians and Gynecologists. 1974. *Standards for obstetric-gynecologic services.* Chicago: American College of Obstetricians and Gynecologists.

Bakketeig, Leiv S.; Seigel, Daniel G.; and Sternthal, Phyllis M. 1978. A fetal-infant life table based on single births in Norway, 1967–1973. *American Journal of Epidemiology* 107:216–25.

Borkowf, H.I.; Grausz, J.P.; and Delfs, E. 1979. The effect of a perinatal center on perinatal mortality. *Obstetrics and Gynecology* 53:633.

Chard, T. 1974. The fetus at risk. *Lancet* 2:880–82.

Chase, Helen C., ed.; Erhardt, Carl L.; and Nelson, Frieda G. 1973. A study of risks, medical care, and infant mortality. *American Journal of Public Health* 63(Supp.):1–56.

——. 1974. Perinatal mortality: overview and current trends. *Clinics in Perinatology* 1:3–17.

——. 1977. Time trends in low birth weight in the United States. In Dwayne M. Reed and Fiona J. Stanley, ed., *The epidemiology of prematurity.* Baltimore and Munich: Urban & Schwarzenberg.

Cunningham, George C.; Hawes, Warren E.; Madore, Carol; Norris, Frank D.; and Williams, Ronald L. 1976. Intrauterine growth and neonatal risk in California. Santa Barbara: University of California, mimeo.

David, H.A., and Moeschberger, M.L. 1978. *The theory of competing risks.* Griffin's Statistical Monograph Series, No. 39. London: Charles Griffin & Company, Ltd.

Drillien, C.M. 1957. The social and economic factors affecting the incidence of premature births. Part I, Premature births without complications of pregnancy. *Journal of Obstetrics and Gynecology of the British Empire* 64:161–84.

Eastman, N.J. 1947. Prematurity from the viewpoint of the obstetrician. *American Practice* 1:343–52.

Gortmaker, Steven L. 1979. The effects of prenatal care upon the health of the newborn. *American Journal of Public Health* 69:653–60.

Gruenwald, Peter. 1966. Growth of the human fetus. Part I, Normal growth and its violation. *American Journal of Obstetrics and Gynecology* 94:1112.

——.1974. Pathology of the deprived fetus and its supply line. In *Size at birth,* Ciba Foundation Symposium 27 (new series). Amsterdam: North-Holland.

Habicht, Jean-Pierre; Lechtig, Aaron; Yarbrough, Charles; and Klein, Robert E. 1974. Maternal nutrition, birth weight, and infant mortality.

In *Size at birth,* Ciba Foundation Symposium 27 (new series). Amsterdam: North-Holland.

Harris, T.R.; Isaman, J.; and Giles, H.R. 1978. Improved neonatal survival through maternal transport. *Obstetrics and Gynecology* 52:294.

Hasselmeyer, Eileen G. et al. 1980. Pregnancy and infant health. In *The health consequences of smoking for women, a report of the surgeon general.* Washington,: U.S. Department of Health and Human Services.

Hellman, L.M. 1953. The prevention of premature births. In *Prematurity, congenital malformation and birth injury.* New York: Association for the Aid of Crippled Children.

Jacobson, Howard N. 1980. A randomized controlled trial of prenatal nutritional supplementation (editorial). *Pediatrics* 65:835–36.

Jacobowitz, S., and Grossman M. 1980. Determinants of variations in infant mortality rates among counties of the United States: the roles of social policies and programs. Presented at World Congress on Health Economics, Leiden University, The Netherlands, 8–11 September 1980.

Johnson, Norman L., and Kotz, Samuel. 1972. *Distributions in statistics: continuous multivariate distributions.* New York: John Wiley.

Kane, S.H. 1964. Significance of prenatal care. *Obstetrics and Gynecology* 24:66–72.

Kessner, David M.; Singer, James; Kalk, Carolyn E.; and Schlesinger, Edward R. 1973. *Infant death: an analysis by material risk and health care.* Washington: National Academy of Sciences, Institute of Medicine.

Kitchen, W.H., and Campbell, D.G. 1971. Controlled trial of intensive care for very low birth weight infants. *Pediatrics* 48:711–14.

Kleinman, Joel; Kovar, Mary G.; Feldman, Jacob J.; and Young, Cecelia A. 1978. A comparison of 1960 and 1972–74 early neonatal mortality in selected states. *American Journal of Epidemiology* 108:454–69.

Lancaster, Tony. 1979. Econometric methods for the duration of unemployment. *Econometrica* 47:939–59.

Lee, Kwang-Sun; Paneth, Nigel; Gartner, Lawrence M.; Pearlman, Mark A.; and Bross, Leslie. 1980. Neonatal mortality: an analysis of the recent improvement in the United States. *American Journal of Public Health 70:15–21.*

Lewit, Eugene M. 1977. Experience with pregnancy, the demand for prenatal care, and the production of surviving infants. Ph.D. diss., City University of New York.

Lubchenco, Lula O. 1975. Assessment of weight and gestational age. In Gordon B. Avery, ed., *Neonatology.* Philadelphia: J.B. Lippincott.

Mellin, Gilbert, W. 1972. Fetal life tables: a means of establishing perinatal rates of risk. *Journal of the American Medical Association*
180:91–94.
Morris, N.M.; Udry, J.R.; and Chase, C.L. 1975. Shifting age-parity
distribution of births and the decrease in infant mortality. *American
Journal of Public Health* 65:359–62.
Niswander, Kenneth R., Gordon, Myron et al. 1972. *The women and
their pregnancies.* Collaborative Perinatal Study, DHEW Publ. No.
(NIH) 73–379. Washington: National Institute of Neurological Dis-
eases and Stroke.
Oppenheimer, E. 1961. Population and changes and perinatal mortality.
American Journal of Public Health 51:208–16.
Pakter, Jean, and Nelson, Frieda. 1974. Factors in the unprecedented
decline in infant mortality in New York City. *Bulletin of the New York
Academy of Medicine* 50:839–68.
————; Rosner, H.J.; Jacobziner, H.; and Greenstein, R. 1961. Out-of-
wedlock births in New York City. Part II, Medical aspects. *American
Journal of Public Health* 51:846–65.
Rush, David; Stein, Zena; and Susser, Mervyn. 1980. A randomized
controlled trial of prenatal nutritional supplementation in New York
City. *Pediatrics* 65:683–97.
Russell, Louise B., and Burke, Carol S. 1975. Determinants of infant and
child mortality: an econometric analysis of survey data from San Juan,
Argentina. Report prepared for the Agency for International De-
velopment. Washington: National Planning Association.
Shah, Farida K., and Abbey, Helen. 1971. Effects of some factors on
neonatal and postneonatal mortality: analysis by a binary variable
regression method. *Milbank Memorial Fund Quarterly* 49:33–57.
Shapiro, Sam; Schlesinger, Edward R.; and Nesbitt, Robert E.L., Jr.
1968. *Infant, perinatal, maternal, and childhood mortality in the United
States.* Cambridge: Harvard University Press.
Shearman, Rodney P.; Shutt, Donald A.; and Smith, Ian D. 1974. The
assessment and control of human fetal growth. In *Size at birth*, Ciba
Foundation Symposium 27 (new series). Amsterdam: North-Holland.
Schmidt, Peter, 1981. Constraints on the parameters in simultaneous
tobit and probit models. In Daniel McFadden and Charles Manski,
eds., *Structural analysis of discrete data with econometric applications.*
Cambridge: M.I.T. Press (forthcoming).
Shwartz, Samuel. 1962. Prenatal care, prematurity, and neonatal mortal-
ity. *American Journal of Obstetrics and Gynecology* 83:591–98.
————, and Vinyard, J. H. 1965. Prenatal care and prematurity. *Public
Health Reports* 80:237–48.
Slesinger, Doris P., and Travis, Harry P. 1975. A study of infant mortal-

ity in Wisconsin, 1969, from linked birth and death records: an application of log-linear models. Working Paper 75–15, Center for Demography and Ecology, University of Madison, Wisconsin.

Stern, Leo. 1976. The high-risk neonate. In William N. Spellacy, ed., *Management of the high-risk pregnancy*. Baltimore: University Park Press.

Susser, Mervyn; Marolla, Francis A.; and Fleiss, Joseph. 1972. Birth weight, fetal age, and perinatal mortality. *American Journal of Epidemiology* 96:197–204.

Taylor, William F. 1970. The probability of fetal death. In F. Clarke Fraser and Victor A. McKusick, eds., *Congenital malformations*. Proceedings of the Third International Conference, The Hague, 1969. Amsterdam: Excerpta Medica Foundation.

Terris, Milton, and Glasser, Marvin. 1974. A life table analysis of the relation of prenatal care to prematurity. *American Journal of Public Health* 64:869–75.

———, and Gold, E. 1969. An epidemiologic study of prematurity. *American Journal of Obstetrics and Gynecology* 103:371–79.

U.S. National Center for Health Statistics. 1965. Weight at birth and survival of the newborn, United States, early 1950. *Vital and Health Statistics,* series 21, no. 3.

U.S. National Center for Health Statistics. 1972. A study of infant mortality from linked records: comparison of neonatal mortality from two cohort studies. *Vital and Health Statistics,* series 20, no. 13.

———. 1977. *Vital Statistics of the United States*. Volume II, Mortality, Part A. Washington: U.S. Goverment Printing Office.

———. 1978. Prenatal care: United States, 1969–1975. *Vital and Health Statistics,* series 21, no. 33.

———. 1979. Provisional statistics, annual summary for the United States, 1978. *Monthly Vital Statistics Report* 27:1–28.

———. 1980*a*. *Health, United States, 1979*. DHEW Publication No. (PHS) 80–1232. Washington. U.S. Government Printing Office.

———. 1980*b*. Wanted and unwanted births reported by mothers 15–44 years of age: United States, 1976. *Advance Data From Vital and Health Statistics,* no. 56.

Usher, R. 1977. Changing mortality rates with perinatal care and regionalization. *Seminars in Perinatology* 1:309.

Wells, Henry B.; Greenberg, Bernard G.; and Donnelly, James F. 1958. North Carolina fetal and neonatal death study. Part I, Study design and some preliminary results. *American Journal of Public Health* 48:1583–95.

Williams, Ronald L. 1975. Intrauterine growth curves: intra- and international comparisons with different ethnic groups in California. *Preventive Medicine* 4:163–72.

2   The Behavior of Mothers as Inputs to Child Health: The Determinants of Birth Weight, Gestation, and Rate of Fetal Growth

Mark R. Rosenzweig and T. Paul Schultz

The characteristics infants show at birth appear to play important roles in their subsequent growth, morbidity, and survival.[1] Such characteristics—birth weight, length of the gestation period, and rate of fetal growth—are affected by parental behavior, which usually is modified to favorably influence birth characteristics and which may also unknowingly condition the health of the newborn.[2] In recognition of the importance of these birth characteristics, many studies of health production focus on the relationship between the behavior of the pregnant mother and the subsequent characteristics of her newborn. Other studies examine the relationships between parental socioeconomic characteristics and/or access to health services and infant mortality (one indicator of infant health), as well as the relationship between parental socioeconomic characteristics and the mother's utilization of those prenatal medical services that are presumed to affect child health. Most studies suffer, however, from one or a combination of problems—the use of a choice-based sample, such as mothers visiting a subsidized clinic; the lack of control for other health-related behavior or inputs beyond the one studied; the use of implausible econometric specifications of health production relations; or the inattention to the possible importance of population heterogeneity in unobserved characteristics which may affect child health and condition parental health production behavior.

In this paper, we attempt to deal with many of these problems by specifying and estimating a simple model of the parental production of

Mark R. Rosenzweig and T. Paul Schultz are at Minnesota and Yale University, respectively. The research in this paper was supported in part by a grant from NIH, Center for Population Research, HD 12172. Able research assistance was provided by Cynthia Arfken. Useful comments on an earlier version were received from members of the Economics Workshop at SUNY Stonybrook, and from participants at the NBER conference.

child health. The model illustrates the need for examining jointly (1) the determinants of the demand for health production inputs, or parental behavior, including both scioeconomic and health program variables, and (2) the parameters of the technical-biological health production function—the relationship between behavioral inputs and the newborn's health characteristics, the output. Estimates of the production function and the input demand equations are needed to understand and interpret the reduced-form demand equations for birth characteristics, while knowledge of the factors conditioning parental behavior is generally required to obtain consistent estimates of the health production function. These estimates also provide information on the importance of socioeconomic factors compared to the availability of medical services in determining the initial conditions of an infant's life, as well as which type of parental behavior has serious consequences for child health and development.

In the first section of the paper, a model is formulated which embeds a health production function in a utility maximizing framework, distinguishing among goods which have no effect on child health but are desired for their own sake, goods which affect child health but are not desired for the direct utility they provide, and goods or behavior which both augment parental satisfaction directly and affect birth outcomes that indirectly affect parent utility. Implications are derived from the model regarding the demand for these three types of goods and the estimation of the health production function when families differ in either their genetic health endowments or their "caring" for child health. The model also indicates that even when a particular behavior decreases child health or well-being, a tax on such an activity may decrease child health even while resulting in a reduction of the activity.

In the second part we apply the framework to a national probability sample of approximately 10,000 legitimate live births from the National Natality Followback Surveys in the years 1967–1969. Based on the sample socioeconomic information and merged geographic information on such per capita variables as medical doctors, health expenditures, hospital beds, and family planning services, we present estimates of the relationships between birth weight, gestation, and the rate of fetal growth and four inputs: the mother's cigarette consumption while pregnant, her use of prenatal medical services, her age at the infant's birth, and her number of births. Our estimates are based on general functional forms for the health production function and on linear approximations to the input demand equations. Estimates are reported of the effects of father's income, mother's education, and regional medical service and price variables on the three measures of birth outcomes and on the derived demands for the four health inputs. The sensitivity of these estimates to changes in functional form and estimation is discussed. The final section compares our findings with those of other studies and considers alternative interpretations of the differences in birthweight among black and white women.

The Model

Child Health Production and the Demand for Child Health and Inputs

Assume that a family derives satisfaction from three types of goods—the health of each of its children, H; consumer goods, Y, which affect H (health-related goods, such as smoking or number of children); and consumer goods, X, which are health-neutral (have no effect on H, such as books). The health of children is affected by the level of Y goods, as well as other purchased or family inputs, Z, which are bought or allocated only because they contribute to child health (medical services, for example). Thus, the utility function of the family is

$$(1) \qquad U = U(X, Y, H).$$

The relationship between child health and the levels of Y and Z is described by a production function,

$$(2) \qquad H = F(Y, Z, \mu), \; F_y, \; F_z, \; F_\mu \neq 0,$$

where μ is "endowment" health, that component of child health due either to genetic or environmental conditions uninfluenced by parental behavior, but known to them.[3] Distinctions between the perceived production function and the true production function are discussed later, as is the role of schooling.

The family maximizes (1), given (2), which is assumed to be known, and subject to the budget constraint, given by (3)

$$(3) \qquad I = XP_x + YP_y + ZP_z$$

where P_x, P_y, P_z are the prices of the health-neutral and health-related consumption goods and child health investment goods, respectively, and I is income.

The important features of this model are that (a) health cannot be purchased directly; rather, other goods must be bought or utilized to influence health in a way described by (2), and (b) the family does not maximize child health, but looks at child health as one utility-augmenting "good" for which it must sacrifice other goods. Since the X or Y goods can include the number of children, the model also accommodates family choices regarding family size and child health and any trade-offs between them, as in the Becker-Lewis-Tomes interactive model.[4]

The first-order maximization conditions are

(4) $U_x = \lambda P_x$,

(5) $U_y + U_H F_y = \lambda P_y$,

(6) $U_H F_z = \lambda P_z$,

where λ is the Lagrangian multiplier.

While condition (4), applying to the health-neutral good, is conventional, expression (5) indicates the dual role of the health-related consumption good Y in augmenting utility directly and indirectly by its effect on H, through (2). The health investment good Z is demanded, as shown in (6), only because child health contributes to utility. Note, however, that even if Y had no effect, or an adverse effect, on H ($F_y < 0$), Y might still be consumed. The marginal product of Y in health production is an implicit tax ($F_y < 0$) on or subsidy ($F_y > 0$) of the Y good.

The model yields three demand equations for the three goods in terms of prices and income:

(7) $X = D_x(P_x, P_y, P_z, I, \mu)$,

(8) $Y = D_y(P_x, P_y, P_z, I, \mu)$,

(9) $Z = D_z(P_x, P_y, P_z, I, \mu)$.

The effects of changes in the prices of the three types of goods on the level of child health can be derived from these equations, noting that

(10) $dH = F_y \, dY + F_z \, dZ + F_\mu \, d\mu.$

From (2), these effects can be written as:

(11) $\dfrac{dH}{dP_x} = F_y \dfrac{dY}{dP_x} + F_z \dfrac{dZ}{dP_x}$,

(12) $\dfrac{dH}{dP_y} = F_y \dfrac{dY}{dP_y} + F_z \dfrac{dZ}{dP_y}$,

(13) $\dfrac{dH}{dP_z} = F_y \dfrac{dY}{dP_z} + F_z \dfrac{dZ}{dP_z}$,

since $d\mu / dp_i = 0$, $i = x, y, z$. Expressions (11), (12), and (13) indicate that price effects on child health depend on the effects of changes in prices on the demand for health production inputs as well as on the marginal products of these inputs in the production of health. The equations also suggest that changes in the prices of health-neutral goods will also affect the level of child health. It is essential, however, to appreciate what the expressions cannot predict without additional restrictions. For example, assume that it is known that the higher the consumption of the Y good the lower is child health ($F_y < 0$) and that $F_z > 0$. While the model predicts that a rise in P_y will reduce the consumption of Y, ignoring income effects

$(dY/dP_y < 0)$, the sign of (12) cannot be predicted since dZ/dP_y is not signed. For example, assume that smoking by the mother while pregnant is known to adversely affect the newborn child (we test for this later). A rise in the price of cigarettes because of taxation, while decreasing cigarette consumption, might also lower H if smoking and H were complements in the utility function, or if smoking and labor force participation were complements and the latter augmented health.

The model thus indicates that we must know the parameters of the health production function as well as the price effects of goods in order to predict how changes in prices will affect child health. We cannot know a priori whether a tax on or subsidy of a health-related or health-investment good will actually improve child health, even if it does lead to a predicted change in the consumption of the taxed good and even if we have information on the technical or biological relationships between child health and the consumption of the good or health input. The estimation of such technical relations, i.e., the characteristics of the production function (2) which enable the measurement of F_y and F_z, is considered next.

Population Heterogeneity and the Estimation of the Health Production Functions

Information on the technological or biological relationships between behavioral variables and child health outcomes, i.e., knowledge of (2), is useful for predicting and assessing the effects of health-related policies, but such information is also useful for helping potential parents efficiently attain their desired child health goals. Unfortunately, the opportunity to perform controlled experiments to ascertain the partial, causative effects of any one behavioral variable on birth outcomes, while controlling for all other factors, is minimal. We now show that the observed population associations between behavioral and child health variables, even when all commonly observed factors are held constant, are unlikely to provide the correct estimates of the $F_i, i = y, z$ as long as there are observed factors known to the parents but not to the researcher (μ), and even if such family-specific factors are randomly distributed in the population and unaffected by behavior. Knowledge of the determinants of the health production inputs, however, can enable us to obtain consistent estimates of the relevant parameters of the health production function.

To simplify the discussion, assume that function (2) has only one factor in addition to the unobserved health endowment or environmental variable, i.e., $F_y = 0$, and that Y and X are treated as a single variable, X. Then, controlling for all prices and income, the relationship between H and the health factor Z in the heterogeneous (in μ) population is

(14) $$\frac{dH}{dZ} = F_z + F_\mu \frac{d\mu}{dZ} \ .$$

The observed population association between child health and the behavioral variable Z thus does not in this case correspond to the technical relationship or marginal product F_z, but is contaminated by the unobserved, random μ factor as long as Z and μ are not uncorrelated. To see that $d\mu/dZ$ or $dZ/d\mu$ is not likely to be equal to zero, assume for simplicity that $F_{z\mu} = 0$. Then it can be demonstrated that

(15) $$\frac{dZ}{d\mu} = F_\mu \left[U_{HH} F_z \frac{dZ}{dP_z} + U_{XH} \frac{dZ}{dP_x} \right]$$

so that, from (14),

(16) $$\frac{dH}{dZ} = F_z + \left[U_{HH} F_z \frac{dZ}{dP_z} + U_{XH} \frac{dZ}{dP_x} \right]^{-1}$$

Expression (16) indicates that in the simple model the population association between H and the input Z, given by an ordinary least squares regression coefficient, for example, is an upwardly biased estimate of the true, technical parameter F_z, because second-order conditions imply that, controlling for income, $dZ/dP_z < 0$ and $dZ/dP_x > 0$ while $U_{HH} < 0$ and $U_{XH} > 0$. In other words, the model suggests that parents who expect to have relatively healthy children, based perhaps on observations on past births or from the birth outcomes of close kin, and/or who reside in relatively healthy environment, will be observed to use less of the variable input Z but to have healthier children than parents who are less well-educated or reside in less healthy family environments. The positive association between Z and H is in part spurious, the result of choices by the parents conditioned by factors, in this case μ, unknown to the researcher. In the more general case in which there is more than one factor in (2), the bias cannot be signed a priori.

While μ affects parental behavior and thus influences the level of child health and input use, it is not presumably correlated with those factors, affecting behavior, the P's. It is thus possible to estimate without bias the effects on H of the inputs, i.e., to purge the variation in μ from the variation in the Z and Y. In the simple model here, it is possible to obtain an unbiased estimate of dZ/dP_z in the presence of μ, since $dP_z/d\mu = 0$. The association between that part of the variation in Z due only to the variation in P_z and the variation in H provides an unbiased estimate of F_z. In econometric terms, to estimate the parameters characterizing the child health production function (2) requires a two-stage procedure in which the first-stage equations, providing unbiased estimates of the dZ/dP_z, correspond to the demand equations for the behavioral variables (7), (8), and (9). The predicted values of these variables based on the first-stage estimates, orthogonal to the μ, are used to estimate the production function parameters. The demand equations (7), (8), (9) for the Z and Y in terms of the P_z, P_y and P_x and I are the reduced-form input demand equations; the health production function (2) is the "structural" equation.

Education, Information, and the Production of Child Health

In the literature utilizing the household production framework, educational attainment is usually treated as an "environmental" variable which affects the marginal products of production inputs.[5] It is assumed that more educated parents or consumers are more efficient producers of commodities providing utility, where efficiency is defined to mean more output for given inputs. Hence, rewriting (2) with e defined as the level of educational attainment:

(2a) $$H = F'(Y, Z, \mu; e)$$
$$F'_{ye}, F'_{ze} > 0$$

Given the first-order conditions (4), (5), and (6), it is easy to see that the demand for all health inputs, as well as the pure utility good X, will be functions of schooling attainment in addition to prices and income. It is not clear, however, how education can actually alter marginal products of inputs or biological processes embedded in (2) unless inputs are omitted from (2). That is, it is doubtful that schooling can affect the production of H without it being associated with some alteration in an input. Instead, education, by augmenting information, may be thought to affect parental *perceptions* of the relationships between inputs and outputs. Parents maximize utility subject to production relations which they think exist; equation (2a) can be thought of, therefore, as the perceived production function. If parents differ in their understanding of the true technical or biological relationships between Y, Z, and H in ways related to educational attainment, as given in (2a), then input demand in any population will be a function of schooling. Education would not, however, appear empirically to affect actual marginal products of the production inputs as long as all of the inputs which varied across families were suitably taken into account.

Indeed, if households vary in their perceptions of the true parameters of health production relations, then it is possible to estimate the "true" production function (2) even if prices or income do not vary across the population, as long as a variable can be found which is related to such perceptions but which itself plays no direct role in production—such as schooling attainment. To obtain predictions from the model when perceptions concerning (2) differ, one must impose some structure on either the relationships between perceptions and observable characteristics or on the distribution of perceptions of health technology.

Empirical Application

The Data and Econometric Framework

The preceding analysis suggests that to understand and predict the effects of changes in medical or health programs which alter the costs of behavior that influences child health, it is necessary to estimate both the technical or biological relationships between behavior and child health (the health production function) and the determinants of the behavioral variables (the input demand equations). Moreover, knowledge of the latter is often useful for obtaining consistent estimates of the former. To apply the model one needs information on birth outcomes that reflects infant well-being, knowledge of parental behavior, or inputs, related to child health production, and the price and/or availability variables which affect such behavior. The 1967, 1968, and 1969 National Natality Follow-back Surveys appear to meet most of these requirements. These national probability samples of approximately 10,000 legitimate births for the three years combined contain information on birth weight and gestation period for each birth, as well as subsequent child mortality, the educational attainment of both parents, the earnings of the husband, three aspects of the mother's behavior during pregnancy which are potentially linked to infant health at birth—smoking, working, and receiving prenatal medical care—in addition to data on age at birth and parity. The survey also provides information on the county of residence of the mother at the time of the birth, enabling us to merge local price and health program variables with the microdata.

We selected for analysis all nonmultiple births, resulting in a sample of 9,621 births. Based on the geographical information we collected and merged county or state level data on hospital beds per capita (BEDS), per capita governmental health expenditures (HEXP), the per capita number of hospitals (HOSPFP) and health departments (HDFP) offering family planning services, medical doctors per capita (MD), the proportion of women aged 15–59 in the labor force who are unemployed (UNEMPR-W), the percentage of persons in service industries which employ a disproportionately large share of women (SERVICE), the cost (including excise taxes but excluding retail sales taxes) of cigarettes (CPRCE), the retail sales tax (TAXSALES) on cigarettes, and the size of the SMSA (SIZE) for inhabitants of SMSAs. The sample characteristics and definitions of all variables are listed in Table 2.1.

The weight of a child at birth has much to do with its prospects for survival (e.g., Susser et al. 1972). During 1964–65 in the United States,

18.6% of infants weighing less than 2,500 grams did not reach their first birthday; among those weighing more than 2,500 grams the proportion dying in the first year was .97%, for a ratio of 19 to 1. Grouping births by parents' economic characteristics yields much narrower differentials: the ratio of infant mortality rates for mothers with eight years education or less compared to those with sixteen years or more is 1.86 to 1, and for families with annual incomes of under $3,000 compared to those with incomes of $10,000 and over the ratio is 1.67 to 1 (MacMahon et al. 1972, Tables 18, 21, and 22).

If low birth weight is a genetically determined factor predisposing to early death, economic analysis of this indicator of child health in a production function framework would not be useful. But the frequency of prematurity, measured by a birth weight of less than 2,500 grams, varies substantially across social and economic groups in the society. It is almost twice as great among mothers with less than nine years of education as among those with sixteen years or more—10.6% versus 5.6%, respectively (Ibid., Table 19). Moreover, the proportion of nonwhite U.S. births thus classified as premature is much higher than for whites, and increasing from about 10% to more than 13% from 1950 to 1967.[6] The overall proportion of underweight births in the United States remains in excess of that recorded in other industrially advanced countries and is frequently linked to the relatively high level and distribution of infant mortality in the United States (Wiener and Milton 1970; Chase and Byrnes 1972; Hemminki and Starfield 1978; Taffel 1980).

For simplicity, birth weight is treated in this study as a linear indicator of good child health. Though deaths are highly concentrated among very low birth weight infants, the inverse relationship between infant mortality rates and birth weight is approximately linear from under 1,000 grams to about 3,000 grams. Slightly elevated mortality levels are also recorded for infants weighing more than 4,500 grams, but these "overweight" births constituted less than 2% of U.S. live births in 1960 (Chase 1969). The analysis of birth weight as a continuous linear indicator of child health has obvious statistical advantages over a dichotomous and relatively infrequent event such as infant mortality.[7]

A second indicator of the newborn's health is its gestational age. Infants of short gestation die much more frequently during the first month of life: in early 1950, 79% of the U.S. births whose periods of gestation were under 28 weeks died, whereas only .88% of those whose gestation was 37 weeks or more died (Shapiro 1965, Table H). However, gestation is not reported on birth certificates in a few states, and some epidemiologists suspect that reported information on gestation is subject to greater error than that on birth weight (Eisner et al. 1979).

Recently, two health effects of prematurity have been distinguished: a relatively transitory trauma associated with leaving the womb and estab-

Table 2.1   Variable Definition, Means, and Standard Deviations

Variable	Definition	Mean	Standard Deviation
Endogenous			
Birth weight	Weight of baby at birth, in grams	3288	568
Gestation Period	Length of pregnancy, in weeks	39.1	2.45
Standardized birth weight	Birth weight/Predicted birth weight based on gestation period (see text)	1.00	.170
DELAY	Number of months of elapsed pregnancy before mother saw a doctor	2.74	1.55
SMOKING	Number of cigarettes mother smoked per day while pregnant	4.71	8.64
AGE	Age of mother at birth in years	24.9	5.61
BIRTHS	Number of live births born to mother including current one	2.54	1.90
Exogenous–Individual			
MGRM	= 1 if mother did not enter high school	.095	.301
MHSI	= 1 if mother attended high school for less than 4 years	.230	.421
MHSC	= 1 if mother completed high school	.445	.497
MCOLI	= 1 if mother attended college for less than 4 years	.142	.350
MCOLC	= 1 if mother completed college	.087	.282

		6132	3785
HINC	Annual income of husband		
SMSA	= 1 if family is located in an SMSA	.700	.458
BLACK	= 1 if mother is black	.190	.392
1967	= 1 if birth occurred in 1967	.332	.470
1968	= 1 if birth occurred in 1968	.330	.470

Exogenous–Area

BEDS	Number of hospital beds per capita	.00466	.00109
HEXP	Governmental health and hospital expenditures in thousands of dollars per capita	.0203	.0226
HOSPFP $(x10^{-8})$	Number of hospitals with family planning program per capita	299.	158.
HDFP $(x10^{-8})$	Number of health departments with family planning per capita	95.0	199
MD $(x10^{-3})$	Number of persons per medical doctor	1.42	.695
UNEMPR-W	Unemployed proportion of women in labor force aged 15–59	.0526	.0104
SERVICE $(x10)$	Percent of persons employed in service industries	77.9	15.3
CPRCE	Price of cigarettes including state and local excise taxes (cents/package)	34.61	3.38
TAXSALES	Retail sales tax on cigarettes (cents/package)	.583	.490
SIZE $(x10^{-3})$	Population of SMSA	1349.6	2087
n	Number of Observations	9621	

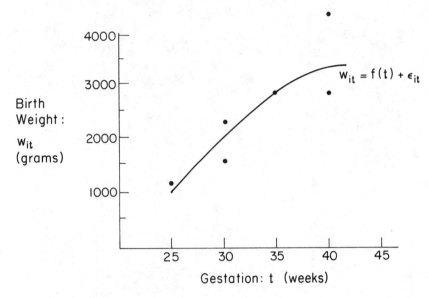

Fig. 2.1   Hypothetical pattern of birthweight by gestation for live births.

lishing viable body functions, primarily respiratory, and more permanent debilities that are more frequently associated with congenital defects and excessive risks of morbidity and mortality continuing beyond the second year of life (Beck and van den Berg 1975). The former transitory health effect is approximated here by short gestation. The latter, more permanent effect is represented by the fetal rate of weight gain to birth, normalized by the average weight gain associated with infants of that gestation.

It is assumed that a biological-technical relationship exists between birth weight and gestation. This is illustrated in Figure 2.1, where the birth weight of individual i at gestation t, w_{it} is represented by a nonlinear function of gestation, $f(t)$, and an individual disturbance, ε_{it}, that could embody random and genetic differences across individuals, variation in behavioral inputs of parents, and errors of measurement. To compare individuals of different gestations, the systematic effect of gestation on birth weight, $f(t)$, must be removed; a measure of individual deviation from the normal fetal growth curve is thereby obtained. The nonlinear fetal growth function is first estimated from our sample as a cubic function of gestation in weeks. The individual's birth weight is then divided by the expected birth weight for the individual's gestation, predicted by the estimated fetal growth function.[8] This measure of normalized birth weight, illustrated in Figure 2.2, represents the more permanent child

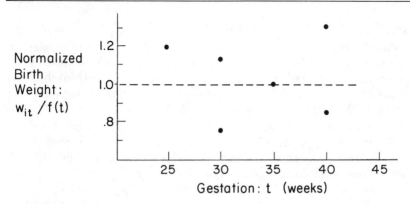

Fig. 2.2   Hypothetical pattern of birthweight normalized for gestation.

health effects of prematurity. The variance of the error associated with this normalized measure of birth weight should also be approximately constant, improving the efficiency of our estimates of a child health production function.[9]

Differences in the distribution of birth weight between distinct ethnic or racial groups might arise for at least two reasons. On the one hand, the demand for health inputs might differ between groups because their income, education, and local prices differ. On the other hand, the biological-technical relationships, such as $f(t)$, may differ between genetic groups, posing a problem of comparability of birth characteristics used as indicators of development or health across such groups.

In this study, and many others (e.g., Chase 1962; Baumgartner 1962), birth weights for blacks and whites differ. Estimates of the production function for birth characteristics and input demands provide a methodology for appraising whether demand for health inputs differs between blacks and whites, and whether birth characteristics differ for blacks and whites given their input demands (Cf. Wiener and Milton 1970). A third approach is to estimate distinct fetal growth functions for black and white births separately, and define the normalized birth weight specific to these race groups.[10] Given the relatively small number of black births in our sample, the entire production function is not estimated for blacks alone, although estimates for only white births are reported in the Appendix for the purposes of comparison.

Thus, three measures of birth outcomes are used in the analysis: birth weight, gestation, and birth weight normalized for gestation, which represents the rate of fetal growth. Birth weight is first normalized for the fetal growth function fitted to the entire sample, and then normalized according to black and white specific growth functions.

The endogenous or behavioral variables considered to be potential determinants of the birth outcomes are the number of months the mother worked while pregnant, the number of months of elapsed pregnancy before the mother visited a medical doctor (DELAY), the number of cigarettes smoked per day by the mother while pregnant (SMOKING), the order of the current live birth (BIRTHS), and the age of the mother at birth (AGE). The mother's age in this context is a choice variable, as it refers to the point in her life cycle at which she is choosing to have a child. In all specifications and tests of the health production function, working by the mother while pregnant never appeared to be a signicant determinant of birth outcomes, and in what follows we consequently do not include this variable. Variables reflecting a part of the health environment as well as possible biological differences are SMSA residence, SMSA size, dummy variables for the year of the child's birth (1967, 1968, or 1969), and whether or not the mother is black (BLACK). The birth characteristics production function in its general form is thus:

(17) $H = F(\text{AGE, DELAY, SMOKING, BIRTHS, SMSA,}$
              $\text{SIZE, 1967, 1968, BLACK; } \mu).$

AGE, SMOKING, and BIRTHS are all health-related goods (Y), providing direct utility to the mother in addition to their impact on child health, whereas DELAY is perceived as only affecting child health (Z).

To estimate the demand for goods potentially affecting the birth characteristics—the endogenous inputs in (17), corresponding to equations (7), (8), and (9)—we utilize both the socioeconomic information from the survey data and the areal program and price variables. Included among the former are school attainment variables of the wife and the annual earnings of the husband as well as the race variable. The area variables correspond to or are determinants of the prices in the model; CPRCE and TAXSALES are components of the price of SMOKING, and should be negatively associated with that activity; UNEMPR-W represents the lack of demand for female work and should be negatively correlated with the value of the mother's time, while we expect SERVICE, a female-intensive industry, to be positively associated with the value of time, one component of the price of both visiting a doctor and the fertility variables. HDFP and HOSPFP, the family planning variables, should be negatively correlated with BIRTHS, as they should be inversely associated with the cost of averting births, and may affect AGE as well; HEXP, BEDS, MD, and HDFP and HOSPFP should all be positively associated with lower costs of medical care, inducing less delay by mothers in seeking prenatal medical care and thus negatively correlated with DELAY. The demand equations will not only enable us to obtain consistent estimates of the effects of the health-related activities on initial infant well-being (17), but allow an assessment of the relative influence of individual characteristics and the local availability of medical services on the mother's input activities which affect the conditions of the child at birth.

Estimating the Infant Health Technology and the Demand for Infant Health Inputs using Approximations.

Because of the difficulty of obtaining exact solutions for the set of input demand equations from a complete parameterization of the household production model (1), (2), and (3) which does not impose implausible behavioral restrictions, we pursue an alternative estimation strategy involving the use of approximations to the demand equations corresponding to (7), (8), and (9) and to the health production function (2). This strategy was also motivated by the rejection by the data of the set of restrictions implied by one completely parameterized demand system involving Cobb-Douglas forms, as reported in Rosenzweig and Schultz (1980). For the approximate demand equations, we do not impose separability (as in the Cobb-Douglas demand system), but allow for the effects of changes in the price or availability of each input to affect other inputs, as implied by the general model. All prices or program variables thus appear on the right-hand side of each child health input demand equation. The equations we estimate, in linear form, are thus:[11]

(18)
through
(21)
AGE, DELAY, SMOKING, BIRTHS = D(MHSI, MHSC, MCOLI, MCOLC, HINC, BEDS HEXP, HOSPFP, HDFP, MD, UNEMPR-W, SERVICE, CPRCE, CPRCE2 TAXSALES, SMSA, SIZE, BLACK, 1967, 1968),

where CPRCE2 is the square of CPRCE.

The functional form used to estimate the infant health production function is the generalized Leontief-Diewert (Diewert 1971). Three specifications are estimated. The first assumes that the relationships between the health inputs and the birth outcome measures are described by a simple linear or Leontief fixed-coefficient model. The second assumes a more general form for these relationships, allowing for substitutions between inputs, but imposes local linear homogeneity. The third, most general parameterization, does not impose linear homogeneity. All specifications assume that birth outcomes are affected linearly by the biological-environmental variables represented by SMSA, SIZE, 1967, 1968, and BLACK. The health production functions we estimate is thus given by:

$$(22) \qquad H = \sum_i \sum_j \beta_{ij} y_i^{\frac{1}{2}} y_j^{\frac{1}{2}} + \Sigma_i \beta_i y_i^{\frac{1}{2}} + \gamma_1 \text{SMSA} + \gamma_2 \text{ SIZE}$$

$$+ \gamma_3 \text{BLACK} + \gamma_4 1967 + \gamma_5 1968 + \gamma_o + \mu$$

where the y_i are AGE, DELAY, SMOKING, BIRTHS, $\beta_{ij} = \beta_{ji}, \beta_{ij} = 0$, $i \neq j$ for the linear model, $\beta_{ij} \neq 0$, $i \neq j, \beta_i = 0$, for the more general linear model, and $\beta_i \neq 0$ for the general case in which local linear homogeneity is not imposed.

This flexible functional form, which can be considered a second-order approximation to any production function, can be used to test the three models against each other and to compute elasticities of substitution between the inputs, measures of the degree to which each input can substitute for another in the production of infant well-being.[12] Such elasticities are assumed to equal one in the Cobb-Douglas case.

Because, as we have shown, the error term μ is likely to be correlated with the y_i, ordinary least squares (OLS) estimates of the β's (22) may be inconsistent. Two-stage least squares estimates are required, utilizing exogenous determinants of the input demand equations for the four behavioral variables y_i in the first stage. OLS estimates of (22) are also reported in order to evaluate the importance of heterogeneity.[13] The first-stage equations contain, in addition to the variables specified, interactions of the education and race dummies and husband's income with all of the price and program availability variables.

Child Health Input Demand Equation Estimates: Linear Specifications

The four linear health production input demand equations are reported in Table 2.2 In all equations, both the sets of socioeconomic variables and the regional health input availability and price variables contribute significantly to explanatory power. While in most cases parameter estimates are precise and conform to expectations and/or findings from prior household-level studies, the R^2's are relatively low, ranging from .03 for the SMOKING equation to .15 for BIRTHS.

The demand estimates for DELAY indicate that women with more education and women in high income families seek prenatal care earlier, and that black mothers postpone such care by just over a half-month more than do white mothers with similar personal and regional characteristics. Among the variables representing the availability of medical services, two variables are associated with mothers obtaining early prenatal care: residence in an SMSA and in counties where more public health facilities include family planning services. Over the sample three-year period, prenatal care was sought earlier during the later years, particularly between 1968 and 1969.

While mothers with husbands who have high levels of earnings appear to smoke more while pregnant, there is a clear negative relationship between the mother's school attainment and the number of cigarettes per day she smokes while pregnant. On average, black women smoke half as much while pregnant as do white mothers, other things equal.[14] Where female unemployment rates are high, mothers appear to smoke less,

Table 2.2   **Linear Input Demand Equation Estimates**

Independent Variable	AGE	DELAY	SMOKING	BIRTHS
MHSI	−3.44	−.561	1.49	−1.06
	(17.06)	(9.48)	(4.46)	(15.33)
MHSC	−2.56	−1.08	−.426	−1.68
	(13.45)	(19.30)	(1.35)	(25.70)
MCOLI	−2.37	−1.25	−1.01	−1.95
	(10.57)	(18.96)	(2.71)	(25.29)
MCOLC	−.873	−1.27	−1.66	−2.21
	(3.42)	(16.87)	(3.91)	(25.19)
HINC$(x10^{-3})$	.548	−.041	.127	.122
	(35.28)	(9.03)	(4.91)	(22.85)
BEDS	258.2	19.16	83.35	60.07
	(4.53)	(1.14)	(0.88)	(3.06)
HEXP	−7.25	−.296	2.65	−1.92
	(2.18)	(0.30)	(0.48)	(1.68)
HOSPFP	29697	−3679	17838	−39247
	(0.84)	(0.35)	(3.04)	(3.23)
HDFP	−1002	−6781	28316	−5646
	(0.12)	(2.66)	(1.96)	(1.89)
MD$(x10^{-5})$	3.71	−.518	.298	−4.00
	(0.47)	(0.22)	(2.27)	(1.47)
UNEMPR-W	−11.20	3.06	−22.68	.948
	(1.86)	(1.73)	(2.27)	(0.46)
SERVICE	−.0094	.0023	−.012	−.00010
	(2.21)	(1.87)	(1.64)	(0.04)
CPRCE	−.226	.054	−.031	.295
	(0.80)	(0.65)	(0.07)	(3.02)
CPRCE2	.0040	−.00083	.0011	−.0045
	(0.92)	(0.65)	(0.15)	(3.00)
TAXSALES	.095	−.042	−.273	−.028
	(0.72)	(1.10)	(1.25)	(0.61)
BLACK	1.16	.661	−2.35	1.03
	(8.13)	(15.77)	(9.90)	(20.96)
SMSA	.090	−.141	.719	−.187
	(0.53)	(2.82)	(2.54)	(3.36)
SIZE$(x10^{-8})$	2.78	−.205	.150	−1.40
	(0.82)	(.205)	(2.65)	(1.20)
1967	.686	−.172	.857	.171
	(5.34)	(4.56)	(4.01)	(3.87)
1968	.222	−.162	.396	.021
	(1.75)	(4.33)	(1.86)	(0.50)
CONSTANT	26.47	2.74	4.20	−2.82
	(5.80)	(2.04)	(0.62)	(1.80)
R^2	.170	.130	.031	.146
F Statistic	98.17	71.70	15.58	82.13

Absolute value of t statistics in parentheses.

although the number of doctors per capita and the availability of family planning services in the local area are positively associated with female smoking, as are SMSA residence and city size. The year dummy coefficients suggest a decline in cigarette consumption by pregnant women by 18% from 1967 to 1969.

The AGE equation coefficients suggest a U-shaped relationship between school attainment of mothers and age at infant's birth. While mothers with less than nine years of schooling (the omitted category) appear to be older on average, among women with at least some high school education those with more schooling have their children at older ages. The earnings of the husband appear to be positively associated with delay in childbearing, while in regions of high female unemployment, fertility appears to occur at younger ages. Family planning programs do not appear to affect the timing of births, although local health expenditures per capita are negatively associated with childbearing age of mothers, and the number of hospital beds per capita is positively correlated with this variable. The year dummy coefficients suggest a temporal decline in the average age of childbearing.

The estimates of the BIRTHS equation are consistent with findings of many prior studies of fertility behavior—more educated women tend to have fewer births, husband's earnings and cumulative fertility are positively correlated, and black women have on the average almost one more birth than white women. Mothers in urban environments have lower fertility. Most interesting, while local family planning programs do not appear to influence the timing of births, i.e., affect AGE, the BIRTHS equation indicates that family planning programs are effective in reducing cumulative fertility—the coefficients of both HOSPFP and HDFP are negative and statistically significant. Public health expenditures per capita also appear to reduce total fertility, although public and private hospital BEDS and BIRTHS are positively correlated. Finally, as would be expected in the sample years, fertility displays a decline, by almost one-fifth of a child in the 1967–1969 period.

Birth Characteristics Production Function Estimates: Linear
and Generalized Leontief-Diewert Specifications.

Estimates for the three specifications of the production function relating the behavioral variables to birth weight and gestation are reported in Table 2.3 and to birth weight normalized for gestation in the total population and within race groups in Table 2.4. The results suggest that the neglect of population heterogeneity in unobserved health characteristics affects (biases) the estimates of the effects of health input activities on the health characteristics of the newborn: the two-stage least squares (TSLS) and ordinary least squares (OLS) estimates of the production parameters differ substantially. For example, the OLS estimates of the

Leontief model suggest that the mother's delay in seeking prenatal care is an unimportant determinant of birth weight, while use of the more defensible TSLS procedure indicates that such a delay would lower birth weight. This pattern of differences is anticipated, if women who have had problems with their prior pregnancies are more likely to seek early prenatal care and deliver low birth weight infants. These biological factors that are unobserved by the researcher but known to some degree by the woman are responsible for the heterogeneity bias. The direct association between DELAY and birth weight captured in the OLS estimates includes this heterogeneity effect, whereas the TSLS estimates are purged of these effects and confirm that across otherwise comparable women, those who seek medical care earlier in their pregnancy have heavier babies.

The production function estimates also suggest that while the more generalized functional specifications do not yield precise TSLS estimates because of the collinearity among the many transformations of the input variables, the linear (Leontief) specification of the production relationship appears to mask relatively important and anticipated interactions among the designated inputs and our measures of child health.

The marginal products, F_i, of the four input activities evaluated at the sample means are summarized in Table 2.5 for the various functional specifications of the production relationships and for the OLS and TSLS estimates. Discussion focuses here on the TSLS estimates of the marginal productivities of inputs obtained from the generalized Leontief-Diewert functional form. These estimates indicate that delay in seeking prenatal care appears to reduce both birth weight and gestation, and has little residual effect on birth weight normalized for gestation—our proxy for the more permanent health consequences of prematurity (Table 2.5). A delay of six months in obtaining prenatal care is estimated to reduce birth weight by 45 grams or about 1%, and to reduce gestation by 1.6 weeks, or 4%, with a net effect of increasing birth weight normalized for gestation. Direct epidemiological correlational studies have not always found an effect on birth weight of the timing of prenatal care (Eisner 1979).

Smoking while pregnant, on the other hand, notably reduces birth weight but is linked to longer gestation. Smoking is related, therefore, to lower birth weight normalized for gestation. Although other estimates of the effect of smoking on birth characteristics are not precisely comparable to those reported here, the direct correlational evidence of many epidemiological studies as summarized by the recent Surgeon General's report on smoking is that "babies born to women who smoke during pregnancy are, on the average, 200 grams lighter," U.S. Department of Health and Human Services 1980, p. 225). By comparison our direct (OLS) estimates of the fixed coefficient (Leontief) linear model suggest smokers (a third of our sample of mothers) would have babies weighing

Table 2.3 **Birth Characteristics Production Function Estimates:**
Linear and Generalized Leontief-Diewert

Independent Variable	A. Birth weight					
	(1)		(2)		(3)	
	OLS	TSLS	OLS	TSLS	OLS	TSLS
AGE	3.58 (2.79)	1.83 (0.38)	−1.48 (0.64)	−32.8 (1.54)	−59.5 (2.81)	−206 (1.32)
DELAY	−1.56 (0.42)	−39.6 (1.71)	−44.3 (3.05)	−177 (1.16)	−37.6 (1.68)	−129 (0.62)
SMOKING	−10.1 (15.4)	−16.2 (3.49)	5.48 (2.47)	−1.80 (0.06)	5.74 (2.54)	−9.76 (0.32)
BIRTHS	20.9 (5.34)	43.3 (2.31)	−14.7 (1.64)	128 (0.79)	−74.2 (3.18)	43.9 (0.24)
$(AGE \cdot DELAY)^{1/2}$			27.7 (2.56)	193 (1.79)	−8.65 (0.27)	155. (0.58)
$(AGE \cdot SMOKE)^{1/2}$			−13.5 (4.65)	12.1 (0.34)	• −9.19 (1.26)	−44.1 (0.61)
$(AGE \cdot BIRTHS)^{1/2}$			10.8 (1.79)	43.8 (0.41)	83.09 (2.29)	236 (0.93)
$(DELAY \cdot SMOKE)^{1/2}$			−3.74 (0.58)	21.2 (0.27)	−1.30 (0.17)	20.7 (0.24)
$(DELAY \cdot BIRTHS)^{1/2}$			22.5 (1.52)	−276 (1.20)	58.7 (1.79)	−213 (0.76)
$(SMOKE \cdot BIRTHS)$			−3.66 (0.87)	−100 (1.28)	−6.99 (0.87)	−80.8 (0.98)
$AGE^{1/2}$					533 (2.66)	1568 (1.00)
$DELAY^{1/2}$					86.5 (0.53)	−77.5 (0.05)
$SMOKING^{1/2}$					−20.0 (0.58)	296 (0.80)
$BIRTHS^{1/2}$					−178 (1.11)	−809 (0.72)
BLACK	−252 (16.8)	−257 (11.1)	−245 (16.3)	−234 (8.16)	−244 (16.1)	−229 (6.54)
SMSA	−20.8 (1.55)	−18.9 (1.31)	−21.0 (1.57)	−17.3 (1.16)	−21.8 (1.63)	−16.4 (1.08)
$SIZE(x10^{-8})$	465 (1.54)	525 (1.67)	475 (1.60)	388 (1.15)	482 (1.62)	300 (0.86)
1967	18.1 (1.32)	19.8 (1.36)	22.4 (1.64)	31.9 (1.89)	23.7 (1.73)	30.8 (1.56)
1968	14.8 (1.08)	14.2 (0.99)	19.6 (1.43)	25.2 (1.53)	19.9 (1.45)	25.7 (1.48)
CONSTANT	3263 (95.0)	3360 (24.0)	3267 (91.9)	3190 (18.1)	1943 3.84	−205 0.05
R^2	.053	—	.061	—	.062	—
F	—	29.46 (10,9611)	—	17.53 (16,9605)	—	13.82 (20,060)

In parentheses are the absolute values of the t and asymptotic t statistics for the OLS and TSLS coefficients, respectively.

B. Gestation Period ($x10^2$)

(1)		(2)		(3)	
OLS	TSLS	OLS	TSLS	OLS	TSLS
−6677	1.46	−1.34	14.6	−28.4	−166
(1.20)	(0.70)	(1.32)	(1.54)	(3.03)	(2.28)
−2.25	−8.23	−19.4	91.1	−16.9	233
(1.38)	(0.82)	(3.03)	(1.33)	(1.72)	(2.44)
−.784	1.45	.398	−14.7	.236	−19.6
(2.72)	(0.72)	(0.41)	(1.13)	(0.24)	(1.37)
.174	−5.26	1.01	102	6.15	34.6
(0.10)	(0.65)	(0.25)	(1.42)	(0.60)	(0.41)
		8.97	−53.9	10.49	31.5
		(1.88)	(1.12)	(0.74)	(0.25)
		−1.30	19.9	−3.51	−5.17
		(1.01)	(1.25)	(1.09)	(0.15)
		−6.03	−45.3	−5.32	94.6
		(2.28)	(0.96)	(0.33)	(0.80)
		.086	−6.39	.385	18.2
		(0.03)	(0.18)	(0.12)	(0.45)
		16.8	−75.9	11.5	−125
		(2.57)	(0.74)	(0.80)	(0.96)
		.458	−3.01	2.45	9.62
		(0.25)	(0.09)	(0.69)	(0.25)
				282	1497
				(3.19)	(2.05)
				−14.1	−855
				(0.20)	(1.28)
				7.99	99.5
				(0.52)	(0.58)
				−17.6	−401
				(0.25)	(0.77)
−71.5	−53.6	−70.7	−62.3	−69.7	−64.1
(10.8)	(5.31)	(10.7)	(4.87)	(10.4)	(3.94)
.996	−4.56	1.13	−4.93	.677	−5.08
(0.17)	(0.72)	(0.19)	(0.74)	(0.11)	(0.72)
−282	−354	−283	−376	−290	−418
(2.15)	(2.59)	(2.16)	(2.50)	(2.21)	(2.56)
54.5	52.7	55.0	44.5	56.2	42.8
(9.05)	(8.28)	(9.12)	(5.90)	(9.31)	(4.65)
11.1	11.1	12.0	3.15	12.8	3.69
(1.85)	(1.78)	(1.99)	(0.43)	(2.12)	(0.46)
3927	3896	3922	3969	3222	1153
(261)	(63.9)	(250)	(50.3)	(14.4)	(0.58)
.024	—	.025	—	.027	—
—	24.94	—	14.21	—	10.76
	(10,9611)		(16,9605)		(20,9601)

Table 2.4 **Production Function Estimates of Birth Weight Normalized for Gestation: Linear and Generalized Leontief-Diewert**

Independent Variable	A. Total Population Normalization ($x10^2$)					
	(1)		(2)		(3)	
	OLS	TSLS	OLS	TSLS	OLS	TSLS
AGE	.112	−.057	−.017	−1.68	−.802	.315
	(3.04)	(0.39)	(0.25)	(2.57)	(1.26)	(0.07)
DELAY	−.623	−1.03	−.795	−7.99	−.803	−12.1
	(0.56)	(1.48)	(1.83)	(1.70)	(1.20)	(1.89)
SMOKING	−.275	−.563	.177	.766	.194	.793
	(14.1)	(4.03)	(2.67)	(0.85)	(2.87)	(0.84)
BIRTHS	.600	1.57	−.398	.518	−2.33	1.45
	(5.12)	(2.80)	(1.48)	(0.10)	(3.34)	(0.25)
$(AGE \cdot DELAY)^{1/2}$			.637	7.80	−.611	3.54
			(1.97)	(2.40)	(0.64)	(0.43)
$(AGE \cdot SMOKE)^{1/2}$			−.409	−.395	−.144	−.529
			(4.70)	(0.36)	(0.66)	(0.24)
$(AGE \cdot BIRTHS)^{1/2}$			.467	3.81	2.62	2.12
			(2.61)	(1.17)	(2.42)	(0.27)
$(DELAY \cdot SMOKE)^{1/2}$			−.0773	1.73	.0200	.970
			(0.40)	(0.72)	(0.09)	(0.36)
$(DELAY \cdot BIRTHS)$			.102	−8.05	1.47	−5.68
			(0.23)	(1.14)	(1.50)	(0.66)
$(SMOKE \cdot BIRTHS)^{1/2}$			−.0818	−4.57	−.249	−4.62
			(0.65)	(1.90)	(1.04)	(1.81)
$AGE^{1/2}$					6.16	−10.7
					(1.03)	(0.22)
$DELAY^{1/2}$					3.86	32.3
					(0.80)	(0.73)
$SMOKING^{1/2}$					−1.26	1.56
					(1.22)	(0.14)
BIRTHS					−5.16	1.69
					(1.07)	(0.05)
BLACK	−5.16	−5.97	−4.95	−4.68	−4.95	−4.69
	(11.5)	(8.55)	(11.0)	(5.32)	(10.9)	(4.32)
SMSA	−.815	−.522	−.821	−.458	−.828	−.416
	(2.02)	(1.20)	(2.05)	(1.00)	(2.06)	(0.88)
SIZE ($x10^{-8}$)	30.9	35.8	31.3	30.7	31.8	30.8
	(3.48)	(3.79)	(3.53)	(2.97)	(3.59)	(2.83)
1967	−1.64	−1.52	−1.52	−.820	−1.51	−.699
	(4.01)	(3.46)	(3.71)	(1.58)	(3.70)	(1.14)
1968	−.073	−.094	.052	.529	.036	.569
	(0.18)	(0.22)	(0.13)	(1.05)	(0.09)	(1.06)
CONSTANT	99.1	105	99.2	95.8	838	94.9
	(97.0)	(24.8)	(93.3)	(17.7)	(5.54)	(0.72)
R^2	.0398		.0468		.047	
F		16.88		10.39		8.04

In parentheses are the absolute values of the t and asymptotic t statistics for the OLS and TSLS coefficients, respectively.

B. Race-Specific Normalization ($\times 10^2$)

(1)		(2)		(3)	
OLS	TSLS	OLS	TSLS	OLS	TSLS
.115	−.078	−.148	−1.62	−.982	.275
(3.00)	(0.40)	(1.33)	(2.50)	(1.54)	(0.06)
.101	−1.04	−.592	−7.96	−.705	−11.4
(0.88)	(1.50)	(1.13)	(1.70)	(1.06)	(1.81)
−.275	−.562	.188	.709	.202	.705
(14.1)	(4.04)	(2.83)	(0.80)	(2.98)	(0.75)
.592	1.57	−1.94	.700	−2.20	1.44
(5.03)	(2.80)	(3.16)	(0.14)	(3.14)	(0.26)
		.233	7.62	−.424	4.33
		(0.54)	(2.31)	(0.44)	(0.53)
		−.384	−.343	−.196	−.647
		(3.71)	(0.31)	(0.90)	(0.29)
		1.53	3.55	2.45	2.12
		(3.39)	(1.10)	(2.26)	(0.27)
		−.0853	1.70	.0226	.933
		(0.42)	(0.72)	(0.10)	(0.35)
		.905	−7.62	1.33	−5.44
		(1.17)	(1.09)	(1.35)	(0.64)
		−.162	−4.53	−.252	−4.50
		(0.74)	(1.89)	(1.05)	(1.78)
				8.00	−11.5
				(1.33)	(0.24)
				2.91	25.6
				(0.60)	(0.58)
				−1.04	2.51
				(1.00)	(0.22)
				−4.57	1.17
				(0.94)	(0.03)
1.81	1.94	−1.12	.686	−1.08	−.633
(2.89)	(2.80)	(2.47)	(0.78)	(2.38)	(0.59)
−.718	−.505	−.723	−.441	−.733	−.409
(1.77)	(1.17)	(1.79)	(0.97)	(1.81)	(0.88)
30.4	35.5	31.1	30.4	31.2	30.1
(3.42)	(3.77)	(3.51)	(2.96)	(3.52)	(2.79)
−1.53	−1.48	−1.43	−.806	−1.40	−.731
(3.73)	(3.38)	(3.50)	(1.57)	(3.40)	(1.20)
−.034	−.058	.062	.544	.081	.565
(0.08)	(0.14)	(0.15)	(1.08)	(0.20)	(1.06)
97.5	104	97.0	95.4	78.4	102
(99.7)	(24.7)	(97.2)	(17.7)	(5.17)	(0.78)
.0318		.0386		.0389	
	7.06		4.91		3.83

Table 2.5 **Estimates of Marginal Products of Inputs at Sample Means on Birth Characteristics**

	Marginal Products (F_i)			
Model specification and estimation techniques	AGE (years)	DELAY (months)	SMOKING (cigarettes per day)	BIRTHS (number)
Leontief (input-output coefficient)				
OLS	3.58	−1.56	−10.1	20.9
TSLS	1.83	−39.6	−16.2	43.3
Leontief-Diewert				
Locally linear				
Homogeneous				
OLS	1.91	5.80	−12.82	11.41
TSLS	8.83	−4.79	−16.42	−15.14
Leontief-Diewert				
Generalized				
OLS	3.58	8.32	−12.50	25.8
TSLS	4.48	−7.54	−13.95	−6.35
Gestation (weeks x 10^2)				
Leontief (input-output coefficient)				
OLS	−.677	−2.25	−.784	.174
TSLS	1.46	−8.23	1.45	−5.26
Leontief-Diewert				
Locally Linear				
Homogeneous				
OLS	−1.09	2.24	−0.896	0.631
TSLS	2.77	−30.76	4.64	−10.41
Leontief-Diewert				
Generalized				
OLS	−.0662	0.424	−0.914	−0.484
TSLS	2.85	−25.8	7.88	−1.63
Race-Specific Standardized Birth Weight ($x10^2$)				
Leontief (input-output coefficient)				
OLS	.115	.101	−.275	.592
TSLS	−.078	−1.04	−.562	1.57
Leontief-Diewert				
Locally Linear				
Homogeneous				
OLS	.0506	.138	−.346	.814
TSLS	.135	.978	−.695	−.794
Leontief-Diewert				
Generalized				
OLS	.0946	.188	−.347	.721
TSLS	.0405	.856	−.753	−.769

Source: Derived from tables 1, 3, and 4.

144 grams less than nonsmokers (i.e., $- 10.1 * 4.71 * 1/.33$). The generalized Leontief-Diewert approximation to the production function implies that this average level of smoking of fourteen cigarettes a day lowers birth weight by 179 grams, based on direct (OLS) partial correlations. When population heterogeneity is taken into account, the impact of smoking is increased further to 195 grams ($- 13.95 * 14$).[15]

The epidemiological evidence based on direct correlations is that smoking only minimally reduces gestation by about two days (Ibid., p. 229), which is not inconsistent with our Leontief OLS estimate of a reduction of about one day ($- .784$ weeks$* 14 \div 100$). However, when population heterogeneity is taken into account in the TSLS estimates, babies of smokers are found to have 1.1 weeks longer gestation, leading to our new finding that for birth weight normalized for gestation the impact of smoking is substantially increased. The generalized TSLS estimates imply that the average consumption of cigarettes by smokers is related to an 11% reduction in birth weight normalized for gestation ($- .753 * 14$). The retardation in the fetal growth rate attributable to average smoking levels is, therefore, larger than has heretofore been estimated.

The effects of age and fertility of the mother appear to be nonlinearly related to birth weight in other studies using quite different analytical techniques (Eisner et al. 1979), and thus considering only the average effect of these variables may obscure their effects in particular segments of the population. At the means of the sample, the effect of age is to increase birth weight slightly and to increase more strongly the gestation of the newborn. No substantial average effect of age is noted, therefore, on normalized birth weight. The number of births the mother has had slightly decreases birth weight, but may decrease the period of gestation, with a consequent negative effect on normalized birth weight.

Interactions between inputs, particularly with AGE (Tables 2.3 and 2.4), appear quantitatively important in several cases, confirming the cluster of characteristics that describe subpopulations which are at high risk of having premature babies. Births to very young mothers and to women who have already had many births tend to be particularly low in weight. Moreover, the AGE and BIRTHS interactions with DELAY suggest that delay in seeking prenatal care is more critical for younger mothers and for high-fertility mothers, whether or not birth weight is normalized for gestation. Moreover, the deleterious effects of smoking on birth weight and birth weight normalized for gestation are increased for older mothers as well as for mothers having many births. The positive birth weight effect of the AGE-BIRTHS interaction suggests that delaying childbearing (or childspacing) enhances, on balance, the health prospects for the newborn. The one interaction that is hard to interpret is the positive birth weight effect of smoking and delaying prenatal medical care.

The estimates of the health production function also indicate that once fertility, age at birth of the mother, health-related activities, and the presence of heterogeneity are taken into account, there remains a two-thirds of a week difference in average gestation period between black and white mothers. There is also a difference in birth weight by race—even after taking into account differences in input behavior, represented here by fertility, age, smoking, and the timing of prenatal care. There is a statistically significant 229 gram differential in birth weight between the babies of black and white mothers, and about a 5% difference in the total population rate of uterine growth (normalized birth weight, Table 2.4). Further investigation shows that this racial difference in birth weight does not appear to be a function of racial differences in the sex ratio at birth—while female infants appeared to have a slightly lower birth weight than did male infants, there is not a statistically significant higher propor-tion of female infants among blacks than among whites in the sample. However, when race-specific birth weight-gestation functions are esti-mated and employed to normalize birth weight in Table 2.4-B, the black-white difference disappears in the TSLS estimates of the Leontief-Diewert production function. These findings suggest that there may be distinct black-white differences in the biological-technical relationship between birth weight and gestation. It is possible, moreover, that distinct scaling of these birth characteristics by genetic group would improve their predictive value as indicators of future child health across a mixed population. In the Appendix Tables 2.A.1 and 2.A.2 we report the estimates for all three birth characteristic production functions based only on births of white mothers.

Birth Characteristics, Socioeconomic Variables and Health Programs: Linear Reduced Forms

Table 2.6 presents estimates of the reduced-form equations relating the socioeconomic variables and those variables representing the availability of health services and programs to the three birth characteristics. These estimates contain several puzzles. For example, the relationship between the schooling level of the mother and birth weight is U-shaped; mothers with only some high school education have babies with the lowest birth weight, whether or not standardized for gestation period, while mothers with less than nine years of schooling bear children of about the same weight as mothers with at least high school educations. Family planning programs associated with hospitals (HOSPFP) appear to reduce birth weight significantly, as does residing in an SMSA. In contrast, husband's income (HINC) and the unemployment of women are positively associ-ated with birth weight. The estimates of the behavioral and technical relationships of Tables 2.2, 2.3, and 2.4 and the computed sample mean marginal products should help account for these findings, however, since

Table 2.6 **Birth Characteristics Reduced Form Demand Equations**

Independent Variable	Birth weight	Birth weight $(x10^2)^*$	Gestation Period
MHSI	−60.28	−2.15	.104
	(2.71)	(3.27)	(1.09)
MHSC	−16.62	−1.01	.175
	(0.80)	(1.63)	(1.94)
MCOLI	−11.58	−1.11	.231
	(0.47)	(1.52)	(2.18)
MCOLC	−12.85	−1.26	.253
	(0.46)	(1.51)	(2.09)
HINC$(x10^{-2})$	5.45	.1410	.0010
	(3.20)	(2.78)	(0.14)
BEDS	10590	358.3	−18.08.
	(1.78)	(1.93)	(0.67)
HEXP	427.86	8.60	1.72
	(1.17)	(0.79)	(1.09)
HOSPFP	−125758	−243276	−24882
	(3.25)	(2.11)	(1.49)
HDFP	−227338	−16314	663.1
	(0.03)	(0.58)	(0.16)
MD$(x10^{-5})$	−1063.7	31.76	1.83
	(1.23)	(1.23)	(0.49)
UNEMPR-W	2105.1	96.77	−2.93
	(3.20)	(4.94)	(1.03)
SERVICE	−1.62	−.048	.001
	(3.48)	(3.46)	(0.60)
CPRCE	38.16	1.51	−.069
	(1.23)	(1.64)	(0.52)
CPRCE2	−.518	−.022	−.0014
	(1.09)	(1.60)	(0.66)
TAXSALES	−5.51	.685	−.247
	(0.38)	(1.61)	(4.00)
BLACK	−184.98	−3.35	−.642
	(11.83)	(7.20)	(9.52)
SMSA	−50.62	−1.49	−.093
	(2.71)	(2.68)	(1.16)
SIZE$(x10^{-8})$	−76.70	16.53	−4.05
	(0.21)	(1.49)	(2.52)
1967	20.79	−1.59	.547
	(1.48)	(3.79)	(9.02)
1968	14.98	−.124	.063
	(1.07)	(0.30)	(2.09)
Constant	2627.6	74.00	40.21
	(5.25)	(4.97)	(18.64)
R^2	.030	.021	.027
F	14.84	10.38	13.09

*Normalized for gestation within total population.

the reduced-form birth characteristics equations reflect the marginal products of the health-related activities as well as the effects of the socioeconomic and program variables on the levels of input activities demanded.

The estimates of the production functions presented in Tables 2.3 and 2.4 indicated that of the activities considered, delay in seeking prenatal medical care, smoking during pregnancy, and birth order had significant effects on child health, with such effects somewhat dependent on the age of the mother. At the sample means, however, birth weight appeared to be most sensitive to levels of smoking—Table 2.5 indicates that while a delay in seeking medical care of six months would lower birth weight by 45 grams, an increase of one pack of cigarettes per day during pregnancy lowers birth weight by 279 grams or by 8.5%. The estimates of Table 2.2 suggested that the health-related activities were importantly but differently related to both the income and educational level of the father and mother, respectively, as well as to the program and health services variables. These findings together imply that the nonlinear effects of education on birth weight are the result of the differential effects of schooling on the several input activities. For example, women with incompleted high school educations (MHSI) appeared to have the second highest fertility of all the educational groups, to smoke more when pregnant than all other women, and to delay more in seeking prenatal medical care than did women with higher levels of schooling. This combination of behavior is consistent with the finding reported in Table 2.6 that this educational group has the lowest birth weight children. The birth weight of women with higher schooling levels, however, appears to differ only modestly from that of women with less than a high school educations, mainly because of only small differences in smoking habits between these groups.

Because of the impact on birth weight of the timing of prenatal medical care, the relatively strong effects of HINC in hastening the utilization of prenatal medical services appears to account for the net positive association between husband's earnings and birth weight. These effects are evidently only partly offset by the tendency of mothers with higher-income husbands to consume more cigarettes while pregnant and to have higher fertility.

The negative effect (marginal product) of birth order on birth weight stands in contrast to the significant negative effect of hospital family planning programs on birth weight—such programs, which appear to be successful in reducing family size, should increase, through the BIRTHS effect, average birth weight levels. However, while BIRTHS appears to be lower in urban settings, such environment appears to be associated with significantly greater cigarette consumption by expectant mothers; because of the large effect of smoking, birth weight tends to be lower in

SMSAs, even though such areas appear to provide better access to and thus encourage earlier use of prenatal medical services.

Finally, we have seen that differences in health-related behavior of mothers do not account for all of the difference in average birth weight between the black and white children, although such behavioral differences account for more of the difference in gestation by race. Differences [between black and white women] in input activities affecting newborn health appear to have an ambiguous net impact on birth weight and gestation: while black mothers postpone seeking prenatal medical care, they smoke significantly less than do white mothers while pregnant, and have larger families. The net effect of this behavioral combination on gestation length is minimal. However, controlling for socioeconomic characteristics and variables representing the availability of health services and programs at the county level, the black-white birth weight differential remains 185 grams, and controlling for the health-related input behavior of the mother that differential is of similar magnitude, namely 229 grams. This suggests that the net impact of black-white differences in measured behavior does not account for the noted birth weight differential between these racial groups. Normalizing birth weight for period of gestation, moreover, reduces the black-white differential only modestly (Table 2.4). Black infants weigh 5–6% less than whites, given gestation and the measured health input behavior of the mother. But if the relationship between birth weight and gestation is fit separately for white and black births in the sample, the TSLS estimates of a race-specific normalized birth weight production function exhibit no statistically significant black-white differences.

Conclusion

In this paper we have formulated an economic model of the household in order to estimate (1) the determinants of activities (inputs) affecting the production of the weight of children at birth and length of gestation, and (2) the biological-technical relationships between parental behavior and birth outcomes in the presence of population heterogeneity. The theoretical model was used to illustrate the advantages of estimating jointly the health production technology and the determinants of the activities potentially affecting infant health, particularly when households differ (are heterogenous) with respect to factors affecting health which are known to the households but not to the researcher. The empirical analysis, based on a probability sample of over 9,000 legitimate births in the United States between 1967 and 1969 combined with geographical information on prices and health programs, considered four endogenous health-related inputs—smoking while pregnant, timing of prenatal medical care, mother's age at birth and birth order—and, initially, two dimensions of prematurity at birth—birth weight and gestational age.

Experimentation with functional forms for the birth outcome production function indicated that estimates of the impact of household input activities on birth characteristics of children are more sensitive to whether or not the estimates account for heterogeneity than to the choice of the functional form. In particular, heterogeneity appeared to almost completely mask a negative impact on child health of the mothers' delay in seeking medical care. Estimates of the production functions also indicated that smoking by the mother while pregnant had the largest (negative) impact on birth weight and on the rate of fetal growth of all the inputs considered while work by the mother during pregnancy did not appear to affect the birth outcomes. Significant interactions were also found among birth order, the timing of births, prenatal care, and smoking; however, the estimated production functions indicated that the four behavioral inputs are more important in the determination of birth weight than of gestation, suggesting that variation in gestation may be less affected by economic and social conditions and more a reflection of biologically exogenous variability.

Since it has been suggested that babies who are underweight relative to other infants of the same gestation exhibit weight deficiencies that persist into later childhood and, after the first month of life, are sick and die more frequently, a normalization procedure was also developed to isolate these more permanent impairments of prematurity related to the rate of fetal growth. Widely noted, but infrequently analyzed, differences in the distribution of birth weight by gestation between white and black births led us to also perform this standardization procedure within each sample for black and white births separately, and then combine these normalized birth weight values in estimating the total sample child health production function. In some instances we found that the effects of an input on birth weight and gestation cancel in terms of their permanent effects on normalized birth weight, as in the case of the mother's age, or are magnified, as in the case of smoking, indicating that the effects of smoking by the mother while pregnant may have a more lasting effect on the child's health. The impact of smoking on the rate of fetal growth (birth weight normalized for gestation) was doubled by taking account of population heterogeneity.

Our treatment of the heterogeneity problem used information on local market prices and health programs both to estimate input demand equations and to identify the child health production functions. We think it unlikely that the demand for health input activities would be independent of latent population characteristics that affect child health production and are known to households. The appropriate treatment of this form of population heterogeneity is crucial for obtaining consistent estimates of underlying health production functions and deriving sound causal conclusions that might be useful for policy.

The next step in such an analysis is to ask whether the identifying program and price variables are themselves independent of our heterogeneous population characteristics, i.e., μ. Government health programs may be established to serve groups in the population that are known by the government to have distinctly different health endowments or environments, or in our notation different values of μ. Alternatively, individuals may themselves migrate to regions with lower prices for preferred inputs and/or available programs; in other words, individuals are drawn selectively to certain regions according to their own perceived health endowments or preferences. In either instance, the source of identifying information required to obtain consistent estimates of the child health production function may prove more difficult to observe. Estimates of input productivities and price and program effects based on regional price and program information could in this case be inconsistent, for the regional variables would no longer be independently distributed with regard to heterogeneous population characteristics.

Notes

1. See, for example, Baumgartner (1962), Beck and van den Berg (1975), Chase (1969), Chernichovsky and Coate (1979), Eisner et al. (1979), and Shapiro (1965).
2. Examples of behavioral correlates of early child health indicators, based on univariate associations, are medical care (Shah and Abbey 1971, Rosenwaike 1971, and Iba et al. 1973), cigarette smoking by mothers (Hobel et al. 1971) and wife's work (Coombs et al. 1969).
3. We abstract from uncertainty, or alternatively, assume that parents are risk-neutral. Under the latter assumption random effects on health outcomes unknown to the family decision-makers at the time when decisions are made will not enter the process of optimization. Variations in μ, however, do effect decisions and, as shown below, have important econometric implications. See also Mundlak and Hoch (1965).
4. Becker and Lewis (1973) and Becker and Tomes (1974). For a discussion of the predictive content of models which assume interactions between family size and investments in children, see Rosenzweig and Wolpin (1980).
5. See, for example, Michael (1973) and Grossman (1972). The conventional assumption that education is exogenous to adult demand behavior might also require reconsideration here. Some young women become pregnant unexpectedly and therefore terminate their schooling at an earlier stage than they would otherwise. If these women also tend to have low birth weight babies, part of the association between mother's low education and low birth weight would be generated by unplanned pregnancies and the endogeneity of the mother's educational attainment. This effect may be reduced by the exclusion of illegitimate births from the natality followback survey files.
6. Victor Fuchs noted that this development might be explained by the increasing proportion of nonwhite births occurring in hospitals in this period, where (low) birth weight was more accurately reported. (See Querac and Spratley 1978, Fig. 6.) In 1950 the nonwhite

"prematurity" rate was 10.2% and by 1967 had increased to 13.6%, while the rate for whites was 7.1% in both years (Chase and Byrnes 1972). In the mid–1960s, 8% of all U.S. births were under 2,500 grams, but these births accounted for 62% of the deaths occurring in the first year of life (MacMahon et al. 1972). It is not surprising, therefore, that some investigations have found birth weight alone explains an overwhelming share (90%) of the variance in perinatal mortality (Susser et al. 1972).

7. The authors plan subsequent research to explore nonlinear transformations of birth weight and mortality outcomes as well.

8. The estimates are

total sample: birth weight = 10107 − 1042 weeks + 37.8 weeks^2 − .398 weeks^3
                            (7.72)   (9.95)   (10.44)   (10.90)
       $R^2 = .227$, $n = 9763$
whites: birth weight = 13416 − 1354 weeks + 47.3 weeks^2 − .492 weeks^3
                      (8.48)   (9.13)   (10.4)   (10.9)
       $R^2 = .201$, $n = 7896$
blacks: birth weight = 9188 − 937 weeks + 34.4 weeks^2 − .366 weeks^3
                      (4.39)   (4.57)   (5.26)   (5.39)
       $R^2 = .273$, $n = 1867$

where the absolute values of t statistics are reported in parentheses beneath the regression coefficients, and n is the sample size. For additional evidence of this relationship, see Querec and Spratley (1978, Fig. 2).

9. The unexplained variation of individual birth weights around the estimated fetal growth function is undoubtedly heteroscedastic; that is, the absolute magnitude of this variation increases systematically with the level of birth weight expected on the basis of gestation, or $f(t)$. If the variance of these individual deviations increased in proportion to $f(t)^2$, our normalization measure of birth weight controlling for gestation would exhibit a constant variance error, and standard estimation procedures would then be efficient. Heteroscedasticity would, on the other hand, reduce the efficiency of our estimates, but not affect their consistency or probability limits in a large sample.

10. Infant mortality rates in the United States in 1960 were 41.4 per thousand nonwhite births and 22.2 per thousand white births. Also, 12.9% of nonwhite births weighed less than 2,500 grams, whereas only 6.8% of the white births were so classified. Yet when periods of infancy are distinguished, mortality rates for whites exceed those for nonwhites in each of these periods within the high mortality weight categories below 3000 grams (Chase, 1962). This might suggest that nonwhite births have a lower distribution of birth weights than do whites, given similar health inputs. Differences between races in pelvic structures might rationalize such a difference in birth weight. Also, more rapid postnatal skeletal growth has been noted in nonwhite than in white U.S. populations. Regardless of the origin or function of possible racial differences, separate normalizations of birth weight for gestational age are explored since the size of the nonwhite sample population did not permit us to estimate with any confidence the parameters of the production function for each racial group separately.

11. We set *DELAY* equal to the sample mean gestation period (39 weeks) if no prenatal medical care was sought, and to 4 weeks if "immediate" care was received upon learning of the pregnancy.

12. The formula for computing elasticities of substitution between any two inputs y_i and y_j (σ_{ij}) based on production functions which are linear in parameters (Fuss and McFadden 1978, Chapter II.1) is

$$\sigma_{ij} = \left[- F_{ii}/F_i^2 + 2(F_{ij}/F_iF_j) - F_{jj}/F_j^2 \right] \left[(y_iF_i)^{-1} + (y_jF_j)^{-1} \right]^{-1}$$

where it is assumed that the quantities of other inputs and output are held constant.

13. An alternative strategy which could provide consistent estimates of the health production function in the presence of heterogeneity would make use of differences in birth outcomes and parental behavior between births within the same family. To implement such a technique would require longitudinal data or good retrospective information on prior births and would necessitate the assumption that (perceived) μ is constant across all births in the same household, ruling out modifications in expectations through experience. This technique can only be applied, of course, to families with at least two live births and would suffer from the imprecision of estimates obtained from most individual fixed effects models.

14. In 1978 black women over the age of 17 were less likely to be smokers than white women, 39.8% versus 45.6% (U.S. Department of Health and Human Services, 1979, Table 3). Moreover, white women over the age of 17 reported smoking more cigarettes per day: twice the percentage of black as white female smokers reported smoking less than fifteen cigarettes daily, whereas five times as many white as black female smokers reported smoking twenty-five cigarettes or more daily (Table 5). These estimates based on the National Health Interview Survey for 1978 are similar to those published in earlier years, but rarely are the black-white differences reported in greater detail, by age and sex and in particular by pregnancy status.

15. Analysis of current population survey data collected in June 1966 (Ahmed and Gleeson 1970) confirms roughly similar levels of cigarette consumption as found in the 1967–69 NNFS, assuming that about one-third of the smokers stop smoking during pregnancy. For example, among women aged 25–44, 42.9% were currently smokers in June 1966. This percentage fell to 38.8% by 1970 (U.S. Department of Health and Human Services, 1979, Table 1) and to 35.9% in 1978. From the 1966 survey (Table 6), one can estimate that among smokers 16.4 cigarettes were smoked per day, implying an average for the total female population aged 25–44 of 7.04 cigarettes daily. If one-third of the smokers stopped smoking while pregnant, but those continuing to smoke continued to smoke 16.4 cigarettes daily, the average consumption for pregnant women would have been 4.7 cigarettes. This compares with our estimate for legitimate births in the three subsequent years of 1967–69 of 4.71 cigarettes per day.

References

Ahmed, P.I., and Gleeson, G.A. 1970. Changes in cigarette smoking habits between 1955 and 1966. *Vital and Health Statistics,* series 10, no. 59. Rockville, Maryland: U.S. Department of Health and Human Services.

Baumgartner, L. 1962. The public health significance of low birth weight in U.S.A. *Bulletin of the World Health Organization* 26: 175–82.

Beck, G.J., and van den Berg, B.J. 1975. The relationship of the rate of intrauterine growth of low birth weight infants to later growth. *Journal of Pediatrics* 86: 504–11.

Becker, G., and Lewis, H.G. 1974. On the interaction between quantity and quality of children. *Journal of Political Economy* 82: S279–S288.

————, and Tomes, N. 1976. Child endowments and the quantity and quality of children. *Journal of Political Economy* 84: S143–S162.

Chase, H.C. 1969. Infant mortality and weight at birth: 1960 United States birth cohort. *American Journal of Public Health* 59: 1618–28.

————, and Byrnes, M.E. 1972. Trends in prematurity: United States, 1950–1967. *Vital and Health Statistics,* series 3, no. 15. Rockville, Maryland: U.S. Dept. of Health, Education, and Welfare.

Chernickovsky, D., and Coate, D. 1979. An economic analysis of diet, growth, and health of young children in the United States. Working Paper No. 416. Cambridge: National Bureau of Economic Research.

Coombs, L.; Freedman, R.; and Namboothiri. 1969. Inferences about abortion from foetal mortality data. *Population Studies* 23: 247–65.

Diewert, W.E. 1971. An application of the Shepherd duality approach: a generalized Leontief production function. *Journal of Political Economy* 79, no. 3: 481–507.

Eisner, V.; Brazie, J.V.; Pratt, M.W.; and Hexter, A.C. 1979. The risk of low birth weight. *American Journal of Public Health* 69: 887–93.

Fuss, M., and McFadden, D. 1978. *Production economics: a dual approach to theory and applications,* vols. 1 and 2. Amsterdam: North-Holland.

Grossman, M. 1972. On the concept of health capital and the demand for health. *Journal of Political Economy* 80:223–55.

Hemminki, E., and Starfield, B. 1978. Prevention of low birth weight and preterm birth: literature review and suggestions for research policy. *Milbank Memorial Fund Quarterly–Health and Society* 56: 339–61.

Hobel, R.; Entwisle, G.; and Tayback, M. 1971. A risk adjustment technique for comparing prematurity rates among clinic populations. *HMSHA Health Reports* 86:946–52.

Iba, B.Y.; Niswander, J.D.; and Woodville, L. 1973. Relation of prenatal care to birth weights, major malformations, and newborn deaths of American Indians. *Health Services Reports* 88: 697–701.

MacMahon, B.; Kovar, M.G.; and Feldman, J.J. 1972. Infant mortality rates: socioeconomic factors in the United States. *Vital and Health Statistics,* series 22, no. 14. Rockville, Maryland: U.S. Dept. of Health, Education, and Welfare.

Meyer, M.B.; Jonas, B.C.; and Tonascia, J.A. 1976. Perinatal events associated with maternal smoking during pregnancy. *American Journal of Epidemiology* 103: 464–76.

Michael, R.T. 1973. Education in nonmarket production. *Journal of Political Economy* 81: 306–27.

Mudlak, Y., and Hoch, I. 1965. Consequences of alternative specifications in estimation of the Cobb-Douglas functions. *Econometrica* 33: 814–28.

Querec, N.A., and Spratley, E. 1978. Characteristics of births: United States, 1973–1975. *Vital and Health Statistics,* series 21, no. 30. Hyattsville, Maryland: U.S. Department of Health, Education, and Welfare.

Rosenwaike, I. 1971. The influence of socioeconomic status on incidence of low birth weight. *HMSHA Health Reports* 86: 641–49.

Rosenzweig, M.R., and Schultz, T.P. 1980. Birth weight, the production of child health, and input demand. Discussion Paper 352, Yale Economic Growth Center.

———, and Wolpin, K.I. 1980. Testing the quantity-quality fertility model: the use of twins as a natural experiment. *Econometrica* 48: 227–40.

Shah, F.K., and Abbey, H. 1971. Effects of some factors on neonatal and postneonatal mortality. *Milbank Memorial Fund Quarterly* 49:33–57.

Shapiro, S. 1965. Weight of birth and survival of the newborn: United States, early 1950. *Vital and Health Statistics,* series 21, no. 3. Washington: U.S. Department of Health, Education, and Welfare.

Susser, M.W.; Marolla, F.A.; and Fleiss, J. 1972. Birth weight, fetal age, and perinatal mortality. *American Journal of Epidemiology* 96: 197–204.

Taffel, S. 1980. Factors associated with low birth weight: United States, 1976. *Vital and Health Statistics,* series 21, no. 37. Hyattsville, Maryland: U.S. Department of Health, Education, and Welfare.

U.S. Department of Health and Human Services. 1980. *The health consequences of smoking for women: a report of the Surgeon General.* Washington: Office of the Assistant Secretary for Health, Office of Smoking and Health.

U.S. National Center for Health Statistics. 1979. Changes in cigarette smoking and current smoking practices among adults: United States, 1978. *Advance data from Vital and Health Statistics,* no. 52. Hyattsville, Maryland: U.S. Department of Health, Education, and Welfare.

———. 1980. Selected demographic characteristics of teenage wives and mothers. *Advance data from Vital and Health Statistics,* no. 61. Hyattsville, Maryland: U.S. Department of Health and Human Services.

Valanis, B.M. 1979. Relative contribution of maternal social and biological characteristics to birth weight and gestation among mothers of different childhood socioeconomic status. *Social Biology* 26: 211–25.

van den Berg, B.J. 1968. Morbidity of low birth weight and/or preterm children compared to that of the 'mature'. *Pediatrics* 42: 590–97.

———, and Yerushalmy, J. 1966. The relationship of the rate of intrauterine growth of infants of low birth weight to mortality, morbidity, and congenital anomalities. *Journal of Pediatrics* 69: 531–97.

Werner, T. and Milton, T. 1969. Demographic correlates of low birth weight. *American Journal of Epidemiology* 91, no. 3.

Yerushalmy, J.; van den Berg, B.J.; Erhardt, C.L.; and Jacobziner, H. 1965. Birth weight and gestation as indicies of 'immaturity'. *American Journal Dis. Child* 109: 43–57.

Appendix

Table 2.A.1   **Birth Characteristics Production Function Estimates for White Population: Linear and Generalized Leontieff-Diewert.**

Independent Variable	A. Birthweight					
	(1)		(2)		(3)	
	OLS	TSLS	OLS	TSLS	OLS	TSLS
AGE	2.72 (1.94)	2.10 (0.42)	−8.01 (1.84)	−49.1 (1.83)	−56.1 (2.38)	−286 (1.70)
DELAY	−2.52 (0.54)	−30.54 (1.26)	−31.4 (1.49)	−274 (1.61)	−24.2 (0.89)	−363 (1.57)
SMOKING	−10.5 (15.6)	−17.6 (4.11)	5.74 (2.42)	13.9 (0.49)	6.14 (2.52)	6.82 (0.22)
BIRTHS	24.7 (5.29)	44.9 (2.11)	−60.6 (2.37)	349. (1.45)	−63.0 (2.18)	300 1.06
$(AGE \cdot DELAY)^{1/2}$			17.9 (1.04)	367 (2.82)	7.18 (0.19)	12.4 (0.03)
$(AGE \cdot SMOKE)^{1/2}$			−10.4 (2.80)	−2.44 (0.06)	−6.37 (0.82)	−64.1 (0.88)
$(AGE \cdot BIRTHS)^{1/2}$			55.0 (3.02)	−2.28 (0.02)	78.2 (1.83)	176 (0.54)
$(DELAY \cdot SMOKE)^{1/2}$			−6.85 (0.90)	14.7 (0.16)	−3.73 (0.44)	−4.95 (0.05)
$(DELAY \cdot BIRTHS)^{1/2}$			16.4 (0.50)	−591 (2.10)	12.2 (0.30)	−441 (1.23)
$(SMOKE \cdot BIRTHS)^{1/2}$			−12.3 (1.54)	−97.3 (1.16)	−14.7 (1.68)	−84.6 (0.95)
$AGE^{1/2}$					474 (2.14)	2730 (1.59)
$SMOKING^{1/2}$					−23.7 (0.64)	351 (0.93)
$BIRTHS^{1/2}$					−104 (0.55)	−947 (0.71)
$DELAY^{1/2}$					34.7 (0.18)	1894 (1.04)
SMSA	−14.9 (1.02)	−13.2 (0.86)	−13.9 (0.96)	−13.3 (0.81)	−14.5 (0.99)	−8.48 (0.50)
SIZE ($x10^{-8}$)	172 (0.54)	258 (0.77)	191 (0.60)	105 (0.29)	178 (0.55)	−.038 (0.00)
1967	25.3 (1.70)	26.7 (1.71)	29.3 (1.97)	48.6 (2.52)	31.4 (2.11)	60.3 (2.67)
1968	9.39 (0.63)	7.57 (0.49)	13.8 (0.92)	23.4 (1.18)	14.8 (0.99)	27.3 (1.33)
CONSTANT	3259 (91.1)	3334 (23.2)	3234 (88.9)	3067 (16.0)	2086 (3.73)	−4749 (0.98)
R^2	.0386		.0468		.0475	
F		5.60		3.90		3.11

t-values in parentheses.

B. Gestation Period ($x10^2$)					
(1)		(2)		(3)	
OLS	TSLS	OLS	TSLS	OLS	TSLS
−.365 (0.63)	2.74 (1.32)	−1.86 (1.04)	11.4 (1.05)	−19.4 (1.99)	−88.5 (1.33)
−.649 (0.34)	.078 (0.01)	−28.0 (3.22)	24.6 (0.35)	−22.5 (2.00)	10.6 (0.12)
−1.03 (3.67)	.178 (0.10)	.020 (0.02)	−3.95 (0.35)	−.144 (0.14)	−4.73 (0.38)
−1.82 (0.95)	−9.76 (1.12)	2.62 (0.25)	121 (1.25)	3.56 (0.30)	74.6 (0.67)
		17.7 (2.48)	−.377 (0.01)	19.7 (1.27)	−138 (0.96)
		−1.62 (1.05)	10.7 (0.71)	−3.81 (1.19)	−9.02 (0.31)
		6.63 (0.88)	−68.9 (1.25)	−2.45 (0.14)	53.2 (0.41)
		−1.77 (0.56)	−28.4 (0.75)	−2.56 (0.73)	−30.5 (0.73)
		8.01 (0.59)	−51.6 (0.46)	1.41 (0.08)	17.6 (0.12)
		3.71 (1.13)	12.4 (0.37)	4.64 (1.28)	14.2 (0.40)
				175 (1.90)	1060 (1.56)
				11.5 (0.75)	102 (0.69)
				−15.9 (0.20)	−571 (1.09)
				−16.7 (0.21)	640 (0.88)
3.00 (0.50)	−6.05 (0.96)	−2.87 (0.48)	−8.00 (1.22)	−3.20 (0.53)	−6.01 (0.89)
−239 (1.80)	−284 (2.07)	−240 (1.81)	−304 (2.13)	−248 (1.87)	−335 (2.29)
51.3 (8.35)	50.9 (7.96)	52.5 (8.52)	46.9 (6.06)	53.1 (8.59)	50.6 (5.64)
8.50 (1.38)	8.81 (1.39)	9.95 (1.61)	5.08 (0.64)	10.2 (1.66)	6.32 (0.78)
3925 (266)	3861 (65.6)	3917 (259)	3899 (50.5)	3489 (15.0)	1099 (0.57)
.0127		.0144		.0151	
	10.88		6.20		4.94

Table 2.A.2   Birthweight Production Function
Estimates for White Population: Linear and Generalized Leontief-Diewert

Independent Variable	(1)		(2)		(3)	
	OLS	TSLS	OLS	TSLS	OLS	TSLS
AGE	.0790 (1.94)	−.082 (0.55)	−.168 (1.34)	−2.12 (2.62)	−1.20 (1.75)	−5.62 (1.11)
DELAY	.00592 (0.04)	−.891 (1.26)	.0829 (0.14)	−9.86 (1.91)	.0866 (0.11)	−12.7 (1.83)
SMOKING	−.287 (14.7)	−.586 (4.69)	.189 (2.76)	.743 (0.86)	.202 (2.86)	.467 (0.49)
BIRTHS	.756 (5.59)	1.65 2.65	−1.58 (2.14)	8.23 (1.13)	−1.68 (2.00)	8.52 (1.00)
$(AGE \cdot DELAY)^{1/2}$			.0117 (0.02)	12.5 (3.19)	−.509 (0.47)	6.87 (0.63)
$(AGE \cdot SMOKE)^{1/2}$			−.323 (2.99)	−.666 (0.59)	−.187 (−0.83)	−2.28 (1.04)
$(AGE \cdot BIRTHS)^{1/2}$			1.71 (3.23)	2.51 (0.61)	2.31 (1.86)	3.26 (0.33)
$(DELAY \cdot SMOKE)^{1/2}$			−.0734 (0.33)	2.64 (0.92)	.0154 (0.06)	1.80 (0.57)
$(DELAY \cdot BIRTHS)^{1/2}$			−.107 (0.11)	−20.0 (2.35)	.0102 (0.01)	−17.5 (1.62)

Standardized for Gestation ($\times 10^2$)

	(1)	(2)	(3)	(4)	(5)	(6)
(SMOKE · BIRTHS)$^{1/2}$			-.429 (1.86)	-4.62 (1.83)	-.503 (1.99)	-4.10 (1.53)
AGE$^{1/2}$					10.3 (1.61)	44.4 (0.86)
SMOKING$^{1/2}$					-.772 (0.72)	9.85 (0.87)
BIRTHS$^{1/2}$					-2.94 (0.54)	-8.18 (0.20)
DELAY$^{1/2}$					2.36 (0.43)	35.4 (0.64)
SMSA	-.361 (0.85)	-.161 (0.36)	-.334 (0.79)	-.077 (0.16)	-.344 (0.81)	-.0102 (0.02)
SIZE (x10^{-8})	17.1 (1.83)	22.1 (2.26)	17.7 (1.90)	17.1 (1.59)	17.4 (1.87)	14.5 (1.31)
1967	-1.22 (2.83)	-1.13 (2.48)	-1.13 (2.62)	-.225 (0.39)	-1.08 (2.50)	-.023 (0.03)
1968	-.0702 (0.16)	-.133 (0.29)	.0153 (0.03)	.497 (0.83)	.0391 (0.09)	.567 (0.92)
CONSTANT	98.2 (94.8)	104 (24.7)	97.6 (92.6)	93.2 (16.1)	72.0 (4.44)	-44.4 (0.31)
R^2	.0375		.0455		.0460	
F		6.27		4.50		3.50

t-values are in parentheses.

Table 2.A.3   **Statistical Appendix: Level of Aggregation, Year and Source for Area Variables**

Variable Name	Aggregation Level and Year	Source
BEDS	State, 1965	*Hospital, Journal of the American Hospital Association: Guide Issue* American Hospital Association, 1965
HEXP	State or SMSA, 1965	*County and City Data Book*, Bureau of the Census 1967
HOSPFP	State, 1969	*Need for Subsidized Family Planning Services: United States, Each State and County*, Center for Family Program Development, 1969
HDFP	State or SMSA, 1969	*Need for Subsidized Family Planning Services: United States, Each State and County*, Center for Family Program Development, 1969
MD	State or SMSA, 1969	*Need for Subsidized Family Planning Services: United States, Each State and County*, Center for Family Program Development, 1969
UNEMPR-W	State, 1970	*Census of Population 1970*, U.S. Bureau of the Census, 1974
SERVICE	State, 1970	*County and City Data Book*, Bureau of the Census, 1972
CPRCE	State or Town, 1967–1969	*Tax Burden on Tobacco*, Tobacco Tax Council, Inc., Richmond, VA, 1975
TAX SALES	State or Town, 1967–1969	*Tax Burden on Tobacco*, Tobacco Tax Council, Inc., Richmond Va 1975
SIZE	SMSA, 1970	*Census of Population 1970*, U.S. Bureau of the Census, 1974

3 Time Preference and Health: An Exploratory Study

Victor R. Fuchs

This paper reports the results of an exploratory effort in a new area—the relationship between intertemporal choice, health behavior, and health status. Intertemporal choice (or time preference) is, of course, a subject much discussed by economists and psychologists. (See Maital and Maital 1978.) There is also a large literature on individual behavior (e.g., cigarette smoking, diet, exercise) and health status. This paper, however, seems to be the first to attempt to bring these subjects together and to test empirically for possible interrelations.

In the first section of the paper I briefly review some of the considerations that suggest that an investigation of time preference might throw light on health behavior and health status. These include empirical studies of the relation between schooling and health, epidemiological investigations of the health effects of cigarette smoking, diet, exercise, and the like, and theoretical issues concerning investment in human capital, imperfections in capital markets, and optimizing behavior.

The second section considers the critical problem of the measurement of time preference and reviews some recent efforts by other investigators to measure time preference in contexts other than health. I then describe a pilot questionnaire given to 500 men and women and present the results

Victor R. Fuchs is professor of Economics at Stanford University and a research associate at the National Bureau of Economic Research. This research was supported by grants from The Robert Wood Johnson Foundation and The Henry J. Kaiser Family Foundation. Phillip Farrell provided research assistance and made many valuable suggestions. The participants in the Stanford University Interdisciplinary Seminar in Decision Analysis offered stimulating comments, and at an early stage I benefited from discussions with Martin Seligman and Richard Thaler. Helpful comments from the participants in the NBER Conference "Economic Aspects of Health" are also gratefully acknowledged. The contributions of many other colleagues are indicated in the references and notes. The research reported here is part of the NBER's research in the Health Economics Program. Any opinions expressed are those of the author and not those of the National Bureau of Economic Research.

of correlation and regression analyses of their replies. The paper concludes with a discussion of questions raised by this exploratory research.

Background

Empirical considerations

Cross-sectional studies of the determinants of health status in the United States usually report a strong association between health and years of schooling. This result typically appears regardless of whether health is measured objectively (e.g., mortality rates) or subjectively (e.g., self-evaluation), and is equally robust in studies of differences across groups (e.g., states or cities) or across individuals (e.g., household survey data). Simple correlations between health and years of schooling are usually significant in both the statistical and the practical sense. Furthermore, the relation remains strong after controlling for other variables such as income.

Probably the most thorough investigation of this relationship has been carried out by Michael Grossman in "The Correlation between Health and Schooling" (1975). This study of middle-aged men is particularly notable for two reasons.

First, a statistically significant effect of schooling on health remains after controlling for a large number of other variables, including family background, health status in high school, income, job satisfaction, and scores on physical and mental tests taken by the men when they were in their early 20s.

Second, each of the men had at least a high school diploma; the mean level of schooling was over fifteen years. Grossman's finding that the favorable effects of additional schooling persist even at high levels of schooling is in sharp contrast to the relation between income and health, which is positive at low levels of income but seems to be much weaker or nonexistent at average or high levels (Auster, Leveson, and Sarachek 1969).

While the relationship between schooling and health seems well established, the mechanisms through which schooling affects health are less clear. Grossman has interpreted the empirical results as support for a household production function model; additional years of schooling make the individual a more efficient producer of health. This efficiency may arise through wiser use of medical care or, what is more likely, through differences in cigarette smoking, diet, and other elements of "life style."

The view that "the greatest potential for improving the health of the American people . . . is to be found in what people do and don't do to and for themselves" (Fuchs, 1967) has gained widespread acceptance in recent years as the result of numerous studies by epidemiologists and social scientists interested in health.[1] These studies report significant differences in health status and in life expectancy associated with such factors as cigarette smoking, diet, and exercise. Not only is a statistical correlation well established, but in many instances there is some understanding of the causal mechanisms as well, e.g., the role of diet and exercise in the prevention of atherosclerosis. What is not understood at all well is the cause of individual variation in health-related behavior.

From an economic point of view many of these behaviors have a common characteristic—they involve trade-offs between current costs and future benefits. The costs may be purely psychic, such as the loss of pleasure from passing up a rich dessert or a cigarette. They may involve time, such as jogging, or they may involve other costs including financial and nonfinancial resources. The expected benefits typically take the form of reductions in the probability of morbidity and mortality from one or more diseases sometime in the future.

Theoretical considerations

The acceptance of a current cost for a future benefit constitutes an investment. Becker's development of the theory of investment in human capital (Becker 1964) and Grossman's application of this theory specifically to health (Grossman 1972) provide a convenient framework for thinking about these health behaviors. Suppose individuals differ in their willingness or ability to undertake investments, i.e., they have different time preferences. Such differences might help to explain variations in cigarette smoking, diet, and the like. Furthermore, this approach suggests possible links with the health-schooling relationship that has been found by so many investigators.

There are at least two ways that individual variation in time preference could explain the correlation between schooling and health.[2] First, suppose that differences in time preference are established early in life, are relatively stable, and do affect subsequent behavior.[3] These differences might be due to differences in the education or income of parents, the stability of the family, the values associated with different religions, or to other background characteristics. Given variation in time preference, it would not be surprising to observe that individuals with low rates of time discount would invest in many years of schooling and would also invest in health-enhancing activities. According to this view schooling has no direct effect on health; the observed correlation is due to both schooling and health as depending upon time preference.

A second possibility (the two explanations are not mutually exclusive) is that schooling actually affects time preference; those with more schooling are more willing to invest at a lower rate of return.[4] Thus more schooling could result in better health by increasing investments in health. The empirical portion of this paper, based on a single cross-section survey, cannot distinguish between these two hypotheses, but we can test for possible relations between schooling and time preference.

Empirical investigation of time preference through survey questions designed to elicit marginal rates of time discount depends critically on capital markets being "imperfect." If capital markets were perfect (i.e., if individuals could borrow and lend without limit at a single market rate of interest) marginal rates would be equal for all regardless of time preference. Differences across individuals in time preference might still result in differences in nontradeable health-related activities, but these would not be predictable from the replies to interest rate questions. However, if capital markets are not perfect (an assumption of this paper), individuals may well have different rates of interest at the margin, and these may be related to health behavior and health status.

Let us imagine a two-period world. Suppose utility in each period depends upon consumption of goods (G). Utility in the first period also is a function of some activity C_1 (for simplicity assumed to be free with respect to G) which affects health (and therefore utility) in period two. For example C_1 might be cigarette smoking:

$$U_1 = U_1(G_1, C_1)$$

$$U_2 = U_2(G_2, H_2) \text{ where } H_2 = H(C_1).$$

A wealth compensated increase in the rate of interest (r) will, *ceteris paribus*, alter the allocation of wealth between G_1 and G_2. But if the marginal utility of C_1 depends on the quantity of G_1 (and the marginal utility of H_2 depends on the quantity of G_2), the change in r will also affect C_1 (and H_2). If G_1 and C_1 (and G_2 and H_2) are substitutes, an increase in r will lead to an increase in C_1 and a decrease in H_2. If the relationship is complementary (which seems less plausible to me), the reverse would be true.

It should be emphasized that (given imperfect capital markets) differences across individuals in marginal rates of interest can be the result of differences in underlying preference functions (indifference curves) or differences in opportunities to borrow and lend.[5] In general, it will not be possible to distinguish between these sources empirically, although controlling for family income (as a proxy for "opportunities") may move the analysis somewhat closer to a focus on preference functions per se.

Because time preference is probably only one of many factors affecting the demand for cigarettes, jogging, or other health-related behaviors, we can hardly expect perfect correlation among these activities. Differences in time preference across individuals, however, should result in some positive correlations among these behaviors.

Measurement of Time Preference

In recent years there have been several attempts to measure time preference through household survey techniques. The objectives of the investigators have varied greatly, but the general approach has been similar: the respondent is confronted with a hypothetical situation involving different sums of money at different points in time and is asked to express a preference which will implicitly reveal a rate of time discount.

Thomas and Ward (1979)

Psychologists Ewart A. C. Thomas and Wanda E. Ward were interested in relations between time preference and various psychological measures of temporal orientation[6] and measures of optimism or pessimism. They were also interested in possible effects of time preference on saving and spending behavior. Their sample consisted of 63 college students who were asked 24 open-ended time preference questions of the following type:

If offered $100 now or X dollars in six months, what would be the *smallest* amount of money (X dollars) you would accept rather than the immediately available $100?

Some questions gave the future amount and asked the respondent to choose a current value; others gave both amounts and asked for the time period that would make them commensurate. Still others were formulated as payments rather than as receipts, and some were expressed in terms of goods rather than dollar amounts.

Implicit discount rates were found to be negatively correlated with future time orientation and positively correlated with "big spending." The group results were considered satisfactory, but the measurement of time preference was "disappointing" to the authors because of the "high instability of parameter estimates for individual subjects."

West (SRI) (1978)

Economists involved in the Seattle-Denver income maintenance experiment were interested in time preference because the bias introduced by the finite length of the experiment (compared to a national program of indefinite life) would vary depending upon the household's rate of time discount (Metcalf 1974). The families in the experiment (more than 1,500 in each city) were asked a large number and variety of time preference questions. Some were open-ended, similar to those of Thomas and Ward. Some were "cascades" of the following type:

Suppose you had a choice between a cash bonus of $100 today and $200 a year from now; which would you choose?

If the respondent chooses $200, the question is repeated, with $175 substituted for $200, and so on until the respondent chooses $100. Some cascade questions go up instead of down; some involve payments rather than receipts; and some involve different time periods.

The mean interest rates implicit in the replies of these low income respondents were typically quite high, but the correlation between questions was typically low ($r =$ about .1 or .2). The author, Richard W. West, expressed some concern that "the measures are not reliable" (p. 23).

Maital and Maital (1978)

A paper by an economist and a psychologist, Shlomo Maital and Sharona Maital, reviews some of the economic and psychological literature on time preference and reports the results of a survey of 515 Israeli adults. The Maitals' focus is on the role of time preference in the intergenerational transmission of income inequality. They asked one cascade question involving choice between a sum of money now and higher sums one year from now. A similar question in which gift certificates for a week's shopping at a supermarket were substituted for money was asked in an attempt to measure the real as opposed to the nominal implicit rate of interest.

The implicit interest rate was negatively correlated with years of schooling ($r = -.08$) and with a dummy variable which took a value of 1 if the subject and the subject's father were born in Israel ($r = -.12$). The nominal rate was negatively correlated with income ($r = -.14$), but the real rate was not. The authors concluded that the ability to defer gratification is part of the process of socialization and that "after adolescence the propensity to delay gratification is quite stable" (p. 192). This may be correct, but it is not clear that the conclusion follows from their results.

Thaler (1979)

In a questionnaire administered[7] to approximately 75 college students, Richard Thaler posed a large number of open-ended money choices primarily to learn how the implicit interest rate varies with the amount of money involved, the time period, the starting point of the comparison, and whether the choice involves receipt or payment. He found that the implicit rate was lower the larger the amount of money and the longer the time period. Also, choices involving two points both in the future typically invoked a smaller implicit interest rate than choices involving the present versus the future. He concluded that there is a "psychic *fixed* cost" to waiting, as well as a cost that varies with amount and time.

I included a few questions on health status in the Thaler questionnaire and found a significant negative correlation between health and median implicit interest rate across individuals. This result led me to undertake the larger pilot survey described in the next section.

The Pilot Survey

In November 1979, Stephen and Ann Cole conducted a survey measuring time preference, health status, and health behavior as well as a large number of family background and current socioeconomic variables.[8] Telephone interviews approximately twenty minutes in length were conducted with 508 individuals living in Nassau and Suffolk Counties (on Long Island just east of New York City). Respondents were selected through a random sample of telephone numbers;[9] interviews were completed with 58% of the eligible respondents. The characteristics of the respondents conformed closely to census data for those two counties, but the possibility of selection bias remains, especially with respect to some of the family background variables.

The sample was restricted to individuals aged 25–64, and interviewers were instructed to obtain an approximately equal distribution between female and male respondents. The respondents differ from a national sample with respect to religion (55% Catholic and 17% Jewish), race (3% black), and schooling (about one year above the national average). They are also somewhat more affluent and in slightly better health. Allowing for the predominantly suburban middle-class character of the two counties, the distributions of replies on the health, health behavior, family background, and socioeconomic variables conform closely to those obtained in national surveys.

The principal approach to the measurement of time preference was through a series of six questions asking the respondent to choose between a sum of money now and a larger sum at a specific point in the future,[10] e.g., "Would you choose $1,500 now or $4,000 in five years?" The amount and the time period varied, as did the interest rate implicit in each question. The lowest implicit rate was 10.1% per annum (continuously compounded); the highest was 51.1%. This dichotomous choice type of question was used because it was deemed simpler for the respondent than the open-ended or cascade type questions discussed previously.[11]

In addition to the implicit interest rate series of questions, a cascade type question with an explicit interest rate (beginning at 6% and rising to 50%) was asked. The survey also included four attitudinal questions, e.g., "Do you agree or disagree with this statement: It makes more sense to spend your money now rather than save it for the future." Also, each respondent was asked to choose an expected rate of change of prices for the coming year. The final time preference questions dealt with the respondent's use of credit during car purchases or through unpaid balances on bank credit cards.

Empirical Results

One of the purposes of the pilot survey was to determine whether respondents would, in a brief telephone interview, give sensible answers to hypothetical money choice questions when the interest rates implicit in the questions are far from transparent. The data presented in Table 3.1 suggest that many respondents do give sensible replies; some do not. The six implicit interest rate questions ask the respondent to choose between taking a smaller prize now or waiting for a larger prize. A priori we expect the fraction of respondents taking the prize now to diminish as the implicit interest rate rises. Table 3.1 shows that this did occur. For the sample as a whole, 76% chose "now" for the question with an implicit interest rate of 10.1% per annum; only 33% did so when the implicit interest rate was 51.1%.

Not only do the group results conform to a priori expectations, but almost two-thirds of the respondents gave replies which were internally consistent for each individual. A set of replies was defined as consistent if the respondent never answered "now" to a question with an implicit interest rate that was higher than the rate in another question to which the answer was "wait."[12] The last three columns of Table 3.1 show results for the sample divided into three groups: those with consistent answers, those whose answers would be consistent if one reply were reversed (about one-fourth of the sample), and those respondents whose replies require two or three reversals in order to achieve consistency (about 10% of the sample).[13] The relation between the fraction taking the prize now and the implicit interest rate is much weaker for those respondents with inconsistent answers and much stronger for those with consistent answers. Most of the results reported here are based on analyses limited to those respondents with consistent replies.

Table 3.2 presents the results of regressions in which each question to each individual is treated as an observation. When the regressions are run OLS, the dependent variable is dichotomous, taking a value of 1 if the

Table 3.1   Mean Probability of Taking Prize Now

Question number	Implicit compound interest rate (% per annum)	All respondents ($N = 504$)	Number of inconsistent answers		
			0 ($N = 329$)	1 ($N = 124$)	2 or 3 ($N = 51$)
30	10.1	.76	.78	.75	.61
32	15.7	.61	.66	.56	.34
28	19.6	.58	.59	.60	.41
29	30.5	.52	.52	.48	.61
33	40.2	.34	.35	.28	.41
31	51.1	.33	.25	.37	.71

Table 3.2   **Regressions of Probability of Taking Prize Now on Interest Rate Variables**

	All respondents	Number of inconsistent answers		
		0	1	2 or 3
N	2952	1956	719	277
R^2	.106	.158	.082	.026
Intercept	.733	.783	.733	.414
	(.022)	(.026)	(.046)	(.074)
Question compound implicit interest rate (% per annum)	−.0073**	−.0111**	−.0037	.0106*
	(.0012)	(.0014)	(.0024)	(.0040)
	[−.0071]	[−.0126]	[−.0034]	[.0135]
Question simple implicit interest rate (% per annum)	−.0017**	−.0008	−.0032**	−.0042*
	(.0006)	(.0007)	(.0011)	(.0019)
	[−.0020]	[−.0007]	[−.0037]	[−.0053]
Respondent explicit interest rate (% per annum)	.0054**	.0068**	.0020	.0010
	(.0008)	(.0009)	(.0019)	(.0025)
	[.0064]	[.0090]	[.0019]	[.0010]

Notes: Regressions based on person-question observations. The OLS regression coefficients are shown first with their standard errors in parentheses below. The marginal effects (at mean probability) from the logistic regressions are in brackets.

*$p < .05$
**$p < .01$

reply is "now" and 0 if it is "wait." The right side variables are the *compound* interest rate implicit in each question, the *simple* implicit interest rate, and the individual's *explicit* interest rate given in reply to the cascade question mentioned in the previous section. We see that the probability that a given individual will reply "now" to a given question falls sharply as the interest rate implicit in the question rises, and rises rapidly as the individual's explicit interest rate rises. These results hold for the entire sample and are particularly strong for those respondents classified as consistent, but do not hold for the other respondents. Logistic regressions estimated by a maximum likelihood procedure give similar results when evaluated at the mean probability of taking "now." (See marginal effects in brackets.)

The contrast between the compound interest rate and the simple interest rate coefficients, depending upon the consistency class, suggests one possible reason why some respondents give inconsistent replies.[14] The two interest rates are, of course, highly correlated, but not perfectly so. Those giving consistent replies seem to have been influenced by the implicit compound rate, while those with the most inconsistent replies seem to have been influenced primarily by the simple rate. We also see that there is a close connection between the explicit rate and the probability of choosing "now" for the consistent individuals, but not for those whose replies to the implicit rate questions were inconsistent.

Inasmuch as these results are based on replies to only six questions, they can only be suggestive, not definitive. (It would be desirable to see if the distinction between the compound and simple interest rate holds up in a survey based on a large number of questions.) For this sample, this distinction gives stronger results than do regressions based on Thaler's hypotheses about the effects of length of time or amount of money on the willingness to wait.

Table 3.3 resports the results of regressions similar to those in Table 3.2, but designed to measure the effects of individual characteristics on the probability of the individual choosing "now" in response to the implicit interest rate questions. The regressions are limited to respondents with consistent replies and are run separately for females and males because preliminary analysis revealed significant interaction effects for some variables. A brief discussion of the additional variables follows:

AGE: Respondents placed themselves in one of four age categories: 25–34, 35–44, 45–54, or 55–64. The midpoint of each category was used to construct a continuous variable. There was no a priori expectation for this variable. Maital and Maital had found a positive correlation between age and the "real" interest rate ($r = .10$), but no relation with the nominal rate.

PARED: Parents' education is the mean of the years of schooling of the respondent's mother and father. The separate schooling variables are highly correlated, and do not yield any significant information when included separately. A priori I expected a negative coefficient for *PARED*, at least prior to inclusion of other variables that are also affected by PARED, e.g., the respondent's own years of schooling.

LIVPAR: This is a dummy variable taking a value of 1 if the respondent lived with both parents until age 16; 0 otherwise. Some of the psychological literature suggests that this coefficient should be negative, i.e., should work much the same way as PARED.

CATH, JEW: These are dummy variables taking a value of 1 if the respondent is Catholic (or Jewish), and 0 if Protestant or other.

EXINFL: Expected inflation is a continuous variable derived from the respondent's reply to the question about expected price change during the coming year. A positive coefficient is expected when the implicit interest rate is held

Table 3.3   Regressions of Probability of Taking Prize Now on Socioeconomic Variables

	Females (N=969)[a]					Males (N=939)[a]				
	(1)	(2)	(3)	(3) S.E.	(3L)	(1)	(2)	(3)	(3) S.E.	(3L)
Question compound implicit interest rate (% per annum)	-.011**	-.011**	-.011**	(.001)	[-.014]	-.013**	-.013**	-.013**	(.001)	[-.016]
AGE	.002	.001	.002	(.002)	[.003]	-.003**	-.002*	-.002*	(.001)	[-.002]
PARED	-.003	.007	.013**	(.005)	[.016]	-.031**	-.029**	-.030**	(.006)	[-.037]
LIVPAR	.066	.091*	.105**	(.042)	[.138]	.061	.049	.058	(.048)	[.065]
CATH	-.046	-.057	-.078*	(.033)	[-.089]	-.033	-.017	-.018	(.038)	[-.006]
JEW	-.222**	-.164**	-.137**	(.046)	[-.197]	-.064	-.081	-.086	(.045)	[-.110]
EXINFL	.015**	.013**	.013**	(.003)	[.017]	.004	.004	.005	(.003)	[.003]
≤12YRS		.116**	.087*	(.036)	[.111]		.129**	.142**	(.042)	[.170]
≥16YRS		-.134**	-.138**	(.040)	[-.161]		.164**	.161**	(.039)	[.218]
ADJINC			-.016**	(.003)	[-.019]			.004	(.003)	[.004]
Intercept	.647	.566	.648	(.125)		1.257	1.115	1.063	(.129)	
R^2	.155	.186	.210			.176	.192	.194		

Note: Regressions based on person-question observations.
The coefficients from the OLS regressions are in columns 1–3.
The marginal effects (at mean probability) from the logistic regressions are in column 3L.
[a]Consistent respondents only.

*p < .05

**p < .01

constant. At any given nominal rate, the respondent should be less willing to wait if prices are expected to rise rapidly because the implicit "real" rate of interest is lower.

≤12YRS These are dummy variables for the respondent's own
and years of schooling. The omitted class is those with 13 to
≥16YRS: 15 years. A positive coefficient is expected for ≤12YRS, and a negative one for ≥16YRS, for reasons discussed in the first section of this paper.

ADJINC: Adjusted family income is a continuous variable derived as follows. The respondent placed total family income in one of the following categories: under $15,000, $15,000 to $25,000, $25,000 to $35,000 or over $35,000. Values of 10, 20, 30, and 40 were assigned to each category. Sixty of the respondents did not answer the income question. An income category was assigned to them on the basis of their reply to a social class question and a regression of income on social class. Total family income was divided by adult equivalents to create adjusted family income. "Adult equivalents" is the weighted sum of the number of adults and the number of children in the household with the following weights: respondent = 1; each additional adult = .8; first child = .5; second child = .4; each additional child = .3. A negative coefficient was expected for ADJINC both because of a possible effect of income on time preference, and an effect of time preference on income.[15]

Three alternative OLS specifications (for each sex) allow us to look first only at the background variables (controlling for the implicit interest rate and expected inflation), then at the effects of schooling (which is probably affected by the family background variables and may be a route through which they affect time preference), and finally at the effect of family income. The regressions were also estimated in logistic form by maximum likelihood; the results are similar to those for OLS. The coefficients from the logistic version of the third specification, converted to marginal effects at the mean probability of taking "now" are shown in column (3L).

In the first specification, AGE and PARED are statistically significant for males in the expected direction, while JEW is highly significant for females. A coefficient of − .22 indicates that, ceteris paribus, a Jewish female respondent has .22 lower probability of answering "now" than does a Protestant or other female. The sign of the LIVPAR coefficient is opposite to that expected, perhaps because of sample selection bias. It may be that most persons from broken homes do have high rates of time discount, but those who "make it" to a middle class suburban community are probably atypical and may have low rates of time discount.

The schooling variables behave as expected for females and are highly significant. For males, the ≤12YRS coefficient is as expected, but the ≥16YRS coefficient has the wrong sign and is statistically significant. It is not obvious why men with 16 years of schooling or more should be, *ceteris paribus*, more eager to take the prize now than men with 13 to 15 years; possibly the former have better opportunities to invest the money.

The income variable works as expected for females and is significant; it has the wrong sign for males but is not significant. In the fullest specification, LIVPAR and PARED are statistically significant for females with signs opposite to that expected. Some of the background and socioeconomic variables are highly correlated with one another (see Appendix Table 3.A.1 for the zero order correlation matrix) and multicollinearity may explain some of the perverse results. EXINFL is statistically significant in the expected direction and has approximately the same effect as the nominal implicit interest rate on the probability of taking the prize now.

The model underlying the regressions reported in Table 3.3 treats time preference (as reflected in the choice between "now" and "wait") as dependent on years of schooling. As previously discussed, some writers believe that differences in time preference are established early in life and are stable. They would treat years of schooling as dependent on time preference. Table 3.4 presents the results of regressions in which years of schooling is regressed on time preference and other variables. The new variables:

IMPINT: An implicit interest rate is calculated for each respondent who gave consistent answers to the six implicit interest rate questions. Those respondents who answered "now" to some questions and "wait" to others were assigned a rate equal to the mean of the highest implicit rate to which they answered "now" and the lowest to which they answered "wait."[16] Those respondents who always chose to "wait" were assigned a rate of 5% and those who always chose "now" were assigned 60%. The higher the respondent's IMPINT, the lower should be the years of schooling. The variable EXINFL should work in the opposite direction.

HSRANK: The respondent's scholastic performance in high school was inferred from replies to the question: When you were in high school were you (percent of sample in each category shown in parentheses)
1) an excellent student (10%)
2) an above average student (28%)
3) an average student (57%)
4) a below average student (5%).

Table 3.4   Regression of Years of Schooling on Implicit Interest Rate and Other Variables

	Females (N=162)[a]				Males (N=157)[a]			
	(1)	(2)	(3)	(3) S.E.	(1)	(2)	(3)	(3) S.E.
AGE	-.066**	-.035**	-.038*	(.016)	-.045*	-.035	-.043*	(.017)
IMPINT	-.024**	-.019*	-.014	(.008)	-.004	.003	-.000	(.009)
EXINFL	-.036	-.032	-.031	(.029)	.104*	.106*	.107**	(.040)
PARED		.223**	.150**	(.056)		.137	.091	(.074)
LIVPAR		1.252*	1.025*	(.456)		1.398*	1.299*	(.568)
CATH		.082	-.143	(.357)		-1.346**	-1.157*	(.460)
JEW		1.276*	1.077*	(.488)		.899	.730	(.550)
HSRANK			.120**	(.021)			.089**	(.027)
HSHLTH			.130	(.367)			.109	(.403)
Intercept	17.367	12.116	3.562	(1.951)	15.277	12.505	6.426	(2.351)
R^2	.128	.274	.411		.072	.273	.324	

[a]Consistent respondents only.
*p<.05
**p<.01

Grade averages of 95, 85, 75, and 65 were assigned to the four categories respectively, and the variable is treated as a continuous variable. A positive coefficient is expected.

HSHLTH: Health in high school was treated as a dummy variable taking a value of 1 if the respondent recalled his or her health as being "better than most of the other kids" (26%), and 0 if it was "about average" (70%) or "worse than most of the other kids" (4%). A positive coefficient is also expected for this variable.

The results of these regressions again give weak support for the view that there is a relation between time preference and schooling, but leave open the question of the direction of the causality. In the first specification the coefficient of IMPINT is highly significant for females, and is still significant when the family background variables are introduced. EX-INFL has the wrong sign and is not significant. For males the reverse is true: EXINFL is significant with the expected sign, but IMPINT shows no effect.

The background variables work as expected, with PARED and LIV-PAR both raising years of schooling. HSRANK has a very strong effect, but the causality may be partly the reverse of that assumed in this regression, i.e., persons who plan to go on to college may exert more effort to do well in high school. HSHLTH shows practically no effect on years of schooling. In general, this variable has very low correlations with other socioeconomic or health variables, suggesting that it may be poorly measured.

One of the purposes of the pilot survey was to determine the correlation among alternative measures of time preference. These correlation coefficients, shown in Table 3.5, indicate a weak but statistically significant correlation between the implicit and explicit interest rates and between the implicit rate and replies to the two simple attitudinal questions ("spend now" and "don't worry"). The other two attitudinal questions, which are more complex because they introduce considerations such as life insurance and the education of children, do not correlate well with either the implicit or explicit rates, although they are correlated with each other. The fact that the credit card debit and car loan dummy variables are not significantly correlated with the interest rate variables would be disturbing, but given the timing of the pilot survey, there may be an easy explanation. The interest rates on these loans were legally restricted to unrealistically low levels, given the high interest rates prevailing at that time and given the high rates revealed by the respondents in replies to the implicit rate questions.

Explanations aside, the low correlations across time preference questions must be a source of some concern. They suggest the need for further refinement in the survey techniques and the need to understand better how the specific context of a decision affects intertemporal choice.

Table 3.5   Correlation Coefficients[a] among Time Preference Variables ($N = 329$)[b]

	Implicit interest	Explicit interest	Don't sacrifice	Spend now	No life insurance	Don't worry	Credit card debit	Use car loan
Implicit interest	—	.23**	.00	.23**	-.06	.14*	.09	.06
Explicit interest	.23**	—	.02	.11	-.04	.08	-.02	.00
Don't sacrifice[c]	-.01	.03	—	.08	.25**	.09	.07	.12*
Spend now[d]	.23**	.11*	.09*	—	.03	.11	.11	.04
No life insurance[e]	-.06	-.04	.26**	.02	—	-.06	-.07	-.01
Don't worry[f]	.14**	.08	.09*	.10*	-.05	—	.08	.09
Credit card debit	.09	-.03	.07	.11*	-.08	.09*	—	.21**
Use car loan	.06	.00	.13*	.04	-.01	.10	.19**	—

[a]Upper right triangle shows simple correlations; lower left triangle shows partial correlations controlling for age and sex.
[b]Only respondents with consistent answers to implicit interest rate questions.
[c]Disagree with statement in question 35.
[d]Agree with statement in question 36.
[e]Disagree with statement in question 37.
[f]Agree with statement in question 38.
 *p < .05
**p < .01

Investment in Health

Do differences in time preference affect investments in health? Some crude measures of these investments were obtained by asking the respondents about their cigarette smoking, dental visits, exercise, weight (as a proxy for diet), and seat belt usage.

Replies to questions about these behaviors were converted to continuous variables as follows:

		Assigned value	% of sample
SMOKE	Question: Do you currently smoke cigarettes?		
	Replies:		
	1) No.	0	64
	2) Yes, less than a pack a day.	10	12
	3) Yes, about a pack a day.	20	14
	4) Yes, more than a pack a day.	30	10
OVWT	Question: Would you say that you are currently . . .		
	Replies:		
	1) underweight.	0	5
	2) about the right weight.	0	39
	3) about 5–10 pounds overweight	7.5	35
	4) about 11–20 pounds overweight.	15	12
	5) more than 20 pounds overweight.	30	9
DENTDEL	Question: When did you have your last dental checkup?		
	Replies:		
	1) Within the last year.	0.5	72
	2) About one or two years ago.	1.5	19
	3) About three to five years ago.	4.0	5
	4) More than five years ago.	8.0	4
EXER	Question: How often do you exercise for 30 minutes or more?		
	Replies:		
	1) Never.	0	40

2) Once a month or less.	1	9
3) Several times a month.	2.5	9
4) About once a week.	4	10
5) Two to three times a week.	10	16
6) More than three times a week.	18	16

STBELT   Question: When you are in a car, how often do you use seat belts?
Replies:

1) All the time.	1.00	21
2) Most of the time.	.75	7
3) Some of the time.	.30	13
4) Rarely or never.	.05	59

The correlation between favorable health behaviors is positive for every possible pair (reversing signs where appropriate), but the coefficients are quite low and only some are statistically significant (see Table 3.6). The correlations with seat belt usage suggest that individual differences with respect to health in general may be more important than differences in time preference. Moreover, the generally low correlations underscore the fact that even if there is a common factor at work across behaviors, there are also other factors that are specific to particular behaviors. The low coefficients may also be attributable to the rough approximations used to measure the variables.

In order to test for possible effects of time preference, the health behavior variables were regressed on IMPINT, EXINFL, and several other variables. The results for cigarette smoking are reported in Table 3.7. They confirm the expectation that cigarette smoking does increase

Table 3.6   Correlation Coefficients[a] among Health-related Behavior Variables (N = 508)

	SMOKE	OVWT	DENTDEL	EXER	STBELT
SMOKE	—	.01	.06	−.08	−.12**
OVWT	.01	—	.06	−.18**	−.12**
DENTDEL	.05	.06	—	−.01	−.07
EXER	−.08*	−.17**	−.01	—	.09*
STBELT	−.12**	−.12**	−.08*	.09*	—

[a]Upper right triangle shows simple correlations; lower left triangle shows partial correlations, controlling for age and sex.

*p < .05

**p < .01

with higher IMPINT, and decrease with higher EXINFL, but the size of the effect of IMPINT is quite small. We also see an effect of schooling on cigarette smoking as expected; the difference between the coefficients for ≤12YRS and ≥16YRS is statistically significant for males. The overall explanatory power of the regression is low; most of the variation in cigarette smoking is not explained by these variables and the addition of ADJINC was of little value.

Regressions for the other health behaviors were even less statisfactory. The total explanatory power was low, and IMPINT was not statistically significant except for EXER for males, where the sign was the opposite of that expected.

Health Status

In the first section of this paper questions were raised about whether difference in time preference could help explain health status or throw light on the relation between health status and schooling. Table 3.8 reports the results of regressions addressed to these questions. Part A uses as the dependent variable LnHLTH, the same variable used by Grossman (1975) in "The Correlation between Health and Schooling." It is obtained by taking the logarithms of values given to replies to the question: In general, would you consider your health to be . . .

	Assigned value	% of sample
1) Excellent	1.0	43
2) Good	9.8	45
3) Fair	26.4	9
4) Poor	86.7	3

Grossman obtained these values from a regression of work-loss weeks due to illness on self-evaluation of health status.[17]

The results support Grossman's finding of a strong effect of schooling on health and it appears that the effect is equally strong for females and males.[18] The coefficients for IMPINT have the expected negative sign, but are not statistically significant. When time preference and schooling are entered simultaneously, the latter clearly dominates the former. When ADJINC is added to the regression, its coefficient is not significant, and the other results are unchanged.

Three other sets of health status questions were asked in addition to the subjective self-evaluation. One used a checklist of symptoms and diagnoses; a second requested information on utilization of hospitals, drugs, and physicians' services; and the third asked about the respondent's ability to walk or jog a mile. These measures are significantly correlated with each other and with self-evaluation of health status, even after controlling for age and sex (partial correlation coefficients are

Table 3.7   Regression of Number of Cigarettes Smoked Per Day on Socioeconomic Variables

| | Females (N = 162)[a] | | | | Males (N = 157)[a] | | | |
	(1)	(2) Coefficient	(3)	(3) S.E.	(1)	(2) Coefficient	(3)	(3) S.E.
AGE	-.041	-.075	-.081	(.076)	.018	.037	.025	(.080)
IMPINT	.072*	.074*	.063	(.036)	.092*	.098*	.091*	(.043)
EXINFL	-.280*	-.297*	-.292*	(.136)	-.263	-.275	-.155	(.186)
PARED		-.376	-.313	(.268)		.234	.403	(.337)
LIVPAR		.117	-.049	(2.139)		-2.887	-1.326	(2.664)
CATH		-2.325	-2.604	(1.658)		-.617	-1.647	(2.136)
JEW		.092	1.012	(2.300)		-1.224	-.758	(2.537)
≤12YRS			-2.089	(1.814)			5.325*	(2.315)
≥16YRS			-5.568**	(2.045)			-.853	(2.207)
Intercept	8.606	15.284	17.595	(6.097)	5.759	5.577	1.102	(7.018)
R^2	.043	.067	.110		.043	.054	.108	
Dependent variable mean			6.42				6.82	
Dependent variable standard deviation			9.43				10.68	

[a]Only respondents with consistent answers to implicit interest rate questions.

*$p < .05$

**$p < .01$

typically about .20). A composite health status variable MNEXHLTH was calculated from the four measures by assigning a value of .25 to respondents for each of the following:

1) Self-evaluation excellent (44%)
2) Zero symptoms (47%)
3) Very low medical care utilization[19] (64%)
4) Able to jog a mile (61%)

This "mean proportion of excellent health measures" is the dependent variable in the regressions reported in Part B of Table 3.8. They indicate a stronger effect for time preference and a relatively weaker effect for schooling.[20] IMPINT actually achieves statistical significance for males. It appears that the choice of health status measure makes a difference.

Unresolved Questions

This exploratory study leaves unresolved many empirical and theoretical questions concerning time preference, health behavior, and health status. The attempt to measure implicit interest rates through a series of six dichotomous choices between "money now" and "money in the future" produced answers that are clearly not all "noise," but neither are they completely satisfactory. About one-third of the respondents had at least one inconsistent reply. Moreover, one-half of those who were consistent answered all the questions the same way (either all "now" or all "wait"). An extension of the range of the implicit interest rates might yield more information about this group. An increase in the number of questions would be desirable for many reasons, but the directors of the survey believe that six is about all the respondents will tolerate as part of the total telephone interview.

At a time of sharply rising prices, the measurement of "real" vs. "nominal" interest rates presents a major problem which is solved only partially by including a question on expected inflation. The EXINFL variable usually works as expected—opposite to IMPINT—but the coefficients are not always equal, and sometimes the signs are inconsistent.

The mean implicit interest rate in this survey of 30% per annum is substantially lower than the rates reported in surveys by other investigators. This rate is still high, however, compared to current borrowing and lending rates, and high compared to the mean response to the explicit interest rate question (14%). Why the difference? Also, although the implicit and explicit rates are significantly correlated ($r = .23$ for the two-thirds of the sample with consistent replies), why isn't the correlation higher?

The pilot survey confirms our a priori expectation of a correlation between schooling and time preference, but other types of data are needed if we are to learn something about the direction of the causality.

Table 3.8   Regressions of Health Status[a] on Time Preference, Schooling, and Age

	Females					Males				
	IMPINT	EXINFL	SCHOOL	AGE	R^2	IMPINT	EXINFL	SCHOOL	AGE	R^2
Part A										
LnHLTH										
(1)	−.003 (.003)	−.004 (.012)		−.015* (.006)	.045	−.003 (.003)	.018 (.015)		−.021** (.006)	.084
(2)			.059* (.025)	−.010 (.006)	.069			.059* (.027)	−.020** (.006)	.106
(3)	−.002 (.003)	−.001 (.011)	.054* (.026)	−.011 (.006)	.072	−.003 (.004)	.013 (.016)	.054 (.028)	−.020** (.006)	.115
Part B										
MNEXHLTH										
(1)	−.001 (.001)	.001 (.005)		−.007** (.002)	.062	−.002* (.001)	.001 (.005)		−.011** (.002)	.208
(2)			.013 (.010)	−.006** (.002)	.071			.009 (.008)	−.011** (.002)	.189
(3)	−.000 (.001)	.002 (.005)	.013 (.010)	−.006** (.002)	.072	−.002* (.001)	.001 (.005)	.009 (.008)	−.011** (.002)	.214

[a]For definitions and measurement of health status variables, see text.
*p < .05
**p < .01

The effect of time preference on health behavior and on health status is usually in the expected direction, but is not always statistically significant, and even when statistically significant the size of the effect is frequently small. This may be partly the result of errors in the measurement of time preference but may also indicate weaknesses in specification of the model.

For instance, the assumption that investment behavior is affected only by time preference is probably unrealistic. Investments typically involve uncertainty as well as time preference because future values of any variable, whether the price of a stock or the state of health, cannot be known with certainty. Thus, individual attitudes toward risk will also affect investment behavior. The uncertainty element is probably particularly large in the case of investments in health such as giving up cigarettes, eliminating fatty foods, jogging, and the like. Even the best information available indicates only the *average* expected benefit from such health investments; the return to any individual is highly uncertain. Only a minority of cigarette smokers will actually contract lung cancer, while giving up cigarette smoking does not provide a guarantee against the disease. Therefore, individual differences with respect to uncertainty can also affect health investment and health status.

Psychologists Kahneman and Tversky, in their highly original and provocative work on prospect theory (1979), have suggested that most individuals prefer certain to uncertain *gains*, but prefer uncertainty to certainty with respect to *losses*. For example, most individuals, when offered a choice between A) a certain gain of $500 or B) an equal chance to win $1,000 or nothing, will choose A. The same individuals, when offered a choice between A) a certain loss of $500 or B) an equal chance to lose $1,000 or nothing, will choose B.

Such asymmetry in risk aversion, if applicable to health-related behavior, could be important. Consider a person contemplating giving up some current pleasurable activity or undertaking an unpleasant one in return for the chance of an improvement in health status sometime in the future. The immediate action involves a loss with a high degree of certainty, but the future gain is quite uncertain for the individual even though it may be highly predictable, on average, for a large population. Thus, the stronger the individual's asymmetry with respect to uncertainty (as described by Kahneman and Tversky), the less likely will he or she be to undertake the health-enhancing action. This conclusion is unaltered if one reverses the framing of the decision and thinks of the current activity such as cigarette smoking as a "gain" (where certainty is preferred) and the possibility of ill health in the future as the "loss." Thus, individual differences in risk aversion may confound attempts to measure time preference or to analyze the effects of time preference on health.

This survey and the analyses reported here also highlight problems of measurement of health status and health investment. When health is measured by subjective self-evaluation, the results are different from those that are obtained when a composite health measure based on self-evaluation, medical care utilization, symptoms, and physical ability is used. Problems in the measurement of health investment surface when we examine a variable like exercise; it seems that exercise is undertaken for many reasons other than to improve health. These other reasons may swamp an effect of time preference. Perhaps more detailed questions concerning the type and intensity of exercise would help.

I conclude this report of exploratory research on a note of cautious optimism. Crude but useful measures of time preference, health investment, and health status can be obtained, even through very inexpensive telephone interviews. Time preference *is* related to schooling, and also shows some relation to health investment and health status. However, none of the relationships found in these data are particularly strong. Whether improvements in survey design, more accurate measurement of variables, and better specification of models will produce more significant results remains to be determined.

Appendix

Table 3.A.1   Zero-order Correlations among Selected Variables

	SCHOOL	HSRANK	PARED	LIVPAR	ADJINC	IMPINT	EXINFL
SCHOOL	—	.47	.37	.21	.25	−.23	−.05
HSRANK	.33	—	.21	.09	.15	−.11	−.03
PARED	.30	.19	—	.02	.29	−.07	.01
LIVPAR	.20	.10	.15	—	.07	.02	.02
ADJINC	.27	.09	.14	−.04	—	−.23	.01
IMPINT	−.03	.03	−.21	.02	−.02	—	.19
EXINFL	.18	−.01	.03	−.05	−.06	.03	—

Females: upper right triangle.
Males: lower left triangele.
$r \geq |.21| p < .01$
$r \geq |.17| p < .05$

Time Preference Questions

A. Implicit interest rate

Given your present circumstances, suppose you won a tax-free prize at a local bank and were offered a choice between two prizes. I am going to read off pairs of choices and for each pair you tell me which prize you would choose.

28. 1 = $1,500 now, or   DON'T [3 = don't know   ____
     2 = $4,000 in 5 years   READ [9 = refuse   28

29. 1 = $1,000 now, or   DON'T [3 = don't know   ____
     2 = $2,500 in 3 years   READ [9 = refuse   29

30. 1 = $4,000 now, or   DON'T [3 = don't know   ____
     2 = $6,000 in 4 years   READ [9 = refuse   30

31. 1 = $750 now, or   DON'T [3 = don't know   ____
     2 = $1,250 in 1 year   READ [9 = refuse   31

32. 1 = $2,500 now, or   DON'T [3 = don't know   ____
     2 = $4,000 in 3 years   READ [9 = refuse   32

33. 1 = $500 now, or   DON'T [3 = don't know   ____
     2 = $2,500 in 4 years   READ [9 = refuse   33

B. Explicit interest rate

34. Suppose you won a tax-free prize of $10,000 at a local bank. You then had a choice between getting the money now or leaving it in the bank for one year. How much interest would the bank have to pay you in order for you to agree to leave the money in the bank? [CASCADE—STOP READING WHEN CHOICE MENTIONED]

1 = 6%   6 = 30%
2 = 8%   7 = 50%
3 = 10%   8 = take the money
                           now
4 = 15%   DON'T [9 = don't know   ____
5 = 20%   READ   or refuse   34

C. Additudinal questions

Do you agree or disagree with the following statements?
       (Categories for Questions 35 to 38)
   1 = agree   2 = disagree   DON'T [3 = don't know
                        READ [9 = refuse

35. Parents should make financial sacrifices in order to save   ____
     money for their children's education.   35

36. It makes more sense to spend your money now rather than
saving it for the future.

36

37. A working man should have life insurance equivalent to at
least three times his annual income even if paying for this
insurance means he would have to live on a tight budget.

37

38. Most people spend too much time worrying about the future
and not enough time enjoying themselves today.

38

D. Expected inflation

39. In general, during the coming year do you expect prices to:
    1 = decrease
    2 = stay about the same
    3 = increase by about 5 percent
    4 = increase by about 10 percent
    5 = increase by about 15 percent
    6 = increase by about 20 percent
    7 = increase by about 30 percent or more

    DON'T [8 = don't know
    READ [9 = refuse

39

E. Use of credit

54. At the end of each month do you usually pay the balance on all
your outstanding credit cards, or do you have a debit balance
on which you must pay interest?

    1 = pay all balances   DON'T [9 = don't know
    2 = have debit balance   READ   or refuse
    3 = have no credit cards

54

55. When you or your spouse buy a car, do you pay cash or take a
car loan?

    1 = pay cash   DON'T [9 = refuse
    2 = take a car loan   READ
    3 = have done both in
        the past
    4 = never buy cars

55

Notes

1. For an excellent summary of present knowledge in this field as well as many useful
bibliographies, see *Healthy People, The Surgeon General's Report on Health Promotion and
Disease Prevention, Background Papers*, U.S. Department on Health, Education, and
Welfare (PHS) No. 79-55071A, Washington: U.S. Government Printing Office, 1979.

2. There are, to be sure, many other possible explanations for this correlation. For instance, persons with better health endowments may be more efficient in schooling activities, or their expected rate of return to schooling may be higher because of their greater life expectancy. Conversely, the rate of return to investment in health may be greater for those who have had more schooling.

3. "When habits are once formed, they regulate the tenor of the future life, and make slaves of their former masters." John Rae, *The Sociological Theory of Capital*, ed. C. W. Mixtor (1834; reprint ed., New York: Macmillan, 1905) as quoted in Shlomo and Sharona Maital (1978).

4. William Hazlitt wrote in *The Round Table* (1817), "Persons without education . . . see their objects always near, and never in the horizon." And Robert Penn Warren wrote "Without the fact of the past, we cannot dream the future." ("Brother to Dragons," a poem.)

5. I am grateful to Alan Garber and Richard Zeckhauser for helpful comments on this point.

6. Temporal orientation refers to the point in time around which a person's thoughts center and to the volume of those thoughts.

7. The questionnaire was administered by psychologists at Perceptronics in Eugene, Oregon.

8. Stephen Cole also made many contributions to the design of the questionnaire.

9. A digit-raising technique was used to insure inclusion of unlisted numbers.

10. See Appendix A for a list of time preference questions.

11. I am grateful to Amos Tversky for advice on this point.

12. Approximately one-quarter of the respondents classified as consistent chose "now" for all six questions and another one-quarter always chose to wait. Their replies, while not inconsistent, are not as informative about consistency as the replies of those respondents who chose "now" for some questions and "wait" for others.

13. Given six questions, every possible set of replies can be made consistent with a maximum of three reversals.

14. This hypothesis was suggested by Phillip Farrell.

15. *Ceteris paribus*, individuals with low rates of time discount might accumulate more savings, might choose occupations with larger on-the-job investment opportunities, etc.

16. For example, a respondent who answered "now" to the first four questions in Table 3.1 and "wait" to the next two was assigned a rate of 35.35%.

17. A different set of values, based on a regression with a different sample, yielded almost identical results to those reported here.

18. Grossman's regression (for middle-aged males) comparable to Regression 2 in Table 38, Part A, had a coefficient of .035 for schooling and − .017 for age.

19. No hospitalization in past year, no prescription drugs in past week, no medical condition requiring regular visits to physician, and fewer than three visits to physician in past six months. To be sure, medical care utilization may reflect factors such as income and insurance coverage as well as health status.

20. The weak effect of schooling is attributable to the "symptoms" and "utilization" measures of health status. When these measures are used as dummy dependent variables in regressions equivalent to (3) in Table 3.8, schooling is negatively (albeit not significantly) related to good health.

References

Auster, Richard; Leveson, Irving; and Sarachek, Deborah. 1969. The production of health: an exploratory study. *The Journal of Human Resources* 9: 412–36.

Becker, Gary S. 1964; 2d ed. 1975. *Human capital.* New York: Columbia University Press.

Fuchs, Victor, R. 1967. The basic forces influencing costs of medical care. Address given at the National Conference on Medical Care Costs, Washington, D.C., 27 June 1967.

Grossman, Michael. 1972. *The demand for health: a theoretical and empirical investigation.* New York: Columbia University Press for the National Bureau of Economic Research.

———. 1975. The correlation between health and schooling. In Nestor E. Terleckyj, ed., *Household production and consumption.* New York: Columbia University Press for the National Bureau of Economic Research.

Kahneman, Daniel, and Tversky, Amos. 1979. Prospect theory: an analysis of decision under risk. *Econometrica* 47: 263–91.

Maital, Shlomo, and Maital, Sharona. 1978. Time preference, delay of gratification, and the intergenerational transmission of economic inequality: a behavioral theory of income distribution. In Orley Ashenfelter and Wallace Oates, eds., *Essays in labor market analysis.* New York: John Wiley.

Metcalf, Charles E. 1974. Predicting the effects of permanent programs from a limited duration experiment. *The Journal of Human Resources* 9: 530–55.

Thaler, Richard. 1979. Individual intertemporal choice: a preliminary investigation. Research memorandum (mimeographed).

Thomas, Ewart A. C., and Ward, Wanda E. 1979. Time orientation, optimism, and quasi-economic behavior. Stanford University (mimeographed).

U.S. Department of Health, Education, and Welfare. 1979. *Healthy people: the Surgeon General's report on health promotion and disease prevention, background papers.* (PHS) No. 79–55071A. Washington: U.S. Government Printing Office.

West, Richard W. 1978. The rate of time preference of families in the Seattle and Denver income maintenance experiment. Research Memorandum 51, SRI International.

4 Healthiness, Education, and Marital Status

Paul Taubman and Sherwin Rosen

In this paper we begin to explore the interrelationships of a number of health variables with several sociodemographic and economic variables for white men using the Retirement History Survey.

The dependent variables we use are categorical and are analyzed by fitting models with various degrees of interaction to frequency tables. Since nearly all the variables discussed in the text are statistically significant (as judged by likelihood ratio and Chi square tests), we will concentrate on the sign and the magnitude of the differences.

The health variables used in this study ask an individual to compare his health with others of the same age and with himself at the time of the prior survey. We recognize that these are both subjective and not particularly finely grained questions. We think, however, the questions convey much information and are not biased by choices as are questions on days lost from work because of illness.[1] We also think that the pattern of empirical results is consistent with what would be expected from an unbiased, objective measure. The text is organized in terms of the results of each dependent variable. A better feel for the results and a more coherent story can be had by looking at the impacts of the various independent variables.

A person's education can affect his health because education is correlated with income, with consumption and life styles, with decision making ability, and with occupational and residential health risks. Thus it is not surprising that we, like others, find that the more educated are more likely to be in better health. As people age, the percentage in better health falls and the decrease (in terms of percentage points) is larger for the more educated.

Paul Taubman is at the University of Pennsylvania; Sherwin Rosen is at the University of Chicago. Financial support from N.I.A. is gratefully acknowledged. Cheryl Carleton provided able research assistance. The authors are responsible for any errors.

The more educated can be in better health for a variety of reasons. If the effects of education flow through the greater income of the more educated, then we would expect the education effect to vanish when we control for income. Yet the available evidence suggests that the education results are fairly robust to inclusion of other variables, such as 1968 earnings, number of medical visits, amount of doctor bills, marital status, and education. The effect of education on health is reduced only modestly when we control for spouse's education. It is not reduced further when we control for 1968 earnings of the head. When we condition on prior level of health, we are studying health deterioration functions. These functions need not be parallel. Health deteriorates more slowly for the more educated. Education, however, has little impact on improving health.

For married men we have examined the effect of spouse's education. The most educated women are more likely to have mates in better health than the least educated, though the effect of spouse's education is not monotonic. Own education has bigger impacts than spouse's education, and the impacts of spouse's education are changed very little when we condition on prior health and doctor bills.

Economists have often examined the effects of education. Marital status has not received intensive study; nevertheless, one expects marriage to be important. Spouses can provide physical and mental aid to one another. Divorce and widowhood are associated with substantial stress. Of course severely ill people may not be able to marry or remarry. We find strong impacts of marital status on health but smaller effects on health change. Married men are much more likely to remain alive in a worse health condition rather than to die. Divorced men have the worst health prospects.

Model and Data

Our data source is unusual in that it follows people over time, and thus has indicators of change in a person's health status as well as the level of health at each point in time. With this data it is possible to estimate the determinants of the change in health status conditioned on initial health status:

(1) $$\Delta H = H_{t+1} - H_t = f(H_t, X, t)$$

where H_t is the level of health at time t, and X is a vector of personal characteristics.

In principal we can solve this difference equation given an initial condition, H_o, to obtain an equation for H_t.

(2) $$H_t = G(H_o, X, t)$$

Equation (2) is the one usually estimated in a cross-section, with H_o treated as an unobserved random variable. The coefficients on X in (2) may be biased because of the omission of H_o, which is generally not measured, and because some components of X may be partially determined by H_o or intervening health status. Our estimates of (2) are subject to the same difficulties.

Equation (1) can be thought of as a transform of a reduced form production function in which investments in health have been optimized out. Because we control for H, we eliminate a large share of the reverse causality running from H to X. We also control those omitted variables that remain constant from period to period. Since X generally remains constant from period to period, what we are measuring is the effect of X on the change in health, not on its level. Therefore, these estimates are not quite comparable to those in the literature, which estimate equation (2).

On average, health deteriorates with age for different levels of X. This is shown in Figure 4.1. The usual cross-section study measures the distance CD. Our equation (1) measures the difference in the slopes at A and B. It is therefore possible that X has no effect in equation (1) but has an effect in equation (2); that would occur if the deterioration functions were parallel. This would imply that all the effects of X in equation (1) operate via prior health and do not cumulate during the life cycle.

In the work that follows we estimate equations (1) and (2) using data from three years of a panel survey, 1969, 1971, and 1973. While our data include crude indicators of life cycle risks, such as occupation of longest job, we concentrate on the effects of marital status and education here. However, we also examine the effects of spouse's schooling, income, and medical expenditures on the evolution of health status over time.

The Retirement History Survey (RHS) commenced in 1969. In that year a random sample of some 11,000 men and women between the ages of 58 and 63 (inclusive) were interviewed, and data were collected on the participants' current and past labor force activity, current earnings and income, family structure, education, health-related and other expenditures, and health status. The same people or their widows were reinterviewed every second year until 1979. We currently have the 1969, 1971, and 1973 waves.

The health data come in various forms. Several questions are subjective but don't reflect economic choices. For example, in each interview a person is asked how his health compares to others of the same age. In the post 1969 waves, he is also asked how his health has changed during the last two years. There are also several potentially choice-contaminated questions. For example, a person not at work is asked why and may respond "poor health." For our purposes this question can be contaminated because wage rates and available health benefits may influence

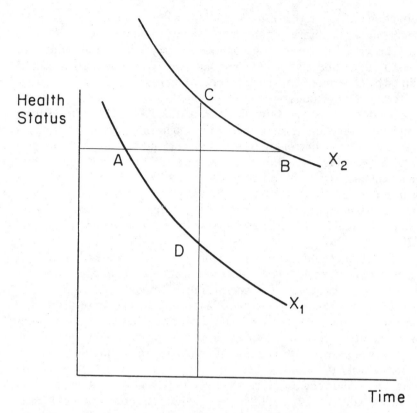

Fig. 4.1   Hypothetical health deterioration functions.

whether a person of a given degree of healthiness chooses to work or to stay home.

The health status variables in level form has four possible responses: health better-than-others (the same age), same-as-others, and worse-than-others, and, for the 1971 and 1973 surveys, deceased. Given the nature of these equations, there are no easy identities in the difference between two successive levels and responses about change in health from one date to the next; therefore, we use both the levels and the changes in health.

With these categorical data the use of conventional regression methods requires arbitrary scaling of categories (better, same, worse, deceased). To eliminate this kind of arbitrary decision, we use instead a linear model based on contingency tables of three or four categories. (See Goodman 1968). Qualitative dependent variables are analyzed by fitting models to frequency tables using the PF3 program in the BMDP package.

Any qualitative model with three variables can be written as:

$$lnF_{ijk} = \alpha\lambda^A + \beta\lambda^{AB} + \gamma\lambda^{ABC}$$

where F_{ijk} is the expected cell frequency, λ^A is a vector of means, λ^{AB} is a vector of first-order interaction terms, and λ^{ABC} is a vector of second-order interaction terms. We can test for interactions of the various factors by restricting parameters to zero. The computational algorithm allows us to estimate the statistical significance of individual variables and their interactions. For the qualitative variables we present a selection of the *estimated* cell means and describe the significance and pattern of the results.

Means and variances of several variables are shown in Table 4.1. It clearly indicates that health worsens with age. It also shows that there are

Table 4.1   Sample Means or Proportions and Variances

	Mean	Variance
Married	.88	.10
Widowed	.04	.04
Divorced	.04	.03
Never married	.05	.04
58 years old	.19	.15
59 years old	.17	.14
60 years old	.16	.14
61 years old	.17	.14
62 years old	.16	.14
63 years old	.15	.13
ED 0–8	.39	.24
ED 9–11	.20	.16
ED 12	.23	.18
ED 13–15	.09	.08
ED 16+	.10	.09
Death (1969–1973)	.15	.12
Number of times received medical care including hospital, 1968	10.03	174.07
Amount of doctor bills, 1968	62.6	289828.4
Amount of doctor bills, 1970	167.5	434808.4
Amount of doctor bills, 1972	89.7	177620.1

Sample Proportions

Health compared to others same age	1969	1971	1973	Health change	1969–1971	1971–1973
Better	.35	.29	.25	Improving	.12	.11
Same	.46	.49	.47	Same	.57	.52
Worse	.19	.18	.17	Worsening	.26	.26
Dead	—	.05	.11	Dead	.05	.11

wide variations in healthiness and medical expenditures. An obvious question, however, is whether the data are sufficiently trustworthy for analysis. In particular, are individuals able to assess and give reasonably accurate accounts of: (1) the level in their health compared to others in the same age group, and (2) the change in their own health? Moreover we must ask if such crude categories as "better" and "worse" convey much information.

In making comparisons with others of the same age, people may well use the mode as the reference value. Since health need not be distributed symmetrically about the mode, there is no reason why the level variable need retain the same distribution over time, and it is not illogical that more people pass to the unhealthy state as they age. Thus it makes sense that the change in health becomes worse over time.

One can also judge the appropriateness of an empirical measure of a theoretical construct by the results obtained in empirical work. In the results that follow, the subjective health variables often act the way one would expect a true health variable to behave. To provide but one example, between 1969 and 1973, 23% of those in worse health in 1969 died, while only 7% of those who were in better health died.

Health Compared to Others of the Same Age

We have fit a variety of models to individuals' 1969, 1971, and 1973 subjective evaluations of their health compared to others of the same age in the particular year.[2] Since the comparison group ages over the time period, the time series comparisons indicate how the distribution of health varies about a changing reference point. Table 4.2 shows that the shape of the health distribution changes systematically with age. Fewer people appear in the better-than-other health category in successive surveys. Apparently people do in fact use the mode as a reference point.

Some estimates of equation (2) are shown in Table 4.2 where the level of health in each survey year is related to education and marital status in 1969. We have used 0–8, 9–11, 12, 13–15, and 16+ as the education categories in our analysis but omit some of these classifications in the tables for ease of presentation. Similarly we have used the marital status categories of married, widowed, divorced, and single in the analysis though each is not always included in the tables. Qualitatively the results for education and marital status are similar to those found by other investigators.

The education and marital status vectors are statistically significant and have independent effects. The effects of education are quite large in each year. Consider, for example, married men (see Table 4.2, panel 1). In 1969, the percentage of white men in better health than others rises from

Table 4.2 Health Compared to Others by Education[a] and Marital Status[b]

Health compared to others same age	Education 0–8				Education 12				Education 16 +			
	Married	Widowed	Divorced	Single	Married	Widowed	Divorced	Single	Married	Widowed	Divorced	Single
1969												
Better	.28	.28	.24	.19	.40	.40	.37	.29	.47	.47	.45	.36
Same	.47	.46	.37	.50	.46	.45	.40	.53	.44	.43	.39	.52
Worse	.25	.26	.39	.30	.14	.14	.23	.18	.09	.09	.16	.12
1971												
Better	.22	.20	.21	.18	.33	.30	.32	.28	.43	.40	.43	.37
Same	.50	.50	.43	.53	.49	.49	.43	.52	.43	.44	.38	.47
Worse	.23	.22	.27	.21	.13	.13	.15	.12	.10	.10	.12	.09
Dead	.04	.08	.09	.08	.05	.08	.10	.08	.04	.07	.08	.07
1973												
Better	.19	.19	.16	.16	.29	.27	.25	.23	.35	.34	.32	.29
Same	.47	.47	.33	.46	.40	.47	.35	.48	.46	.45	.35	.47
Worse	.23	.17	.27	.19	.13	.09	.16	.11	.10	.07	.13	.09
Dead	.11	.18	.23	.19	.10	.17	.23	.18	.08	.13	.19	.14

[a]Education in years.
[b]Marital status as of 1969.

28%to 47% as education rises from elementary school to college completion. Comparable increases occur in the intervening categories. The pattern for worse health and death is the opposite for those in better health. The fraction in worse-than-others falls sharply with education. In 1969 higher education is associated with substantial reductions in the percentage in health worse-than-others, from 25% for married elementary school men to 9% for college graduates. For married men in 1971, the fraction in the educational extremes falls from 23% to 10%. The effect of education is approximately the same in each year as shown in the other two panels of Table 4.2.

Now examine the effects of marital status. In 1969, married men and widowers have very similar distributions at all education level. (We do not know how long men have been widowed or divorced). Single (never married) men are less likely to be in better or in worse health than divorced men, while the latter are a bit less likely to be in better health but substantially more likely to be in worse health than others. The patterns in the other two years are similar except that the disadvantage of single men in better health has narrowed, and married men have a substantially lower death rate even though we suspect more complete reporting of death for this group.

To try to understand better why married men remain alive longer, we have examined that group in more detail. In all three years studied, own and spouse's education have statistically significant and independent impacts on health. Table 4.3, presents some estimated proportions taken from an equation which uses own and spouse's education without interactions.

For a given spouse's education level, own education continues to show substantial positive effects. For example, if the spouse has 12 years of schooling, the percentage in better health in 1969 rises from 30% to 46%, and the percentage in worse health falls from 21% to 8% as own education rises from elementary school to college graduate. These effects are only slightly smaller than those found in Table 4.2.

For a given level of own education there is a definite tendency for the percentage in better health to increase with spouse's education, the jump between elementary and high school being particularly noticeable. There is an even more marked tendency for the percentage of those in poor health to decline as spouse's education increases—generally about 5 percentage points between spouses with elementary school and college education. However, the group with the lowest percentage in worse health are those whose spouse has 13–15 years of schooling (not shown).

An increase in one's own education is much more effective than an increase in spouse's education. For example, in 1969, going from elementary school to college graduate raises the fraction in better health by about 15 points for own education but by 7 points for spouse's

Table 4.3   Married Men's[a] Health Compared to Others by Own and Spouse's Education[b]

Health compared to others	Own Education 0–8			Own Education 12			Own Education 16 +		
	Spouse's Education			Spouse's Education			Spouse's Education		
	0–8	12	16+	0–8	12	16+	0–8	12	16+
1969									
Better	.26	.30	.33	.35	.40	.42	.41	.46	.49
Same	.46	.49	.46	.46	.47	.43	.46	.46	.43
Worse	.28	.21	.22	.19	.13	.14	.12	.08	.09
1971									
Better	.20	.26	.26	.28	.34	.35	.37	.44	.44
Same	.50	.51	.49	.50	.49	.47	.46	.44	.42
Worse	.26	.19	.22	.16	.12	.14	.13	.09	.10
Dead	.04	.04	.04	.06	.05	.04	.04	.03	.03
1973									
Better	.19	.24	.21	.25	.31	.28	.33	.39	.35
Same	.47	.47	.53	.47	.47	.52	.44	.43	.48
Worse	.24	.20	.17	.15	.13	.10	.14	.12	.09
Dead	.10	.08	.09	.12	.10	.10	.09	.07	.07

[a]Marital status as of 1969.
[b]Education in years.

education. Similarly the decline for worse health is about 14 and 6 points respectively.

In 1971, the decrease in percentage points of health better-than-others is approximately the same at all spouse's education levels. There is an increase in the "same" group with worse health down only slightly. The percentage decrease is very small and unrelated to either education variable. In this year, as in 1969, own education has a much larger impact on health than spouse's education. Moreover, the effect of either variable is about the same in both years in percentage point terms.

By 1973, the percentage in better-health-than-others has fallen even more at all education levels. The decrease, however, is more noticeable at higher levels of spouse's education. By 1973, the differential between spouse having 0–8 and 16 or more years of schooling is only about 2 percentage points, while for own education the corresponding differential runs about 14 points. The percentage in worse health has generally declined slightly from 1971. The percentage who have died decreases slightly with either education measure.

Health Levels Conditioned on Previous Health

The results to be discussed next examine variants of equation (1). Adding H_t to both sides of equation (1) gives us an equation relating H_{t+1} to H_t and X. We can then use health compared to others in two surveys. Alternatively we can relate a person's own change in health to prior health compared to others and to X.

Table 4.4 shows 1971 and 1973 health status respectively, cross-classified by education, marital status, and health status in 1969. Table 4.5 conditions on 1971 health status rather than on 1969 health status. Before turning to the detailed results, we may state the general conclusions: the direct effects of schooling are quite strong within given health status classifications; thus, the slopes of the health change functions illustrated in Figure 4 are different. The effects of marital status on the slopes of the health change function are less strong than those of education. However, there are indications that the presence of a spouse prolongs life by keeping an ill mate, who would probably die if the spouse were absent, alive but in a state of ill health.

Let us examine the effects of schooling first. Of those in better health in 1969 the fraction in better health in both 1971 and 1973 increases with the level of schooling (Table 4.4). For example, for married men, the percentages for elementary and college graduates are 47% and 63% in 1971 and 41% and 52% in 1973. Conversely, for those in worse health in 1969, the fraction in worse health or dead in either 1971 or 1973 decreases with the level of schooling. The estimated percentages for the same two groups are 66% and 58% in 1971 and 67% and 60% in 1973. The first of these examples suggests that the effects of education diminish with age. 1969 health status may be a poor conditioning variable for 1973 health. However, when we recomputed using 1971 health as the conditioning variable, the results in Table 4.5 are very similar to those in the top panel of Table 4.4 except for the divorced, who are much less likely to be found in better health in 1973. Furthermore, the effects of schooling on 1973 health conditional on 1971 health is somewhat smaller than the effect of schooling on 1971 health status conditional on the state of health in 1969. One might well expect this, because only the more hardy individuals, whatever their background and circumstances, survive, and so the population distribution changes over time. The much greater differences in levels between the 1969–73 and 1969–71 comparisons shown in Table 4.4 would be expected on purely statistical grounds since random events tend to change individuals' health status classifications as time marches on. Thus, if a married person was in better health in 1969 the probability of remaining in better health in 1971 is about .44. With no state dependence this would imply a probability of remaining in better health in 1973 of about .25 (= .47 × .53). Of course the significantly higher observed proportions of more than .4 suggest more persistence than independent distributions imply, but the point is clear that the proportions should decline over time.

Since deceased is an absorbing state and the other classifications are not, there is some ambiguity in examining the worse-than-others and deceased categories, though surely the latter is the ultimate subclass of the former. These tables indicate a general worsening of health with age. They also suggest that recovery from worse health in 1969 to better-health-than-others in subsequent years occurs very infrequently, though at a slightly greater rate for the more educated. In almost every case the probability of recovery to the better-than-others state given a prior worse-than-others state is smaller than the probability of worse and/or deceased states given prior better-than-others state. For example, for divorced men with elementary school education, the recovery rate in 1971 is 5%, while the deterioration rate (including dead) is 11%. Furthermore, the difference between the off diagonal elements in the transition matrix increases over time. It is interesting to note that the more educated are more likely to recover if they start with worse health, and are less likely to get ill or die if they start in better health.

Let us turn now to marital status differences. In the top panel of Table 4.4 divorced and widowed men have respectively the largest and smallest fractions in better health, given prior better health. For those with elementary school education, the percentages in better health are 50% and 43% respectively. The same pattern occurs in 1973 conditioned on

Table 4.4   Level of Health in 1971 and 1973 Conditioned on 1969 Health

1971

	Married		Widowed		Divorced		Single	
	Better 1969	Worse 1969	Better 1969	Worse 1969	Better 1969	Worse 1969	Better 1969	Worse 1969
Education 0–8								
Better	.47	.04	.43	.04	.50	.05	.45	.05
Worse	.07	.58	.07	.54	.06	.53	.05	.47
Dead	.03	.08	.05	.14	.05	.15	.04	.14
Education 12								
Better	.54	.07	.50	.05	.58	.07	.52	.07
Worse	.05	.48	.05	.44	.04	.43	.03	.37
Dead	.03	.11	.05	.19	.05	.20	.05	.19
Education 16+								
Better	.63	.09	.56	.08	.66	.10	.60	.09
Worse	.04	.47	.04	.43	.03	.41	.03	.36
Dead	.02	.11	.04	.18	.04	.19	.04	.19

Education 0–8								
Better	.41	.04	.40	.04	.40	.03	.37	.03
Worse	.09	.49	.06	.35	.10	.45	.07	.38
Dead	.07	.18	.11	.31	.15	.33	.12	.30
Education 12								
Better	.46	.05	.45	.05	.45	.04	.42	.04
Worse	.06	.38	.04	.26	.06	.34	.05	.28
Dead	.07	.23	.11	.36	.15	.40	.12	.36
Education 16+								
Better	.52	.06	.50	.06	.51	.05	.47	.05
Worse	.05	.39	.04	.26	.05	.35	.04	.29
Dead	.06	.21	.09	.33	.13	.37	.10	.33

Same-as-Others categories excluded. Column sums within each education class sum to 1.0 when Same is included.

Table 4.5 **Level of Health in 1973[a] Conditioned on 1971 Health Relative to Others**

1973 Health Level	Married[b]		Widowed		Divorced		Single	
	Better 1971	Worse 1971	Better 1971	Worse 1971	Better 1971	Worse 1971	Better 1971	Worse 1971
Education 0–8								
Better	.48	.04	.49	.05	.44	.03	.42	.03
Worse	.09	.55	.05	.42	.12	.56	.09	.49
Dead	.04	.12	.05	.20	.10	.23	.07	.20
Education 12								
Better	.54	.06	.55	.06	.50	.04	.48	.04
Worse	.05	.44	.04	.32	.08	.45	.05	.38
Dead	.03	.14	.05	.23	.09	.28	.06	.24
Education 16+								
Better	.58	.08	.59	.08	.55	.05	.52	.05
Worse	.05	.31	.03	.31	.07	.45	.05	.38
Dead	.03	.20	.04	.20	.07	.26	.05	.21

[a]Includes only those who were alive in 1971.
[b]Marital Status Classified as of 1969.

1971 health. In 1971, widowers and divorced men have somewhat larger proportions in worse health or dead, given that their health status was initially worse than that of married or single men. However, by 1973 the widowers are on a par with both single men and married men, while the divorced have significantly more adverse experience.

Married men who start off in worse health have significantly smaller probabilities of subsequent death than other groups. It is well known from other studies that married men have higher survival rates than other men. The findings suggest that the presence of a spouse prolongs life even given illness.

The probability of recovery to better than average health from worse than average health appears to be independent of marital status in all comparisons. On the other hand the probability of going from better than average health to worse than average or dead is much larger for divorced males, as shown in Table 4.5. There is a slight advantage for widowers in the 1971–73 comparison though widowers have worse experience than singles in 1969–71 and exhibit about the same effects in 1969–73.

Married men and more educated men earn more and are generally wealthier than others. Therefore it is possible that the effects of education and marital status work through the effects of wealth and its attendent correlates of medical care and consumption patterns. To check on these possibilities we have examined 1969 health status by education, marital status, medical care, doctors' bills, and earnings. The full set of interactions, too numerous to be reported in detail, revealed: (1) those spending more on doctors tend to be in worse health—while hardly earth-shaking, this is worth mentioning as a remark on the quality of the self-assessment of health status; (2) those with lower incomes tend to be in worse health within any given education-marital status-medical expense category, though this might well reflect the well known fact that ill persons have lower propensities to work than those in good health, as well as the reverse causation; and (3) the effects of schooling and marital status are of the same order of magnitude within medical expense and income categories as between them. In sum, the results suggest that independent life style or knowledge effects exist in addition to pure wealth effects.

The changes in own health during the previous two years are shown in Tables 4.6 and 4.7. In the top panel of Table 4.6 we present some percentages for the change in health for 1969 to 1971 estimated from a model which includes 1969 health compared to others. The probability of health improving is independent of 1969 health level and marital status. The results for health worsening, however, are strongly related to 1969 health and marital status. Those in worse health than others in 1969 are much more likely to have deteriorating health or to die during the following two years. The probability of death by 1971 for the various

Table 4.6 Change in Health 1969–71 and 1971–73 Conditioned on 1969 Level of Health

Education and change in health 69 to 71	Married[a]			Divorced			Single		
	Health in 1969 of others			Health in 1969 of others			Health in 1969 of others		
	Better*	Same*	Worse*	Better*	Same*	Worse*	Better*	Same*	Worse*
Education 0–8									
Improving	.11	.10	.10	.11	.10	.10	.10	.09	.10
Same	.67	.57	.30	.63	.53	.26	.71	.61	.34
Worsening	.19	.29	.51	.21	.31	.50	.15	.24	.42
Dead	.02	.03	.08	.05	.06	.15	.04	.06	.14
Education 16+									
Improving	.14	.14	.15	.14	.13	.14	.12	.12	.14
Same	.72	.64	.38	.68	.60	.33	.75	.67	.41
Worsening	.12	.19	.36	.13	.20	.35	.09	.15	.29
Dead	.03	.04	.10	.05	.07	.18	.04	.06	.17

Education and
change in health
71 to 73

Education 0–8									
Improving	.14	.10	.08	.16	.11	.07	.10	.08	.06
Same	.58	.52	.29	.44	.38	.18	.66	.60	.36
Worsening	.22	.30	.45	.26	.34	.43	.15	.21	.33
Dead	.05	.08	.18	.14	.17	.31	.09	.11	.26
Education 16+									
Improving	.12	.09	.08	.15	.11	.08	.09	.07	.06
Same	.67	.62	.39	.53	.47	.24	.73	.69	.44
Worsening	.15	.21	.35	.18	.25	.34	.10	.14	.24
Dead	.06	.08	.19	.13	.17	.34	.08	.10	.26

^aMarital status as of 1969.
*Health in 1969 as compared to others.

Table 4.7 Change in Health 1971–73 Conditioned on 1971 Level of Health[b]

Education and change in health 71–73	Married[b]			Divorced			Single		
	Better*	Health in 1971 of others Same*	Worse*	Better*	Health in 1971 of others Same*	Worse*	Better*	Health in 1971 of others Same*	Worse*
Education 0–8									
Improving	.13	.10	.10	.16	.12	.09	.10	.08	.08
Same	.62	.55	.28	.47	.40	.17	.70	.63	.36
Worsening	.22	.30	.50	.28	.38	.51	.16	.23	.41
Dead	.03	.04	.12	.08	.10	.23	.04	.05	.15
Education 16+									
Improving	.12	.10	.11	.15	.12	.10	.09	.07	.09
Same	.70	.65	.38	.57	.50	.23	.77	.73	.46
Worsening	.15	.21	.40	.20	.28	.42	.10	.15	.31
Dead	.03	.04	.12	.08	.10	.24	.03	.05	.15

[a]The known Dead in 1971 are not shown. The unknown Dead in 1971 are in the same health as others category in 1971.
[b]Marital status in 1969.
*Health in 1971 as compared to others.

nonmarried groups are nearly identical given 1969 health. The probability of health worsening, however, is greater for divorced men than for widowers or single men. For example, among college graduates in worse health in 1969, the percentages whose health worsens are 35% for divorced and 29% for single men. Interestingly, married men's health generally worsens at the same rate as divorced men's, but married death rates are much smaller. This finding again suggests that spouses can keep sick men alive for some period of time.

The bottom panel of Table 4.6 presents the estimated fractions for the 1971–73 change in a model that conditions on 1969 health level. The corresponding estimates obtained from conditioning on 1971 health are given in Table 4.7. In both instances the probability of one's own health improving is generally smaller than in the 1969–71 period. In contrast to the 1969–71 interval the probability of health improving in the 1971–73 interval is related to prior health status, with those in better prior health more likely to improve. For example, as shown in Table 4.7, for married men who attended elementary school, the percentage with improving health is 13% for those in better health and 10% for those in worse health than others in 1971.

Single men have a slightly smaller fraction than married men with improving health, a much smaller fraction with worsening health, and a larger fraction dying, though the sum of the last two categories is about the same for these marital groups. Divorced men are much more likely to die—about 10 percentage points—than married men, but have the same percentage of worse health.

Tables 4.6 and 4.7 condition change in own health on level of health compared to others. When we condition the 1971–73 change on the change in the prior two years, there is positive serial correlation. Those who improved between 1969 and 1971 are more likely to continue to improve, and those worsening in health are more likely to worsen or die. The improvement rate, however, is much smaller than the deterioration rate. The results by marital status and education are similar to those presented above.[3]

The effects of education are also shown in Tables 4.6 and 4.7. For the improving group the largest differential is only 5 percentage points, and most differentials are smaller. Yet the effect of education on the sum of the worsening and dead category is substantial. For example, in the top panel of Table 4.6, the estimates for married men in worse health in 1969 are 59% for elementary school and 46% for college graduates. For the 1971–73 health change variable, the combined estimates for elementary school and college graduates in worse health in 1969 are 63% and 54% respectively. However, the death rates differ little by education, contrary to most previous findings. Thus schooling primarily affects the conditional probability of health worsening.

In conclusion, we observe that self-assessed health measures apparently yield useful information about the state of a person's health, and that health at one time and its change over time are strongly related to education and marital status, even when controlling for family income, use of medical resources, and previous health.

Notes

1. For example, in work not reported here, those reporting worse health than others are much more likely to be working if they are more educated and presumably have higher wage rates.
2. When the health question is not answered and the person is alive, health is placed in the "same" category.
3. We have also fit a model relating the 1971–73 change to the 1969–71 change and the 1969 level. The results of the second order difference equation are similar to the first order model shown above.

References

Brenner, H. 1976. Estimating the social cost of national economic policy: Implications for mental and physical health and criminal agression. Joint Economic Committee, Congress of the United States. Washington: U.S. Government Printing Office.

Fuchs, V. 1974. Some economic aspects of mortality in developing countries. In M. Perlman, ed., *The economics of health and medical care*. London: Macmillan.

Goodman, L. 1968. The analysis of cross classified data: Independence, quasi-independence, and interaction in contingency tables with missing entries. *Journal of the American Statistical Association* 63: 1091–1131.

Grossman, M. 1972. On the concept of health capital and the demand for health. *Journal of Political Economy* 80: 223–55.

Kitagawa, E., and Hauser, P. 1973. *Differential mortality in the United States*. Cambridge: Harvard University Press.

Rosen, S., and Taubman, P. 1979. Changes in the impact of education and income on mortality in the U.S. *American Statistical Association, Social Statistics Section, Proceedings*, Washington, D.C., Vol. 21.

2 Consequences of Ill Health

5   The Status of Health in Demand Estimation; or, Beyond Excellent, Good, Fair, and Poor

Willard G. Manning, Jr., Joseph P. Newhouse, and John E. Ware, Jr.

Several years ago we were faced with the task of determining how to measure health status for the purpose of estimating demand in the Health Insurance Study (HIS).[1] Indeed, our challenge went further, for we were to ascertain the degree to which variation in the consumption of medical care services affected health status. Although in principle we could collect data on any measurable variable, we found virtually no guidance in the economics literature on efficient ways to measure health status. Some work had been done by health services researchers, but even that literature did not offer an entirely satisfactory way to measure health status.[2]

In this paper we examine some issues pertinent to the measurement of health status for estimating demand equations. Our comments should be of particular interest to those faced with the problem of what data to collect to estimate demand. They are also relevant to the literature on demand estimation. Specifically, we address two questions.

First, what is to be gained by using better measures of health status? We define measures that we believe are better in two respects than those used in the economics literature. Our measures tend to be more reliable: they have less random measurement error. Random measurement error will typically affect not only the coefficients of the variables measured with error, but also the coefficients and t-statistics of all variables not orthogonal to those variable(s). The direction of the inconsistency in other variables and their t-statistics cannot be signed a priori (Cooper and Newhouse 1971). Also, our measures are more comprehensive. Many of

The research reported herein was performed pursuant to a grant from the U.S. Department of Health and Human Services, Washington, D.C. The opinions and conclusions expressed herein are solely those of the authors and should not be construed as representing the opinions or policy of any agency of the United States Government.

the measures in the literature are unidimensional, but health is multi-dimensional (Ware, Davies-Avery, Brook 1980). The gains derived from measuring the various dimensions include reduction in residual variance and potential reduction of omitted variable bias.

Second, what are the consequences of using measures of current health to explain past utilization behavior? Most empirical estimates of the demand curve based on microlevel data have been cross-sectional. Thus, they have asked individuals about their current health and their past utilization of health services, usually during the previous year. The health status measures at the time of the interview are then used to explain past utilization. We will show that the estimated coefficients of the health status variables using this procedure are inconsistent. The inconsistency will, of course, affect the coefficients of other variables that are not orthogonal to health status. The problems occur because the observed health status variables do not really predict utilization; they "postdict" it. We develop a simple model of postdiction in which the estimated coefficient of the health status variable is inconsistent, whether or not medical care affects future health status. If medical care at the margin does not affect health status, the direction of the inconsistency is toward zero; but, in general, the direction of the inconsistency cannot be signed a priori. Because of the ambiguous sign and unknown magnitude of the inconsistency, we investigate empirically its sign and magnitude. We use a data set that has similar measures of health status spaced a year apart, as well as measures of utilization during the intervening year.

Prior Work

The most frequent method used to measure health status in economic literature is the simple question: "Would you say your health, in general, is excellent, good, fair, or poor?"[3] We refer to this as EGFP. This variable has been used to estimate demand functions (sometimes with no other health status variable present) by Acton (1975), Acton (1976), Andersen and Benham (1970), Colle and Grossman (1978), Goldman and Grossman (1978), Grossman (1972), Grossman and Benham (1974), Manning and Phelps (1979), Newhouse and Marquis (1978), Newhouse and Phelps (1974, 1976), and Phelps (1975). In part, the popularity of this variable stems from its inclusion in the 1963 and 1970 Center for Health Administration Studies national probability sample surveys, which have been among the richest sources of survey data for estimating demand functions during the past decade. Indeed, nine of the twelve studies just cited used one or the other of those two surveys. The same question was also included in three other household surveys that economists have analyzed. Coincidentally, all three had New York City residents as subjects: Acton (1975) analyzed a 1965 survey of users of hospital outpatient departments; Acton (1976) analyzed a 1968 survey of two poverty neighborhoods in Brooklyn; and Goldman and Grossman (1978) analyzed a 1965–66 survey of medical care utilization by children in the Bronx. No other measure of health status has been quite so popular, although a number of others have been used. Colle and Grossman (1978), Davis and Reynolds (1976), and Newhouse and Phelps (1976) included restricted activity days as a covariate, and Acton (1976) used bed disability days. Andersen and Benham (1970), Grossman and Benham (1974), Hershey, Luft, and Gianaris (1975), and Manning and Phelps (1979) included the number of symptoms that occurred in some previous time period; Acton (1976), Davis and Reynolds (1976), and Hershey, Luft, and Gianaris (1975) included the number of chronic conditions that the respondent had. Phelps (1975) controlled for the amount of pain felt by the respondent over the past year.

Invariably these studies find health status to be an important variable in the demand function. Health status often explains more variance than any other variable, and controlling for it can make a considerable difference in the magnitude of other estimated coefficients.

The studies just cited have all used the family or individual as the unit of observation; we call them microlevel studies. A number of demand studies in the economics literature, however, use aggregate data; i.e., the dependent variable is some measure of the demand for services in an area such as a state or region. Typically these studies do not include explicit health status measures as covariates (Davis and Russell 1972, Feldstein 1971, 1977), but assume implicitly that health status shows negligible variation across geographic entities. Fuchs and Kramer (1972) did include infant and crude mortality rates as measures of health status in analyzing demand by region, but found these measures unimportant and dropped them from their final specification.

In addition to measures of health status, two studies in the economics literature have used measures of attitude toward medical services to explain demand. Colle and Grossman (1978) used a measure they called taste for medical care consumption, and we call below attitude toward the efficacy of medical care services. They did not find this variable important. Hershey, Luft, and Gianaris (1975) used a measure they called self-reliance, and we call attitude toward the efficacy of self-care. In their study, this variable was significantly related to demand.

Two studies in the literature have some similarities with the present paper, and deserve further discussion. These are Andersen and Benham (1970) and Hershey, Luft, and Gianaris (1975). Both investigate the effect on estimated income elasticities if health status variables are included. In their paper, Andersen and Benham examined the magnitude of the bias in estimated income elasticities if health status, demographic characteristics, health insurance status, the nature of the family's usual source of care, and whether a family member had had a physical examination in the past five years were excluded as explanatory variables. Their dependent variables were physician and dental expenditures. (We focus on their results for physician expenditures because that is approximately what we analyze in this paper.) The authors found that the simple permanent income elasticity (controlling for no other variable) was 0.63 but fell to 0.17 if all the above mentioned characteristics except health status were controlled for. When health status (measured as excellent, good, fair, and poor, and using a symptom count) was also controlled for, the income elasticity was 0.30. If measured income rather than permanent income was used, estimates were one-quarter to one-third lower.

Hershey, Luft, and Gianaris examined similar questions. They analyzed data from the sample of families from a semirural California town (population 12,000) rather than the national probability sample that Andersen and Benham had used. Their study also differs from the earlier report in that they examine the number of physician visits rather than physician expenditure. But estimates we have made suggest that expenditures and visits are highly correlated, so this difference in dependent variables should not seriously affect comparisons between the two studies.

The 1975 paper estimated measured income elasticities as being well under 0.1 (at the mean) and statistically insignificant, in marked contrast to Andersen and Benham's work. Also, the inclusion of health status variables did not cause a notable change in the elasticity estimates. Hershey, Luft, and Gianaris use the individual as a unit of observation and include income per person and family size as explanatory variables, while Andersen and Benham use the family as a unit of observation and control for family size by entering it as an explanatory variable. But the authors of the later paper say that their results are similar when the family is used as a unit of observation and total family income is the explanatory variable. Other than the difference in samples, it is difficult to reconcile these two studies.

Because our focus in this paper is on the measurement of health status, we are interested in determining how more complete and reliable measures of health status affect the estimated coefficients. Our focus differs from that of the papers discussed, which are primarily concerned with how the inclusion of a whole host of covariates affects income elasticities, not with how more complete measures of health affect income elasticities and other variables. The papers just discussed do distinguish, however, between the influence of attitudes and that of health status variables per se.[4]

All the studies in the literature that use the EGFP measure postdict utilization. In the next section we will demonstrate that postdicting can cause inconsistent estimates. In addition, health status covariates that nominally refer to the same period as utilization (e.g., disability days in the past year) leave causality ambiguous: Did one suffer from restricted activity and therefore seek care, or did the physician advise taking it easy? In other words, apparently contemporaneous health status variables may also be endogenous.

A Simple Model of Postdiction

Suppose the true model relating utilization and health status is as follows:

(1) $$U_t = \alpha HS_{t-1} + \gamma P_t + \mu_f + \varepsilon'_t,$$

(2) $$HS_t = \beta U_t + \delta HS_{t-1} + u_t \; ,$$

where U_t = utilization in period t,
  HS_t = health status in period t, with larger values indicating better health,
  P_t = price in period t,
  μ_f = a person or family-specific effect that is time invariant,

and ε'_t and u_t are error terms with standard properties. The intercepts and the subscript indexing individuals have been omitted for convenience.

Suppose time is measured in years, and one has observations on health status at the end of each year (health status is assumed constant during the year) and on utilization in year two. In our data, P_2 is (approximately) orthogonal to all other variables. If (1) is estimated as specified (e.g., U_2 is estimated as a function of HS_1 and P_2), "prediction" occurs.

If, however, HS_2 is used in lieu of HS_1, "postdiction" occurs. We derive the plim of the estimated coefficients in Appendix A. In the general postdiction case the estimated coefficients of price and health status are inconsistent and the direction of the inconsistency cannot be signed. If, however, β equals zero (medical care in the observed range does not affect current health status), the inconsistency in the estimated coefficient of health status, α, is toward zero, and the estimated coefficient of price, γ, is consistent.

Because the sign of the inconsistency is in general not known, nor is the magnitude of the problem, we turn to empirical methods to ascertain the possible magnitude of the problem.

Measures of Health Status, Attitudes, Behavioral Propensities, and Knowledge

The World Health Organization defines health as "a state of complete physical, mental, and social well-being and not merely the absence of disease or infirmity" (WHO 1948). Two aspects of this definition have implications for the comprehensive measurement of health status. First, health is multidimensional with distinguishable physical, mental, and social components. (A fourth dimension, physiological health, is outside the scope of this paper; see Brook, Goldberg, Applegate, et al., [in press] for further discussion and definition). Second, the continuum of health for each of its components should extend beyond the negative states defined by different levels of illness and beyond the absence of illness to include the degree to which levels of positive states are enjoyed.

Construction of Health Status, Attitudinal, and Other Measures

Details of the health status and other measures used below can be found in series of monographs, which are referenced and summarized in a supplement of *Medical Care* (see Brook, Ware, Davies-Avery et al. 1979). In summary, these measures were constructed by using standard psychometric scaling techniques intended to achieve several desirable measurement properties: (a) variability and roughly symmetrical score distributions (as opposed to extremely skewed score distributions), (b) reliability (the proportion of measured variance that is true score, as opposed to random error), and (c) validity (an understanding of what is being measured and how differences in scores should be interpreted).

Variability and Symmetry

Health status and attitudinal measures focus on concepts that vary substantially in general populations. For example, with regard to mental health, the measures emphasize prevalent symptoms of emotional instability (for example, anxiety and depression) rather than psychotic disorders that are relatively rare in general populations.

Reliability

To enhance measurement reliability, the HIS fielded unambiguous questionnaire responses, such as "My health is now excellent" as opposed to "Health is good"; the latter response could refer to either the value placed on health or to the goodness of one's health, and its time frame is ambiguous. Multiple-response, as opposed to dichotomous, choices further improved reliability. For example, respondents were asked: "During the past month, how much of the time have you felt depressed?" Six choices, ranging from "All of the time" to "None of the time," were offered, as opposed to asking "During the past month, have you been depressed?" with responses of "Yes" and "No." Finally, rather than depending on less reliable single-item scales (e.g., the EGFP variable), we constructed our measures to combine items whenever appropriate to form multi-item scales.[5]

Validity

John E. Ware, Jr. has studied the validity of each measure, using both a variety of empirical methods and also an analysis of the content of the items contained in each measure. The primary empirical method employed was construct validation (Ware, Davies-Avery, and Brook 1980).[6] Construct validity studies are based on a theoretical model of how a valid measure should relate to other measured variables. For example, a valid measure of physical health should correlate (a) negatively with age, (b) positively with personal ratings of health status, (c) substantially with other physical health indicators that employ different measurement methods (such as another data source or a different scaling technique), and (d) negatively with medical care consumption.

In this paper we have used four categories of health-related measures to explain medical care consumption: (1) health status, (2) attitudes toward self-care and medical care, (3) behavioral propensities, and (4) sophistication or knowledgeability regarding the medical care delivery system. Tables 5.1 and 5.2 contain summaries of information about each variable, including (a) variable labels used in presenting regression results, (b) the kind of concept defined by each variable, (c) number of questionnaire items used in scoring, and (d) a brief operational definition.

Each variable is scored in such a way that a higher score indicates more of what the variable measures; thus, a higher score on the CURRENT health scale indicates more (better) current health, and a higher score on the WORRY scale indicates more worry. Additional background information on the development and rationale for these measures is briefly summarized below. Appendix B lists items by major category.

Physical Health

We measure the physical component of health in terms of limitations on functional status, a count of chronic diseases, and a count of acute symptoms. Functional status refers to the performance of or capacity to perform a variety of activities that are normal for an individual in good health (Stewart, Ware, and Brook 1981). Our functional status variable (PHYSLIM) measures limits on functional status and combines physical performance and capacity items in three areas: self-care (e.g., feeding, bathing), mobility (e.g., confinement indoors), and physical activities (e.g., walking, running). Because some differences in physical health may increase medical care consumption without affecting functional performance or capacity, we included two other measures of physical health, a count of chronic diseases (DISEASE) and a count of acute symptoms of illness whether treated or untreated (ACSIL). We do not at

Table 5.1   Operational Definitions and Labels Assigned to Health Status Measures

Type of Scale Variable Label	Health Concept[a]	Number of Items	Definition
Single–item scales			
POOR	G	1[b]	1 if health rated poor, zero otherwise
FAIR	G	1[b]	1 if health rated fair, zero otherwise
GOOD	G	1[b]	1 if health rated good, zero otherwise
Multi-item scales			
PHYSLIM[c]	P	9	Acute limitations in self-care, mobility, and physical activities
DISEASE[c]	P	32	Simple count of the number of physical disease conditions (26 possible)
ASCIL[c]	P	27	Simple count of the number of acute physical symptoms, past month
EMOINS	M	19	Emotional instability (anxious, depressed downhearted, tense, worried), past month
PWB	M	8	Positive well-being (in good spirits, cheerful, feeling loved, cared for), past month
SOCACT	S	9	Frequency and nature of social contacts and group memberships
CURRENT	G	9	Rating of health in general, at present
PRIOR	G	3	Rating of past health status
OUTLOOK	G	4	Rating of expected future health status
RESIST	G	4	Perceived bodily resistance to health threats
CONCERN	G	2	Amount of concern over personal health
WORRY	G	2	Amount of worry over personal health
HPQTOT	G	22	Health perceptions summary score; unweighted sum of CURRENT, PRIOR, OUTLOOK, RESIST, and negative of WORRY
LCU[c]	G	20	Life change units indicating stressful events

[a]Physical Health (P), Mental Health (M), Social Health (S), and General Health (G).

[b]Dummy variables based on single-item rating of health in terms of excellent, good, fair, or poor.

[c]In the regressions, the variable was replaced by log (variable + 1) to diminish the effect of skewness as well as to produce homoskedastic error plots.

Table 5.2   **Operational Definitions and Labels Assigned to Measures of Attitude, Knowledgeability, and Behavioral Propensity**

Variable Label	Health Concept[a]	Number of Items	Description
TRSIL[b]	B	27	Simple count of acute physical symptoms that care was sought for, past 30 days
ATGD	A	2	Favorable attitude toward going to the doctor
CONSOPH	K	8	Sophistication or knowledgeability about the medical care delivery system
EFFDOC	A	4	Favorable attitude toward the efficacy of doctors and medical care services
EFFSLF	A	4	Favorable attitude toward self care and home remedies
REJECT	B	4	Conscious avoidance of the sick/patient role

[a]Attitude (A), Behavioral propensity (B), Knowledgeability/Sophistication (K).
[b]In the regressions, the variable was replaced by log (variable + 1) to diminish the effect of skewness as well as to produce homoskedastic error plots.

this time have data on disability days. Thus, even our most comprehensive set of measures is not as comprehensive as possible.

Mental Health

We define the mental component of health in terms of selected phenomena of psychological disorders about which there is considerable conceptual agreement in the mental health literature. In addition we include positive states of well-being that are often ignored in general population studies (Ware, Johnston, Davies-Avery et al. 1979). Psychological disorders include two negative constructs: anxiety and depression. Because these constructs are highly collinear, they were combined into a single indicator of emotional instability (EMOINS). To distinguish between persons not experiencing a psychological disorder, highly correlated measures of positive emotional states and ratings of quality of life were combined to define positive well-being (PWB). All mental health items focus on psychological states, rather than on physiological and somatic ones (such as those measured by ACSIL), because inclusion of the latter in mental health would confound definitions of physical and mental health components.

Social Health

We measure the social component of health status by the frequency of social activities and by ratings of social resources in several distinct categories: (a) visits with friends and relatives, (b) memberships and participation in group functions, and (c) quality of social supports (e.g., having close friends that can help solve personal problems). To minimize the overlap between mental and social health measures found in previous studies (Donald, Ware, and Brook 1978), the social health measure excluded ratings of subjective feeling states related to social well-being (as, for example, feeling cared for and loved). Instead, these feelings are included in the positive well-being measure within the mental health concept. Psychometric studies of social activities have identified a common component, which can be summarized by a single health scale (SOCACT). Moreover, prediction of medical care consumption does not improve if we disaggregate social dimensions.

General Health Perceptions

In addition to the physical, mental, and social components suggested by the WHO definition of health status, ratings of general health perceptions were also tested (Ware, Davies-Avery, and Donald 1978). The health perception measures are distinct from the health status measures discussed above in that they do not focus on any specific health component. Instead, they ask for a personal assessment of health in general. In theory, general health ratings allow people to consider not only the objective information they have about their health but also their evaluation of that information. Measures were defined with respect to time (PRIOR, CURRENT, and OUTLOOK) and three other constructs: resistance-susceptibility to illness (RESIST, WORRY, and CONCERN). A unidimensional health component underlying these dimensions was defined by a summary indicator (HPQTOT), which combined the scales just mentioned excluding CONCERN. (The score for WORRY is multiplied by -1 prior to summing; CONCERN did not load on the same factor as the other five.) We also included the number of life change units (LCU), a method of weighting the stressful life events that befell the individual (Ware, Davies-Avery, and Brook 1980).

For comparison, we also measured health perceptions by the single-item rating of current health in terms of EGFP.[7] EGFP should perform less well than CURRENT; CURRENT, in principle, measures the same construct but should be more reliable because it is a nine-item scale with multiple responses for each item (Ware, Davies-Avery, and Donald 1978).

Other Health-related Variables

In addition to the health status measures discussed above, we examine six measures of attitude (tastes/sentiments), behavioral propensity, and knowledgeability regarding medical care services (see Table 5.2 for a summary of operational definitions). In contrast to health status, these measures focus directly on medical care seeking behaviors, such as whether one does or does not like to go to the doctor (ATGD; Ware 1976) or seeks care conditional upon having symptoms (TRSIL). Self-care attitudes, such as whether one believes in the efficacy of home remedies (EFFSLF) or the efficacy of medical care (EFFDOC), assess sentiments regarding treatment options (Lau and Ware, forthcoming). Consumer sophistication (CONSOPH) assesses knowledge of the medical care delivery system (Newhouse, Ware, and Donald, 1981). It should be a conceptually more appropriate measure of knowledge than education because it measures specific rather than general knowledge. Education was, however, tried and had insignificant effects in every specification.

Data and Nonhealth Status Variables

The data come from the first year of experience in three of the six sites of the Health Insurance Study (Newhouse 1974): Seattle, Washington; Fitchburg, Massachusetts; and Franklin County, Massachusetts. The first site—Dayton, Ohio—is omitted because the measures of health status changed somewhat between those taken at enrollment and those taken at the end of the first year of participation. The fifth and sixth sites, which are in South Carolina, are omitted because complete data from those sites are not yet available.

For this analysis we used a random sample of the population of the three sites, with the following exceptions:
1. Those over 61 at the time of enrollment were not eligible.
2. Those with incomes in excess of $25,000 (1973 dollars) were not eligible. This restriction excludes approximately the upper 5% of the income distribution.
3. The military and their dependents, veterans with service connected disabilities, and the institutionalized population (e.g., those in jails or state mental hospitals) were not eligible.
4. In Seattle, those who belonged to the Group Health Cooperative of Puget Sound (approximately 15% of the Seattle population) are not included in the sample analyzed here.
5. In the two Massachusetts sites, the low-income population was oversampled. Specifically, those families with incomes that were within 150% of the poverty line had a 33% greater chance of being included. We have not reweighted the sample of reflect this oversampling because we are not interested in predicting site means.

The sample we analyze is a subset of the adults (aged 18 and older) enrolled in the three sites. Adults who failed to fill out the health questionnaire at enrollment or after the first year of participation were excluded to avoid problems of missing data with the health status measures.

Individuals who died, attrited, or were suspended for part of the year, typically because they were in military service, were also excluded. The sample consists of 1,557 adults; there were 165 exclusions. Approximately half the exclusions were individuals who died, were suspended, or attrited; the remainder did not return the questionnaire.

Health Status Data-gathering Methods

All data on health status were gathered by means of a standardized questionnaire that was self-administered in each respondent's home. Heads of households each received $20 for completing questionnaires containing up to 531 relevant items; dependents received $5 each. The rate of returned questionnaires approximated 95%. While still in the field, we checked returned questionnaires for missing items; callbacks (in person or by telephone) were initiated whenever more than six items were left blank. This procedure produced very few (less than 1%) missing responses for returned questionnaires.

The Nonhealth Status Variables

In this paper we have confined our analysis to covered annual outpatient expenditures (OUTP) for health care,[8] except those for mental health care, dental care, and drugs and supplies. Outpatient care includes services provided by medical doctors, osteopaths, and some nonphysicians, such as chiropractors, podiatrists, speech therapists, physical therapists, and optometrists. Roughly 90% of the outpatient expenditure, however, is for physician services. Claims filed by the participants, including those for unreimbursed expenses, provide data on the amount and type of expenses.

We have used two variables to specify the coinsurance coverage provided to the participant by the HIS.[9] The first is a logarithmic coinsurance function $LC = \ln(\text{coinsurance percent} + 1)$ for those individuals facing a family coinsurance rate, i.e., where all members of a family face the same coinsurance rate at the same time.[10] The second is an indicator variable for the individual deductible plan (IDP). That plan approximates an outpatient care deductible of $150 per person or $450 per family (actually 95% coinsurance to a maximum of $150 out-of-pocket per person or $450 out-of-pocket per family), with all inpatient care free and outpatient care free beyond the deductible.

The explanatory variables also include three other indicator variables for experimental treatment: whether a household was given a pre-enrollment screening examination (EXAM),[11] whether the family was exempted from having to file biweekly diaries reporting sick days (NOHR);[12] and whether the family was enrolled for three rather than five years(YR3).[13]

The remaining nonhealth status explanatory variables control for variation in socioconomic factors. They include income for the two years prior to enrollment, family size, age, sex, and race. We selected functional forms for the continuous variables that would yield homoskedastic residual plots. Table 5.3 contains the formal variable definitions and Table 5.4 describes the sample characteristics. Data on all of these socioeconomic variables were derived from pre-enrollment interviews.

The Expenditure Model

The distribution of outpatient expenses has three characteristics that require special attention if one is to obtain reliable estimates of the demand for care. First, part of the distribution is clustered at zero; second, the distribution of positive expenditure is highly skewed; and third, the error terms for different family members are positively correlated. In other work (Manning, Morris, Newhouse et al. 1981), we have suggested that an appropriate model for expenditures is one with two parts (or equations) with variance components in the error term. The first equation models the decision to seek care and the second estimates the logarithm of nonzero expenses, conditional upon positive expenditure. The first equation appropriately handles the zero mass. The logarithmic transformation of positive expenses reduces the estimation problems caused by the skewness of positive expenses. In this case the variance components specification closely approximates the pattern of intrafamily correlation.

Here we will use a simpler, more tractable model. Instead of the two-part model, we will use a single dependent variable, the logarithm of expenses plus $5. Five dollars was chosen as the constant that left the data

Table 5.3   **Socioeconomic Variables**

Indicator Variables (0,1)

BLACK	= 1	if race of the head of family is black
FEMALE	= 1	if female
AFDC	= 1	if someone in the family received Aid to Families with Dependent Children
INCMIS	= 1	if information was missing
FITC	= 1	if in the Fitchburg site
FRAN	= 1	if in the Franklin County site

Continuous Variables

LNAGE	= ln	(age)
LINC	= ln	(average of 1973, 1974 family income in constant 1972 dollars)[a]
LFAM	= ln	(family size)

[a]Income was set equal to $1,000 if reported to be less. Individuals with INCMIS = 1 received the site mean LINC.

Table 5.4   Sample Characteristics

Variable	Average	Standard Deviation	Minimum	Maximum
LC	1.58	1.95	0.00	4.56
IDP	0.25	0.43	0.00	1.00
NOHR	0.13	0.33	0.00	1.00
EXAM	0.65	0.48	0.00	1.00
YR3	0.75	0.43	0.00	1.00
LINC	8.88	0.67	6.91	10.01
INCMIS	0.02	0.15	0.00	1.00
LFAM	1.00	0.59	0.00	2.40
BLACK	0.02	0.13	0.00	1.00
AFDC*	0.02	0.14	0.00	1.00
FEMALE	0.53	0.50	0.00	1.00
AGE	35.50	11.80	18.00	62.00
LNAGE	3.52	0.33	2.89	4.13
FITC	0.25	0.43	0.00	1.00
FRAN	0.31	0.46	0.00	1.00
OUTP	129.91	191.13	0.00	2454.16
ln (OUTP + 5)	4.08	1.42	1.61	7.81

*Data on AFDC status collected only in Seattle.

most nearly normal. If the goal of the analysis were to predict expenses, then this simpler model would provide biased estimates of raw means because the size of the zero mass is covariate-related in a manner different from the response in the nonzero expenses. But the inferences that can be drawn from the simpler model appear to be robust in spite of this misspecification in the case of these data. Because our goal is inference rather than prediction, we are willing to make a sacrifice for computational simplicity.

An alternative to the logarithmic transform plus $5 would be to use raw dollar expenses as the dependent variable. Unfortunately, with our sample size, the nature of health expenditure data causes least squares to yield imprecise results. Least squares would be appropriate if expenditure had a normally distributed error term or if there were enough data to rely on the Central Limit Theorem. In either case, the t- and F-statistics would be well behaved and the coefficients would be robust. Unfortunately, neither condition is met. Even sample sizes in excess of 1,000 yield imprecise results given the error distribution of our data. A few very large expenses have an undue influence on the results.

The logarithmic transformation of the expenses provides more robust and more efficient estimates. Nonzero outpatient expenses are very close to lognormally distributed, and so the use of a logarithmic transform reduces the departure from normality. The smaller the departure, the more robust the estimates. Thus, the logarithmic transform lessens the likelihood that a few large expenses will have an undue influence on the coefficients. The use of a logarithmic transformation also reduces the coefficient of variation in the dependent variable. The coefficients will therefore be more precise with the logarithmic transform than with the raw dollar sale if lognormality holds. For the HIS data, the increase in precision with a logarithmic transform is roughly equivalent to a three-to-fivefold increase in sample size.

We have used a random-effects variance-components estimator. With this estimator we can obtain efficient estimates of the regression coefficients and consistent estimates of the standard errors. The data exhibit a nearly constant intrafamily correlation across family sizes. Hence, the residual correlations are similar to those of a variance-components model with a family-specific error term. The expenditure equation is estimated by maximum likelihood, iterating over the coefficients and the proportion of the error variance accounted for by the family component.

Empirical Results

In examining the empirical results obtained from our use of alternative sets of health status variables, we focus on the two questions posed in our introduction. What have we gained in explanatory power by using more comprehensive health status variables than the simple excellent, good, fair, poor (EGFP) question? What are the consequences of using postdictive variables, i.e., of using measures of current health to explain past utilization behavior?

Gains from Comprehensiveness

There are two potential gains from employing more comprehensive health status variables than EGFP. The EGFP measure provides only four responses to a unidimensional concept of health. Alternative measures could reduce the coarseness of the measurement by (a) providing a finer and more reliable division in a unidimensional measure, and (b) providing measures of several dimensions of health.

In comparing EGFP with CURRENT, we can observe the effect of greatly increasing the number of responses. In comparing CURRENT with HPQTOT, we can observe the gains from a broader definition of health still restricted to a scalar measure. Comparing HPQTOT with its components (CURRENT, PRIOR, OUTLOOK, WORRY, and RESIST) provides a test of whether health perceptions are unidimensional or multidimensional. Finally, adding measures of physical, mental, and social health, and attitudes toward the efficacy of medical care extends the number of dimensions of health that may affect overall expenditures.

Our results show that there are indeed gains from using more comprehensive measures. Table 5.5 contains test statistics that compare one

Table 5.5   Tests for Alternative Specifications of the Health Variables

H_0	versus	H_1	Pesaran's N_0^*	F^{**} Value	df
EGFP		CURRENT	−2.56	—	—
CURRENT		HPQTOT	−0.48	—	—
HPQTOT		HPQ components	—	4.79	4,1537
HPQ Components		Full set	—	4.74	14,1523

*Distributed $N(0, 1)$. A negative sign implies a rejection of the null hypothesis in favor of the alternative model.

**The one-percent critical value for $F_{4,1000}$ is 3.34, and for $F_{14,1000}$ it is 2.09.

alternative health specification with another. Two sets of tests are presented. First, for testing nonnested specifications, we provide a statistic N_0 that is a standardized normal variate when the null hypothesis (the first health specification) is true.[14] Second, for nested specifications, the standard F-statistic is calculated. For both types of tests, the data have been transformed to remove the effect of intrafamily correlation. As Table 5.5 indicates, we can reject EGFP in favor of CURRENT at an $\alpha < .01$. However, we cannot reject CURRENT in favor of the broader HPQTOT (scalar) measure.

Further gains come when HPQTOT is disaggregated. At an $\alpha < .001$ one can reject the hypothesis that HPQTOT contains all the behavioral information contained in its components. If a single health perceptions scale HPQTOT were appropriate, then the (unstandardized) coefficients on its components would be equal to each other and to the (unstandardized) coefficient on the scale itself. As the test statistic in Table 5.5 indicates, this equality does not hold. Thus, we can reject the hypothesis that behavior reflects a single health perception.

Further, one can reject the hypothesis that only health perceptions matter. A fuller specification, including physical limitations (PHYSLIM), counts of recent symptoms (ACSIL), attitudes about going to the doctor (ATGD), and the efficacy of self-treatment (EFFSLF), exhibits significantly increased explanatory power. The health perception components as a group are still significant, but the size of their coefficients is now reduced because these variables no longer act as proxies for other omitted health status variables.

Explained variation increases from 0.1292 in a specification with only EGFP to 0.1844 with the full model. Another way to describe this increase is that a more comprehensive measure of health status, if available, will yield a gain in precision at least equivalent to a 7% increase in sample size $[1.07 = \exp (1. - .1292)/(1 - .1844)]$. Seven percent is a lower bound because the more comprehensive measure not only causes the residual variance to fall but also decreases the proportion of error variance that comes from intrafamily correlation.[15] We have calculated the decrease in the confidence interval for a mean individual on the free plan; the decrease equals 12%.

The introduction of more comprehensive health status and attitudinal variables could affect the coefficients on other nonhealth covariates. Any variable that is correlated with the omitted variable will have some bias in its coefficient. Table 5.6 presents the coefficients for selected variables, under alternative specifications. The results are rather mixed. The coinsurance function and individual deductible plan coefficients are, of course, unaffected, because the assignment of the sample to coinsurance plans was designed to leave the plan, for practical purposes, orthogonal to other covariates. The coefficients on income (LINC) and family size (LFAM) are significant and also change little as the specification is enriched.

The coefficient on BLACK moves toward zero (becomes less negative) by about one-third of its standard deviation as the health specification becomes more comprehensive. Thus, blacks appear to have relatively poorer health in the dimensions omitted from the EGFP specification. We caution against overinterpreting this result, however, because there are few blacks in our sample (Table 5.4). The age (LNAGE) coefficient increases as the specification is increased, moving about one-half of its estimated standard deviation. Finally, in the most comprehensive specification, the FEMALE coefficient falls by 1 to 1.5 standard deviations. Note, however, that the FEMALE coefficient is always strongly positive, in contrast to the belief of Hershey, Luft, and Gianaris (1975), who suggest that it will be negative if health status is controlled for.

Predictive Results

The coefficients of the health status and attitudinal variables from the various specifications are given in Table 5.7; to facilitate interpretation, we generally present standardized coefficients. The addition of health, attitudinal, and other covariates generally reduced the coefficients of health perceptions. Consumer sophistication (CONSOPH) is insignificant, but its impact is indeterminant because a sophisticated consumer may consume more efficacious services and fewer inappropriate ones. Physical limitations, chronic disease, and symptoms all have a positive impact on utilization. Favorable attitudes about going to the doctor are mirrored in higher utilization of medical services, whereas individuals who believe in the efficacy of self-treatment use fewer services. This latter result is also found by Hershey, Luft, and Gianaris (1975). We replicate Colle and Grossman's (1978) result on the unimportance of attitudes concerning the efficacy of medical care. There is strong support for the

Table 5.6   Selected Variation in Coefficient Estimates as Specification Changes ($|t|$)

			Coefficient Estimates of Selected Variables				
Specification	LC	IDP	LINC	LFAM	BLACK	LNAGE	FEMALE
EGFP	-.15 (7.20)	-.45 (4.80)	.04 (.62)	-.04 (.56)	-.83 (2.94)	.49 (4.30)	.55 (8.58)
CURRENT	-.15 (7.07)	-.44 (4.71)	.04 (.62)	-.03 (.45)	-.87 (3.10)	.52 (4.69)	.57 (8.92)
HPQTOT	-.15 (7.08)	-.44 (4.68)	.04 (.63)	-.03 (.42)	-.86 (3.08)	.54 (4.84)	.56 (8.83)
HPQ components	-.15 (7.15)	-.44 (4.78)	.05 (.84)	-.03 (.39)	-.82 (2.95)	.57 (4.90)	.58 (8.98)
Full list	-.15 (7.32)	-.43 (4.72)	.04 (.72)	-.03 (.46)	-.77 (2.85)	.54 (4.38)	.46 (6.59)

Table 5.7 **Coefficients for Alternative Health Variables**

Specification	Variable[a]	$\hat{\beta}$	$|t|$
EGFP[b]	GOOD	+.17	2.26
	FAIR	+.67	4.89
	POOR	+.64	1.08
CURRENT	CURRENT	−.20	5.73
HPQTOT	HPQTOT	−.21	6.23
HPQ components	CURRENT	−.13	2.76
	OUTLOOK	+.01	1.99
	PRIOR	−.13	3.55
	RESIST	−.02	0.47
	WORRY	+.10	2.50
Full list	ACSIL	+.08	1.83
	DISEASE	+.08	1.89
	PHYSLIM	+.18	2.07
	EMOINS	+.14	2.82
	PWB	+.13	2.69
	SOCACT	+.05	1.29
	CONCERN	+.06	1.51
	CURRENT	−.07	1.37
	LCU	+.04	1.11
	OUTLOOK	+.06	1.49
	PRIOR	−.10	2.66
	RESIST	−.02	0.44
	WORRY	+.03	0.76
	ATGD	+.11	3.06
	EFFDOC	−.02	0.48
	EFFSLF	−.08	2.36
	REJECT	−.01	0.27
	TRSIL	+.08	2.18
	CONSOPH	−.04	1.11

[a]Except for the indicators for EGFP, all health status variables are in standardized form: $(x_{ij} - \bar{x}_i)/\sigma_{x_i}$.
[b]The standardized coefficients are .08, .18, .04.

notion that individuals with anxiety and depression do use the medical system more. But surprisingly, positive well-being has the wrong sign and is significant.[16] The variable social contacts and support (SOCACT) is positive but insignificant. A medical (contagion) model predicts a positive sign, whereas the psychological support model (the more social support, the less reliance on the medical care system for support) predicts a negative sign.

Postdiction vs. Prediction

As noted earlier, most microlevel studies in the literature have used current health measures to explain or postdict past medical utilization. With the panel data we have, we can test whether the inconsistency that a postdictive model causes is important.

We have used Wu's second and preferred test (1973, 1974) to detect any dependence between the postdictive health variables and the error in the expenditure equation.

Consider the following model of medical behavior:

$$(3) \qquad U_i = Y_i'\beta + Z_i'\delta + \varepsilon,$$

$$(4) \qquad Y_i = \mu_i + v_i, \quad i = 1, \ldots, N,$$

where for person i, U_i is the logarithm of outpatient expenditure plus \$5, Y_i is the $G \times 1$ vector of postdictive health status variables, Z_i is the $K_1 \times 1$ vector of known nonstochastic regressors, and μ_i is a $G \times 1$ vector of unknown constants. The errors ε and v are assumed to be multivariate normal with covariance matrix

$$\Sigma = \begin{bmatrix} \sigma_{\varepsilon\varepsilon} & \delta \\ \delta' & \sigma_{vv} \end{bmatrix}.$$

Wu proposed that if $K_2 (> G)$ nonstochastic variables Z_2 were available, then one test for δ equal to zero [i.e., zero covariance between equations (3) and (4)] is

$$T_2 = \frac{Q^*/G}{(Q - Q^*)/(N - K_1 - 2G)},$$

where

$$Q^* = (b_1 - b_2)'[(Y'A_2Y)^{-1} - (Y'A_1Y)^{-1}]^{-1}(b_1 - b_2),$$

$b_1 = $ OLS estimate of β,

$b_2 = $ instrumental variable estimate of β,

$A_1 = I - Z_1(Z_1Z_1)^{-1}Z_1' = M_{Z_1}$,

$A_2 = Z(Z'Z)^{-1}Z' - Z_1(Z_1'Z_1)^{-1}Z_1'$,

$Z = (Z_1, Z_2)$,

$Q = (U - Yb_1)'A_1(U - Yb_1) = N \cdot$ OLS estimate of $\sigma_{\varepsilon\varepsilon}$.

Under the null hypothesis ($\delta = 0$), T_2 is distributed as an F-statistic with $(G, N - K_1 - 2G)$ degrees of freedom.

The instruments that we used for this analysis were the (predictive) enrollment values for the health variables and the physician visits in the year prior to the one being observed. The data have been transformed by using the postdictive estimate of intrafamily correlation to remove the effect of intrafamily correlation.

The values for Wu's test in Table 5.8 confirm that we can detect in our sample the dependence between the error in the equation and the post-dictive variables. At each level of complexity, ranging from EGFP to the full list of health measures, we can reject the hypothesis that the postdic-tive measures are independent of the error at α levels of 1% or less. Postdicting raises the R^2; depending on the specification, postdicting increases the R^2 from 5% (CURRENT) to 26% (full list) (Table 5.9).

As discussed above, the direction of the inconsistency is, in general, theoretically indeterminant. Empirically, postdicting tends to move the coefficients away from zero. Table 5.10 provides a side-by-side compari-son of predictive and postdictive coefficients. (For the richest specifica-tion, collinearity makes side-by-side comparisons more difficult.) For the EGFP, CURRENT, HPQTOT, and HPQ components specifications, the coefficients of the postdictive variables are larger in absolute value in all but two cases: the indicator for good health and the insignificant RESIST variable. In some cases the differences are very striking. The postdictive coefficient on WORRY in the HPQ components specification is double and the indicator for poor health in the EGFP specification is more than double their respective predictive coefficients. The result on WORRY is even more striking in the full specification, where it increases by a factor of 5. The coefficient of PHYSLIM also doubles in that specification.

Table 5.8   **Tests for Independence of the Error and the Postdictive Variables**

Specification	Wu's T_2	df	Significant at $\alpha \leq$
EGFP	10.26	3,1534	.001
CURRENT	16.46	1,1538	.001
HPQTOT	9.43	1,1538	.010
HPQ components	4.08	5,1530	.010
Full list	2.86	17,1506	.001

Table 5.9 R^2 **For the Predict and Postdict Models**

Specifications	Predict R^2	Postdict R^2
EGFP	.1292	.1415
CURRENT	.1338	.1403
HPQTOT	.1371	.1462
HPQ components	.1480	.1741
Full list	.1844	.2316

The results suggest that frequent use of outpatient services during the past year is associated with worry, physicial limitation, and preoccupation with poor health. Whether this reflects exogenous variation in health status that caused utilization (e.g., an auto accident that resulted in physical limitation and medical treatment) or whether it represents an

Table 5.10   Coefficients for Predictive and Postdictive Health Variables

		Predictive		Postdictive	
Specification	Variable[a]	β	$\lvert t \rvert$	β	$\lvert t \rvert$
EGFP[b]	GOOD	+.17	2.26	+.16	2.15
	FAIR	+.67	4.89	+.73	5.78
	POOR	+.64	1.08	+1.63	4.22
CURRENT	CURRENT	−.20	5.73	−.23	6.70
HPQTOT	HPQTOT	−.21	6.23	−.26	7.47
HPQ Components	CURRENT	−.13	2.76	−.13	2.66
	OUTLOOK	+.09	1.99	+.13	2.97
	PRIOR	−.13	3.55	−.17	4.67
	RESIST	−.02	0.47	−.005	0.12
	WORRY	+.10	2.50	+.20	4.94
Full list	ACSIL	+.08	1.83	−.02	0.37
	DISEASE[c]	+.08	1.89	+.07	1.78
	PHYSLIM	+.08	2.07	+.16	4.32
	EMOINS	+.14	2.82	+.02	0.37
	PWB	+.13	2.69	+.03	0.69
	SOCACT	+.05	1.23	−.01	0.16
	CONCERN	+.06	1.51	+.01	0.34
	CURRENT	−.07	1.37	−.03	0.58
	LCU	+.04	1.11	−.01	0.34
	OUTLOOK	+.06	1.49	+.09	2.01
	PRIOR	−.10	2.66	−.14	3.79
	RESIST	+.02	0.44	+.02	0.39
	WORRY	+.03	0.76	+.16	3.71
	ATGD	+.11	3.06	+.17	4.79
	EFFDOC	−.02	0.48	−.02	0.63
	EFFSLF	−.08	2.36	−.07	2.02
	REJECT	−.01	0.27	+.07	1.95
	TRSIL	+.08	2.18	+.22	6.11
	CONSOPH[c]	−.04	1.11	−.03	0.94

[a]Except for the indicators for EGFP, all health variables are in standardized form: $(x_{ij} - \bar{x}_i)/\sigma_{x_i}$.

[b]The standardized predict coefficients are .08, .18, .03; the standardized postdict coefficients are .08, .22, .14.

[c]Measured only at enrollment.

effect of the use of medical care (e.g., detection of previously undiagnosed disease, greater appreciation of the consequence of poor health habits such as smoking) is an intriguing question that remains for future research.

The use of the postdictive measures can also cause the coefficients of other variables that are not orthogonal to the health variables to be inconsistent. Postdiction generally causes the coefficients of LNAGE to decrease in absolute value and BLACK to increase in absolute value (Table 5.11). The largest changes occur in the Full List specification, where the coefficients for LNAGE and BLACK move by 1.4 and 0.6 standard deviations, respectively. In contrast, postdiction has almost no effect on the insurance coverage variables.

Conclusion

In answer to the first question we posed in this paper, we can say that the gain in explanatory power from using more comprehensive measures of health than those traditionally used is substantial. Compared with the simple EGFP question, the use of our most comprehensive definition of health was equivalent to an increase of around 10% in sample size. Much of this gain could potentially be achieved by sampling from those dimensions that predict utilization instead of employing the entire battery used in the HIS; e.g., one might include only two to four items from the current health scale rather than nine, and drop items related to the efficacy of medical care altogether. In general, the cost of a 10% increase in sample size will exceed the cost of collecting data on the more comprehensive measures of health (it would have greatly exceeded it in the

Table 5.11   Predictive and Postdictive Coefficients For LNAGE and BLACK

Specification	Variable	Predictive		Postdictive	
		β	|t|	β	|t|
EGFP	LNAGE	+.49	4.30	+.45	3.99
	BLACK	−.83	2.94	−.91	3.26
CURRENT	LNAGE	+.52	4.69	+.48	4.30
	BLACK	−.87	3.10	−.88	3.15
HPQTOT	LNAGE	+.54	4.84	+.49	4.45
	BLACK	−.86	3.08	−.84	3.01
HPQ components	LNAGE	+.57	4.90	+.56	4.89
	BLACK	−.82	2.95	−.83	3.06
Full list	LNAGE	+.54	4.38	+.37	3.14
	BLACK	−.77	2.85	−.92	3.46

Health Insurance Study), and so more comprehensive definitions seem cost effective.

In principle, more comprehensive definitions should also reduce omitted variable bias in other coefficients, but in our data these reductions were moderate to small. The estimated effect of coinsurance was essentially unchanged, but coinsurance was constructed to be orthogonal to other variables in our sample at the time of enrollment and so our result would not necessarily replicate in nonexperimental data. Likewise there was little effect on the estimated income elasticity, but in our sample the estimated income elasticity itself was near zero. We caution against generalizing this result; e.g., in the Dayton site, our results (not reported here) indicate an income elasticity of 0.2 to 0.4 in each of the first two years (Newhouse, Manning, Morris, et al., 1981). We did not include Dayton data in this paper because the health status measures prior to enrollment are not the same as those at the end of one year. Had we been able to analyze the Dayton data in a fashion similar to those of the other sites, we might have found that the inclusion of a more comprehensive health status measure did have an effect on the estimated income elasticity.

Including more health status variables has a moderate effect on the coefficient measuring race, but we must point out that there are few blacks in either Seattle or the two Massachusetts sites, and so this result may not replicate. We also found a moderate effect on the variable measuring sex, and we can think of no caveats about this result.

One can show in a simple theoretical model that the use of a health status measure from a later period to predict utilization in an earlier period (postdiction) leads to inconsistent estimates. We can detect this inconsistency in our data. Empirically, postdiction raised both the measured R^2 and the absolute values of the coefficients of the health status variables. Postdiction also increased the absolute value of the estimated coefficient for blacks and decreased it for age.

What practical advice can we offer? Many researchers will not be able to avoid the problem of analyzing health status variables from a period subsequent to their measures of utilization. If possible, one would like to treat such health status variables as endogenous. But it is difficult to think of good instrumental variables; a natural choice might be age, but age appears to have an independent effect on demand. At a minimum one should be aware of the problem.

Furthermore, one should use all the health status variables at hand, but the natural tendency would be to do this anyway, so such advice is not particularly helpful. Perhaps our findings about the gains from more comprehensive measures are most helpful to those who have a chance to influence the data that will be collected. At least for demand estimation— and probably for most other purposes as well—the resources necessary to obtain more comprehensive health status measures than EGFP appear worth the sacrifice in sample size.

What future steps seem indicated in research on health status measures as covariates? We see two. First, the remaining measurement error in the covariates should be accounted for in coefficient estimates. Second, one might consider specifying health status as an unobserved or latent variable, thereby exploiting the covariance of demand and health status when deriving scales.

Appendix A

The Inconsistency of Postdiction

Let the true model be

(A.1) $U_t = \alpha HS_{t-1} + \gamma P_t + \mu_f + \varepsilon'_t,$

(A.2) $HS_t = \beta U_t + \delta HS_{t-1} + u_t,$

where U_t is utilization in time t, HS_t is health status in time t, P_t is the price of medical services in time t, μ_f is a time-invariant family-specific error term and ε'_t and u_t are error terms that are independent of the explanatory variables and are not autocorrelated. Suppose t is measured in units of years and P_2 is orthogonal to HS_1. (This latter supposition is not necessarily true in nonexperimental data.)

Let period 1 be the pre-experimental period; we observe HS at the end of that period and denote it as HS_1. We have another observation one year later, which we will denote as HS_2. The utilization we seek to explain is U_2, i.e., utilization during the year bounded by the two observations on health status. Let all variables be measured as deviations from their means.

Postdicting U_2 means using HS_2 in place of HS_1 when estimating α and γ. Let a and g be estimates of α and γ in a postdictive model.

$$\text{plim} \begin{pmatrix} a \\ g \end{pmatrix} = \begin{bmatrix} \text{var } HS_2 & \text{cov}(HS_2, P_2) \\ \text{cov}(HS_2, P_2) & \text{var } P_2 \end{bmatrix}^{-1} \begin{bmatrix} \text{cov}(HS_2, U_2) \\ \text{cov}(P_2, U_2) \end{bmatrix}$$

$$\text{plim } g = \gamma +$$

$$\frac{\gamma(\beta\gamma \text{ var } P_2)^2 - \gamma(\beta^2 \text{var } P_2 \text{var } U_2) - \gamma(\alpha\beta\delta \text{var } P_2 \text{var } HS_1)}{\text{var } HS_2 \text{var } P_2 - (\beta\gamma \text{var } P_2)^2}$$

If $\beta = 0$ (medical care at the margin does not affect health status), the expression on the right is zero, and plim $g = \gamma$; g is consistent. If $\beta < 0$, the direction of the inconsistency cannot be signed with certainty. If $\beta > 0$, the direction of the inconsistency is toward zero. This can be shown as follows. Consider the fraction on the right side. Because the determinant of a variance-covariance matrix is positive, the denominator is positive. Moreover, the sum of the first two terms in the numerator is positive, since var $U_2 > \gamma^2$ var P_2 (by the definition of U_2) and γ is negative. Because γ is negative and δ is positive, the third term in the numerator has the sign of β; if β is positive (medical care improves health status), plim g will be biased toward zero.

$$\text{plim } a = \frac{\beta \operatorname{var} P_2 \operatorname{var} U_2 + \alpha\delta \operatorname{var} P_2 \operatorname{var} HS_1 - \beta(\gamma \operatorname{var} P_2)^2}{\operatorname{var} HS_2 \operatorname{var} P_2 - (\beta\gamma \operatorname{var} P_2)^2}$$

If $\beta = 0$, this expression becomes

$$\frac{\alpha\delta \operatorname{var} HS_1}{\delta^2 \operatorname{var} HS_1 + \operatorname{var} u} = \frac{\alpha}{\delta} - \frac{\alpha}{\delta}\left(\frac{\operatorname{var} u}{\delta^2 \operatorname{var} HS_1 + \operatorname{var} u}\right)$$

$$= \frac{\alpha}{\delta}\left(1 - \frac{\operatorname{var} u}{\delta^2 \operatorname{var} HS_1 + \operatorname{var} u}\right)$$

Because $0 < \delta < 1$, plim a could be greater or less than α. If $\beta \neq 0$, a term is added to this expression that is positive if β is positive and conversely.

Appendix B

Questionnaire Items Used to Construct Measures of Health Status, Attitudes, Behavioral Propensity, and Knowledgeability

Category		Item
Physical Limitations (PHYSLIM)	1)	Are you able to drive a car?
	2)	When you travel around your community, does someone have to assist you because of your health?
	3)	Do you have to stay indoors most or all of the day, because of your health?
	4)	Are you in bed or a chair for most or all of the day because of your health?
	5)	Does your health limit the kind of vigorous activities you can do, such as running, lifting heavy objects, or participating in strenuous sports?
	6)	Do you have trouble either walking several blocks or climbing a few flights of stairs because of your health?
	7)	Do you have trouble bending, lifting, or stooping because of your health?
	8)	Do you have any trouble either walking one block or climbing one flight of stairs because of your health?
	9)	Are you unable to walk unless you are assisted by another person or by a cane, crutches, artificial limbs, or braces?
Chronic Diseases (DISEASE)	1)	Has a doctor ever said you have glaucoma (increased pressure in the eye)?
	2)	Can you usually hear and understand what a person says, without seeing his face and without a hearing aid, if he whispers to you from across a quiet room?

Appendix B (continued)

Category	Item
	3) Have you ever had hay fever or other allergies to plants and grasses?
	4)* Do you have any natural teeth at all? (Your own teeth, not artificial?)
	5)* Has a dentist ever told you that you have gum problems?
	6) In the past 12 months, have you had trouble with pimples on your face?
	7) Has a doctor ever said you had goiter (GOY-ter) or thyroid trouble?
	8) During the past 12 months, have you had any pain, aching, swelling, or stiffness in your joints—for example, your fingers, hip, or knee? (Do not count problems caused by an injury.)
	9) During the past 12 months, have you ever felt short of breath?
	10)* Has a doctor ever told you that you had an enlarged heart or heart failure?
	11) Has a doctor ever said that you had high blood pressure?
	12)* Has a doctor ever said that you had a heart attack?
	13)* Has a doctor ever said that you have angina? (An-JI-na or AN-ji-na)
	14) Has a doctor ever told you that you had chronic bronchitis (bron-KY-tis) or emphysema (em-feh-SEE-ma)?
	15) Has a doctor ever said that you had tuberculosis (T.B.)? (Tuberculosis pronounced "too-burr-cue-LO-sis")
	16) Has a doctor ever said that you had a peptic ulcer, stomach ulcer, or duodenal ulcer (ulcer of the small bowel)?
	17) Did a doctor ever say you had kidney disease?

18) Has a doctor ever said you have high blood cholesterol?

19) Has a doctor ever said that you had anemia (a-NEE-mee-a) or low blood?

20) Has a doctor ever said to you that you had diabetes or pre-diabetes?

21) Has a doctor ever told you that you had cancer?

22) Have you had hemorrhoids (piles) within the past 12 months? (Hemorrhoids pronounced "HEM-or-royds")

23) Have you had a hernia within the past 12 months?

24) During the past 12 months, have you noticed varicose veins in your legs?

25) Do you have any missing limbs—that is, arms, legs, or fingers that are missing or have been amputated?

26) As far as you know, during the past 12 months, have you had bursitis?

27) As far as you know, during the past 12 months, have you had arteriosclerosis or hardening of the arteries?

28) As far as you know, during the past 12 months, have you had chronic hepatitis or yellow jaundice?

29) As far as you know, during the past 12 months, have you had chronic gall bladder trouble or gallstones?

30) As far as you know, during the past 12 months, have you had phlebitis (thrombophlebitis)?

31) As far as you know, during the past 12 months have (women only) you had any disease of the uterus or ovary?

32) As far as you know, during the past 12 months have (women only) you had any lumps in your breasts?

Appendix B (continued)

Category		Item
Acute Physical Symptoms (ACSIL)	1)	During the past 30 days, did you have a cough, without fever, which lasted at least 3 weeks?
	2)	During the past 30 days, did you have a sore throat or cold, with fever, lasting more than 3 days?
	3)	During the past 30 days, did you have a weight loss of more than 10 pounds (unless you were dieting)?
	4)	During the past 30 days, did you have an upset stomach, for less than 24 hours?
	5)	During the past 30 days, did you have stiffness, pain or swelling of joints, lasting more than 2 weeks?
	6)	During the past 30 days, did you have backaches or sciatica?
	7)	During the past 30 days, did you have trouble falling asleep at night?
	8)	During the past 30 days, did you get up exhausted in the mornings, even with the usual amount of sleep?
	9)	During the past 30 days, did you have a skin rash, or breaking out on any part of the body?
	10)	During the past 30 days, did you have shortness of breath with light exercise or light work?
	11)	During the past 30 days, did you have chest pain when exercising?
	12)	During the past 30 days, did you have a stopped up nose, or sneezing or allergies for 2 weeks or more?
	13)	During the past 30 days, did you have swollen ankles when you woke up?
	14)	During the past 30 days, did you have headaches almost every day?

15) During the past 30 days, did you have a cough without fever, which lasted for less than a week?

16) During the past 30 days, did you have loss of consciousness, fainting, or passing out?

17) During the past 30 days, did you have acid indigestion or heartburn after many meals?

18) During the past 30 days, did you have a sprained ankle, but you could still walk?

19) During the past 30 days, did you have a toothache?

20) During the past 30 days, did you have stomach "flu" or virus (gastroenteritis) with vomiting or diarrhea?

21) During the past 30 days, did you have bleeding (other than nose bleed or periods) not caused by accident or injury?

22) During the past 30 days, did you have an eye infection?

23) During the past 30 days, did you feel nervous or anxious most of the time?

24) During the past 30 days, did you feel depressed or sad most of the time?

25) During the past 30 days, did you (men only) have difficulty passing urine or prostate trouble?

26) During the past 30 days, did you (women only) have difficulty controlling urine, or bladder or kidney problems?

27) During the past 30 days, did you (women only) have irregular periods, or bleeding between periods?

Emotional Instability (EMOINS)

1) How often did you become nervous or jumpy when faced with excitement or unexpected situations during the past month?

2) Did you feel depressed during the past month?

3) How much of the time, during the past month, have you been a very nervous person?

Appendix B (continued)

Category	Item
	4) During the past month, how much of the time have you felt tense or "high-strung"?
	5) During the past month, have you been in firm control of your behavior, thoughts, emotions, feelings?
	6) During the past month, how often did your hands shake when you tried to do something?
	7) How much of the time, during the past month, have you felt downhearted and blue?
	8) How often have you felt like crying, during the past month?
	9) During the past month, how often did you feel that others would be better off if you were dead?
	10) How much have you been bothered by nervousness, or your "nerves," during the past month?
	11) How often, during the past month, have you felt so down in the dumps that nothing could cheer you up?
	12) During the past month, did you ever think about taking your own life?
	13) During the past month, how much of the time have you felt restless, fidgety, or impatient?
	14) During the past month, how much of the time have you been moody or brooded about things?
	15) During the past month, how often did you get rattled, upset, or flustered?
	16) During the past month, have you been anxious or worried?
	17) How often during the past month did you find yourself having difficulty trying to calm down?

18) During the past month, how much of the time have you been in low or very low spirits?

19) During the past month, have you been under or felt you were under any strain, stress, or pressure?

Positive Well-being (PWB)

1) How happy, satisfied, or pleased have you been with your personal life during the past month?

2) During the past month, how much of the time have you felt that the future looks hopeful and promising?

3) How much of the time, during the past month, has your daily life been full of things that were interesting to you?

4) During the past month, how much of the time have you generally enjoyed the things you do?

5) When you got up in the morning, this past month, about how often did you expect to have an interesting day?

6) During the past month, how much of the time has living been a wonderful adventure for you?

7) How much of the time, during the past month, have you felt cheerful, lighthearted?

8) During the past month, how much of the time were you a happy person?

Social Activities (SOCACT)

1) About how many families in your neighborhood are you well enough acquainted with, that you visit each other in your homes?

2) About how many close friends do you have—people you feel at ease with and can talk with about what is on your mind? (You may include relatives.)

3) Over a year's time, about how often do you get together with friends or relatives, like going out together or visiting each other's homes?

Appendix B (continued)

Category	Item
	4) During the past month, about how often have you had friends over to your home? (Do not count relatives.)
	5) About how often have you visited with friends at their homes during the past month? (Do not count relatives.)
	6) About how often were you on the telephone with close friends or relatives during the past month?
	7) About how often did you write a letter to a friend or relative during the past month?
	8) In general, how well are you getting along with other people these days—would you say better than usual, about the same, or not as well as usual?
	9) How often have you attended a religious service during the past month?
	10) About how many voluntary groups or organizations do you belong to—like church groups, clubs or lodges, parent groups, etc. ("Voluntary" means because you want to.)
	11) How active are you in the affairs of these groups or clubs you belong to? (If you belong to a great many, just count those you feel closest to. If you don't belong to any, circle 4.)
POOR, FAIR, GOOD	1) In general, would you say your health is excellent, good, fair, or poor?
Current Health (CURRENT)	1) According to the doctors I've seen, my health is now excellent.
	2) I feel better now than I ever have before.
	3) I am somewhat ill.
	4) I'm not as healthy now as I used to be.
	5) I'm as healthy as anybody I know.

	6)	My health is excellent.
	7)	Doctors say that I am now in poor health.
	8)	I feel about as good now as I ever have.
Prior Health (PRIOR)	1)	I was so sick once I thought I might die.
	2)	I've never had an illness that lasted a long period of time.
	3)	I have never been seriously ill.
Health Outlook (OUTLOOK)	1)	I will probably be sick a lot in the future.
	2)	In the future, I expect to have better health than other people I know.
	3)	I think my health will be worse in the future than it is now.
	4)	I expect to have a very healthy life.
Resistance-susceptibility (RESIST)	1)	I seem to get sick a little easier than other people.
	2)	Most people get sick a little easier than I do.
	3)	I'm as healthy as anybody I know.
	4)	When there is something going around, I usually catch it.
Health Concern (CONCERN)	1)	Others seem more concerned about their health than I am about mine.
	2)	My health is a concern in my life.
Health Worry (WORRY)	1)	I never worry about my health.
	2)	I worry about my health more than other people worry about their health.
Sickness Orientation (ORIENT)	1)	Getting sick once in a while is a part of my life.
	2)	I accept that sometimes I'm just going to be sick.
Stressful Life Events (LCU)	1)	During the past 12 months, have you been fired, or laid off, from any job?
	2)	During the past 12 months, has there been any major change in your responsibilities at work?

Appendix B (continued)

Category	Item
	3) During the past 12 months, has there been any major change in your responsibilities at home?
	4) During the past 12 months, would you say that you have been arguing with each other more than usual, or less than usual?
	5) How about your in-laws—during the past 12 months, would you say you have been arguing with your in-laws more than usual, or less than usual?
	6) During the past 12 months, would you say that you and your girlfriend/boyfriend have been arguing with each other more than usual, or less than usual?
	7) At any time in the past 12 months, did you split up with your girlfriend/boyfriend?
	8) During the past 12 months, have you been arguing with your parents more than usual or less than usual?
	9) During the past 12 months, have there been any major changes in your personal habits—that is, the way you talk, dress, eat, or spend time?
	10) Within the past 12 months, did any close family member die?
	11) Within the past 12 months, did any close friend of yours die?
	12) During the past 12 months, have there been any major changes in your living conditions—like moving to a new place, or the neighborhood getting better or worse, or your house or apartment in better or worse shape?
	13) During the past 5 years, how many different homes (houses, apartments, trailers, etc.) have you lived in, including the one you live in now?

14) During the past 12 months, were you attacked or assaulted in any way by another person—like in a fist fight, or being beaten up or mugged?

15) During the past 12 months, did anyone rob or steal something from you—that is, rob you on the street or take money or property from your home or car?

16) During the past 12 months, were you in any kind of accident which involved property damage, but no personal injuries?

17) During the past 12 months, did you have any legal problems?

18) Did you change to a new school during the past 12 months?

19) Did you have to leave school during the past 12 months?

20) During the next 12 months, do you expect to have any problems making payments on any debts or financial obligations you have—like taxes, mortgage payments, consumer loans or installment debts?

Consumer Sophistication (CONSOPH)

1) Some operations done by surgeons are not really necessary.

2) If you have doubts about your own doctor's advice, it's a good idea to get another doctor's opinion.

3) Stomachaches and headaches are hardly ever caused by your emotions.

4) A medicine prescribed by a doctor can have very different prices, depending on whether or not it has a brand name.

5) If you have to go into the hospital, your doctor can get you admitted to any hospital you prefer.

6) Doctors are checked every few years, before their licenses are renewed.

7) For many illnesses, doctors just don't have any cure.

8) Two doctors who are equally good at their job may still suggest very different ways of treating the same illness.

---

*Combined with one other item to score same disease.

Notes

1. The HIS is a social experiment designed, inter alia, to estimate the response of demand and health status to variation in the price of medical care services.

2. Elsewhere John E. Ware, Jr. has reviewed the literature on various measures of health status (Brook, Ware, Davies-Avery et.al. 1979). See also Aday and Eichorn (1972) and Freeburg, Lave, Lave et.al. (1979).

3. This is the wording in the 1963 Center for Health Administration Studies survey and the Health Insurance Study; the Health Interview Survey prefaces the question with: "Compared to other persons of your age, . . .".

4. Andersen and Benham are interested in the difference between measured and permanent income elasticities. We are interested in this difference as well, but have, at the moment, a relatively poor measure of permanent income. We have averaged two years of income (put in real terms), and so our measure should cut the variance of transitory income by a factor of two. Besides the issues discussed in the text, Hershey, Luft, and Granaris are interested in disaggregated measures of utilization, e.g., patient-initiated visits and check-ups.

5. We have not corrected our estimates for any remaining measurement error in the multi-item scales.

If errors in the responses to individual items are not perfectly correlated, error variance will be a smaller proportion of total variance, the greater the number of items in the scale (Nunnally 1967).

6. Construct validation can be very useful when an agreed-upon criterion variable does not exist or is not available for the measure being validated.

7. EGFP was entered as three indicator variables.

8. These expenditures reflect closely the pattern of visits to physicians.

9. In other analyses of these data, we have also attempted to control for other characteristics of the insurance policy. We dropped those variables for this analysis because they were insignificant. In particular, we had included a variable for the upper limit on out-of-pocket expenditures. The lack of significance does not necessarily mean that a cap on out-of-pocket payments has no effect on expenses; instead, it means that we did not discern such an effect in these annual data.

10. In other analyses we have used an ANOCOVA specification with indicator variables for each of the coinsurance plans (free, 25%, 50%, 95%, and individual deductible). The LC specification can explain more than 90% of the between-plan variation in expenditures.

11. Some families were given a screening exam at enrollment to improve the precision with which changes in physiological health could be measured at the end of the experiment. The results were reported to the family's physician. Because one could expect followup of abnormal results, a random (within plans) one-third were not examined.

12. The HIS mailed a diary to the families biweekly so that they could report disability days and information on medical utilization not contained on claims forms (e.g., telephone visits). Because the diary could stimulate both better reporting of utilization and more true utilization, we compared a random 25% of the Massachusetts sites who did not receive the diary with those who did.

13. The duration of the enrollment period was varied to help determine the effect of the length of enrollment on expenses.

14. Pesaran (1974) and Pesaran and Deaton (1978) proposed this variant of Cox's (1961, 1962) test for choosing among nonnested specifications.

Let $\qquad H_0: y = Xb_0 + u_0 , \quad u_0 \sim N(0, \sigma_0^2 I) ,$

$\qquad\qquad H_1: y = Zb_1 + u_1 , \quad u_1 \sim N(0, \sigma_1^2 I) .$

Then $\qquad N_0 = T_0 / [V(T_0)]^{1/2} ,$

where $T_0 = \frac{n}{2} \ln[\hat{\sigma}_1^2/(\hat{\sigma}_0^2 + \frac{1}{n} b_0' X' M_Z X \hat{b}_0)]$,

$V(T_0) = \hat{\sigma}_0^2 \hat{b}' X' M_Z M_X M_Z X \hat{b}_0/\hat{\sigma}_{10}^4$

$M_X = I - X(X'X)^{-1}X'$, $M_Z = I - Z(Z'Z)^{-1}Z'$,

$E(\sigma_{10}^2) = \sigma_0^2 + b_0' X' M_Z X b_0/(n - k_1)$

15. Comparisions of R^2 are not legitimate when the intrafamily correlation changes. If and only if such correlation is constant, the change in R^2 is a sufficient statistic for a change in the log-likelihood ratio. Note that when retransforming the logarithm of dollars to raw dollars the gain in precision is exponentiated.

16. Recall, however, that mental outpatient care is not included in these expenses. Some of this anomaly may reflect the separation of medical and mental treatment of emotionally related problems.

References

Acton, Jan P. 1975. Nonmonetary factors in the demand for medical services. *Journal of Political Economy* 83: 595–614.

———. 1976. Demand for health care among the urban poor, with special emphasis on the role of time. In Richard N. Rosett, ed., *The role of health insurance in the health services sector*. National Bureau Conferences Series, No. 27. New York: National Bureau of Economic Research.

Aday, Lu Ann, and Eichhorn, R. L. 1972. *The utilization of health services: indices and correlates*. DHEW Publ. No. (HSM) 73–3003. Washington: U.S. Government Printing Office.

Andersen, Ronald, and Benham, Lee. 1970. Factors affecting the relationship between family income and medical care consumption. In H. E. Klarman, ed., *Empirical Studies in Health Economics*. Baltimore: The Johns Hopkins Press.

Brook, R. H.; Goldberg, G. A.; Applegate, L. J.; et al. In press. *Conceptualization and measurement of physiologic health*. R-2262-HHS. Santa Monica, Cal.: The Rand Corporation.

Brook, R. H.; Ware, J. E.; Davies-Avery, A., et al. 1979. Overview of adult health status measures fielded in Rand's Health Insurance Study. *Medical Care* 17 (Supp.): 1–131.

Colle, Ann D., and Grossman, Michael. 1978. Determinants of pediatric care utilization. *Journal of Human Resources* 13 (Supp.): 115–58.

Cooper, Richard V., and Newhouse, Joseph P. 1971. *Further results on the errors-in-the-variables problem*. P-4715. Santa Monica, Cal.: The Rand Corporation.

Cox, D. R. 1961. Tests of separate families of hypotheses. *Proceedings of the Fourth Berkeley Symposium on Mathematical Statistics and Probability, Vol. 1*. Berkeley: University of California Press.

————— 1962. Further results on tests of separate families of hypotheses. *Journal of the Royal Statistical Society, Series B* 24: 406–24.

Davis, Karen, and Reynolds, Roger. 1976. The impact of medicare and medicaid on access to medical care. In Richard N. Rosett, ed., *The Role of Health Insurance in the Health Services Sector*. National Bureau Conference Series, No. 27. New York: National Bureau of Economic Research.

Davis, Karen, and Russell, Louise B. 1972. The substitution of hospital outpatient care for inpatient care. *Review of Economics and Statistics* 54: 109–20.

Donald, C. A.; Ware, J.E.; Brook, R. H., et al. 1978. *Conceptualization and measurement of health for adults in the Health Insurance Study: Vol. IV, Social health*. R–1987/4–HEW. Santa Monica, Cal.: The Rand Corporation.

Feldstein, Martin S. 1971. Hospital cost inflation: a study of nonprofit price dynamics. *American Economic Review* 61: 853–72.

————— 1977. Quality change and the demand for hospital care. *Econometrica* 45: 1681–1702.

Freeburg, Linnea C.; Lave, Judith R.; Lave, Lester B.; and Leinhardt, Samuel. 1979. *Health status, medical care utilization, and outcome: an annotated bibliography of empirical studies*. DHEW Publ. No. (PHS) 80–3263. Washington: U.S. Government Printing Office.

Fuchs, Victor R., and Kramer, Marcia. 1972. *Determinants of expenditures for physicians' services in the United States, 1948–1968*. New York: National Bureau of Economic Research.

Goldman, Fred, and Grossman, Michael. 1978. The demand for pediatric care: an hedonic approach. *Journal of Political Economy* 86: 259–80.

Grossman, Michael. 1972. *The demand for health: a theoretical and empirical investigation*. New York: Columbia University Press.

Grossman, Michael, and Benham, Lee. 1974. Health, hours and wages. In Mark Perlman, ed., *The economics of health and medical care*. New York: John Wiley.

Hershey, John C.; Luft, Harold S.; and Gianaris, Joan M. 1975. Making sense out of utilization data. *Medical Care* 13: 838–54.

Lau, R., and Ware, J. E. Forthcoming. *Refinements in the measurement of health-specific locus of control dimensions*. Santa Monica, Cal.: The Rand Corporation.

Manning, Willard G., Jr.; Morris, Carl N.; Newhouse, Joseph P., et al., 1981. A two-part model of the demand for medical care: preliminary results from the Health Insurance Study. In *Health, Economics and Health Economics*, eds. Jacques van der Gaag and Mark Perlman; Amsterdam; North Holland.

Manning, Willard G., Jr., and Phelps, Charles E. 1979. The demand for dental care. *The Bell Journal of Economics* 10: 503–25.

Newhouse, Joseph P. 1974. A design for a health insurance experiment. *Inquiry* 11: 5–27.

Newhouse, Joseph P., Manning, Willard G., Morris, Carl N. et al. 1981. Some interim results from a controlled trial of sharing in health insurance. *New England Journal of Medicine* 305 (in press).

Newhouse, Joseph P., and Marquis, M. Susan. 1978. The norms hypothesis and the demand for medical care. *Journal of Human Resources* 13: (Supp.): 159–82.

Newhouse, Joseph P., and Phelps, Charles E. 1974. Price and income elasticities for medical care services. In Mark Perlman, ed., *The economics of health and medical care*. New York: John Wiley.

———— 1976. New estimates of price and income elasticities. In Richard N. Rosett, eds., *The role of health insurance in the health services sector*. National Bureau Conference Series, No. 27. New York: National Bureau of Economic Research.

Newhouse, Joseph P.; Ware, John E.; and Donald, Cathy. 1981. How sophisticated are consumers about the medical care delivery system? *Medical Care* 19:316-328.

Nunnally, Jum C. 1967. *Psychometric theory*. New York: McGraw-Hill Book Company.

Pesaran, M. H. 1974. On the general problem of model selection. *Review of Economic Studies* 41: 120–31.

Pesaran, M. H., and Deaton, A. S. 1978. Testing nonnested nonlinear regression models. *Econometrica* 46: 677–94.

Phelps, Charles E. 1975. Effects of insurance on demand for medical care. In R. Anderson et al, eds., *Equity in health services*. Cambridge: Ballinger Publishing Company.

Stewart, A. L.; Ware, J. E.; and Brook, R. H. 1981. Advances in the measurement of functional status: construction of aggregate indexes. Medical Care 19:473–488

Ware, J. E. 1976. Scales for measuring general health perceptions. Health Services Research 11:396–415.

Ware, J. D.; Davies-Avery, A.; and Brook, R. H. 1980. *Conceptualization and measurement of health status for adults in the Health Insurance Study: Vol. VI, Analysis of relationships among health status measures*. R–1987/6–HEW. Santa Monica, Cal.: The Rand Corporation.

Ware, J. D.; Davies-Avery, A.; and Donald, C. A. 1978. *Conceptualization and measurement of health for adults in the Health Insurance Study: Vol V, General health perceptions*. R–1987/5–HEW. Santa Monica, Cal.: The Rand Corporation.

Ware, J. E.; Johnson, S. A.; Davies-Avery, A., et al. 1979. *Concep-*

tualization and measurement of health status for adults in the Health Insurance Study: Volume III, Mental health. R–1987/3–HEW. Santa Monica, Cal.: The Rand Corporation.

World Health Organization. 1948. Constitution. In *Basic Documents.* Geneva: World Health Organization.

Wu, De-Min. 1973. Alternative tests of independence between stochastic regressors and disturbances. *Econometrica* 41:733–50.

――― 1974. Alternative tests of independence between stochastic regressors and disturbances: finite sample results. *Econometrica* 42:529–46.

6 Physical Disabilities and Post-secondary Educational Choices

Robert A. Shakotko and Michael Grossman

There is a well-documented positive correlation between good health, measured in a number of different ways, and high levels of formal education (see, for example, Grossman 1976). Furthermore, it is generally agreed that three potential structural relations could generate this this positive correlation. In the first case, poor early life cycle health may hamper an individual's education, leading to the subsequent observation that individuals in poor health tend to have lower levels of education. A second relationship may be that schooling affects subsequent health outcomes. For example, individuals with higher levels of schooling may be able to work at less hazardous jobs, or may be able to make health investments more efficiently. This could happen in addition to any income effects which might be indirectly due to schooling (see Grossman 1972). Finally, the correlation could be generated not by any structural relationship directly linking schooling and health, but by common underlying variables (observed and unobserved) determining each.

This paper is an empirical investigation of the first relationship mentioned above. We use panel data for a sample of 10,430 individuals who were high school seniors in the spring of 1972, and who were resurveyed in October of each year through 1976. Various health information was collected in the base year of the survey, and we use these base year reports as measures of health which are predetermined with respect to educational behavior in the subsequent five years. We examine individuals' choices of post-secondary activities (which include three different types of post-secondary education and no post-secondary education), and the rate at which individuals leave educational activities, in an effort to determine if the behavior of disabled individuals differs from

Robert A. Shakotko is at Columbia University and the National Bureau of Economic Research; Michael Grossman is at the Graduate School of the City University of New York and the National Bureau of Economic Research.

healthy individuals, and if these differences could be attributable to health problems. We find no firm evidence that the disabled differ significantly in either their choices or their rate of attrition; however, there is weak evidence that the disabled choose certain types of post-secondary education more frequently, and stay in such programs longer. An important caveat should be appended: we find that the disabled score significantly lower on standardized tests, which are also good predictors of educational choices and outcomes. It may be that the effects of a physical disability are already embodied in an individual's skills and abilities by the post-secondary stage, and that subsequent effects may actually be minimal, or may not be observed because of a prior selection process. Finally, we find weak evidence for higher rates of return to education for the disabled.

As in many previous studies, the issue of defining and measuring disability is troublesome. One constraint is the data, which contain no detailed descriptions of health, but do contain several qualitative ratings. For this study, we concentrate on the high school's evaluation of whether or not a student is disabled: individuals with mental or emotional problems were excluded from the sample, and slightly over 1% of the remaining sample were classified as disabled students. The criteria whereby such classifications were made are not known. Nevertheless, there are two advantages to using such an indicator. First, school-reported disabilities are likely to reflect health problems of a more permanent and identifiable nature than, say, self-rated health status. Second, school-reported disabilities would likely be used by the school to apply for federal or state aid for disabled students; in other words, this indicator is likely to have been used to identify a target population for a particular policy, and one might argue that a similar type of indicator would be used to identify problems and target populations for future policy. The disadvantages are that such an indicator may reflect "true health" no better than would self-rated health (or any other measure), and that even school-reported disabilities may be subject to some selection bias on the basis of underlying socioeconomic variables.

Education as Sequential Choice

In human capital models with perfect foresight, or those in which certainty equivalence can be invoked, a direct solution for the optimal amount of a certain type of education can be computed by equating the present costs incurred with appropriately discounted future gains. Costs are typically divided into direct and indirect costs, with the former representing explicit educational expenditures and the latter accounting for the foregone income (or at least the valuation of time) during the educational period. The effects of a physical disability on these costs are not unambiguous. Direct costs will likely be higher per unit of education, relative to those for healthy individuals, and in the absence of special assistance, must account for requirements for special equipment or extraordinary provisions. Indirect costs may be higher or lower: lower opportunity costs for the disabled (because of restricted market opportunities) would encourage higher levels of education, but this may be partially or wholly offset by the greater calendar time required to complete a given level of education. Similarly, the benefits of higher levels of education for disabled persons, compared to those persons without disabilities, are also ambiguous. One must remember that benefits are individual-specific, and are measured by the individual-specific benchmark of earnings had a particular educational choice not been made. If higher education is a substitute for other, more physical aspects of human capital, such as good health, then the rate of return to higher education could be higher for the disabled. Conversely, if higher education is complementary to good health, the rate of return would be lower. In short, while conventional theoretical models are convenient vehicles for illustrating the dimensions of the problem, they provide little guidance as to what one might expect to find in data, so that the question of the effects of a physical disability on educational choices is largely empirical.

A useful extension to these models for analyzing educational decisions is to postulate that post-secondary education is regarded by individuals as a problem in sequential choice, whereby individuals may choose to participate in one of several types of education, or not to participate at all. Such choices may be reevaluated periodically, with the result that education may be commenced after a period of absence, terminated, or continued in some different program. Relative to the initial period, these decisions may be either anticipated or unanticipated, since it is reasonable to assume that decisions will be made conditional on new information (e.g. successes or failures in different alternatives). In terms of utility maximization, a particular alternative A_i will be chosen in a given period if the expected stream of lifetime utility, appropriately discounted, given that A_i is chosen, is greater than the expected stream of utility given that any other alternative is chosen.[1]

Consider the following two-period model with alternatives A_i, $i = 1, 2, \ldots, m$. Let utility in period j under state A_i be denoted

$$V_{ij} = V_{ij}(A_{ij}, X_j, e_{ij}) \ , j = 1, 2 \ ,$$

where X_j is a vector of predetermined variables (which may include previously chosen alternatives and their results, and where e_{ij} is a random component specific to individuals and unrelated to X_j. This representation for utility may be viewed as an indirect utility function embodying the costs and benefits associated with different alternatives. Then, expected lifetime utility, evaluated in the first period and given that A_i is chosen in the first period, is given by

$$(1) \qquad EU(A_{i1}) = V_{i1} + r E \max_k (V_{k2}/A_{i1})$$

where r is a discount factor, and where the second term on the right side is the expected maximal second period utility, given that A_i was chosen in the first period, that a number of alternatives are available in the second period, and that second period utility is random (because of the e_{k2}). It follows that A_{i1} will be chosen if and only if $EU(A_{i1})$ is maximal with respect to the set of first period alternatives. Formulated in this fashion, this choice problem is an example of a discrete time-discrete state dynamic programming problem, which can easily be extended to more than two periods.

Since utility is random (because of the individual-state factors e_{ij}), the choice of A_i for any particular individual is a random event, and the probability that A_i will be chosen is given by

$$(2) \qquad P(A_i) = P[EU(A_i) > EU(A_j), j \neq i] \ ,$$

where the time index is discarded for notational simplicity. The difficulty, however, is that (1) is difficult to parameterize except for a few special cases. In the first instance, the distribution of the random variable $EU(.)$ is difficult to derive. Even under the assumptions that the $V..(.)$ are linear and the e_{ij} are normal, this normality will not be preserved in the random variable max (V_{k2}/A_{i1}). In the second instance, even if the marginal distributions for each of the $EU(.)$ can be derived, the probability given by (2) is the probability of a maximal event, and its evaluation requires the derivation of the joint distribution for the set of random variables $EU(A_k), k = 1, 2, \ldots, m$. These random variables will not in general be independent, even if the e_{ij} are independently distributed across states, because valuations of future period utility under different current states are likely to be correlated.

This illustrative model is intended not so much to show the difficulty of parameterizing the choice problem as to indicate a possible relationship between the choice probabilities and the subsequent hazard rates, due to a self-selection bias. The hazard rate (i.e., the probability of leaving an activity) is determined by the individual's valuation of second period utility in this simple model, and the hazard function would express the relationship of V to the event of leaving the initial state. Leaving, of course, may be anticipated or unanticipated, depending on both observed variables and random effects. The problem is that only a subsample is observed to ever have entered a particular initial state, and that this subsample is self-selected on a basis that may prejudice estimation of the hazard function.

Self-selection is only a problem if the random component of utility is not independent between periods; otherwise, we might think of each period's choices as constituting independent events, after conditioning on the observed variables determining these choices. However, if utility is serially correlated in its random component, the independence of intertemporal choices vanishes. For example, an individual may value a particular alternative highly because of certain predetermined variables X, or because of a particular configuration of the e_{i1}, $i = 1, 2, \ldots, m$. It follows that the expectation of these random variables will not in general be zero, given that A_{j1}, for instance, is chosen: the expectation of e_{j1} is likely to be positive, while the expectations of $e_{k1}, k \neq j$, are likely to be negative. For the subset of individuals who have chosen A_j, if the e_{i}. are serially correlated, then $E(e_{i2}/A_{j1}) \neq 0$. Moreover, it is not hard to see that this conditional expectation may be related to the set of predetermined variables X, so that failure to take account of this nonzero expectation may bias estimation of the hazard function.[2]

Given the difficulty even in this simple two-period case of parameterizing the distributions associated with the events A_j, $j = 1, 2, \ldots, m$, it would seem to be nearly impossible to derive an exact representation for the above conditional expectation. However, a linear (wide sense) conditional expectation in the sense of Doob (1953) is not difficult to write, and has the advantage of being empirically tractable in cases when exact representations are not known.

Let z be a set of sufficient statistics for the choice of first period alternatives $A_{j1}, j = 1, 2, \ldots, m$; then, for the definition of Bayesian sufficiency,

(3) $E(e_{i2}/z) = E(e_{i2}/A_{k1})$ for all j, k.

Assuming that the underlying distribution generating the events A_{k1} is regular in the sense of Dynkin,[3] then by Dynkin's lemma the log likelihood function is a sufficient statistic for the event A_{k1}, for each observation.[4] Letting L denote the log likelihood function for a particular individual, the linear conditional expectation can be written

(3') $\bar{E}(e_{i2}/A_{k1}) = a + bL$,

where a and b are in this case unknown parameters. While (3') may not be a completely accurate representation of the "true" conditional expectation (3), it is computationally convenient, especially in cases of nondichotomous or nonnormal selection rules. Furthermore, since L is a sufficient statistic for the prior selecting event, a Taylor series expansion of (3) is equivalent to a polynomial function in L, and (3') can be viewed as the special case where only the first two terms are included.

Data

The data used for this study is a subset of the National Longitudinal Study of the High School Class of 1972. In this panel survey, approximately 21,000 high school seniors were surveyed in the spring in 1972 just prior to graduation, and resurveyed in October of each year through 1976. The criteria for inclusion in the sample analyzed here are that the individual be a nonminority student and that relevant information from all panel waves exist. In addition, students with reported mental or emotional handicaps are excluded. The final sample size is 10,430.

Several health questions were asked in the base year survey, although a professional evaluation of the student's health was not part of the survey. Limited health information (as it related to post-secondary activities) was also collected in the follow-up surveys, but since this study aims at estimating the effect of poor health on post-secondary activities, we ensure that our measures of health are predetermined with respect to these activities by using base year measures only. For the reasons mentioned earlier, primary emphasis is on a school-reported disability indicator, which also includes limited information on the nature of the disability. Table 6.1 presents descriptive statistics for selected variables for the sample as a whole, and for those subsets of the sample which are school-reported disabled and self-reported disabled.

Self-reported disabled is defined as the student's positive response to the question of whether poor health interferes with his/her education. Not surprisingly, a significantly higher proportion of students report a disability than are officially disabled according to school records. This may be indicative of transitory health problems, or perhaps a self-reporting bias induced by other school-related difficulties and not actual health problems. What is more surprising is that the two categories are only mildly correlated: only 34% of those who are school-reported disabled classify themselves as disabled. This may be a reflection on the validity and accuracy of self-reported health data.

Aside from their post-secondary activities, the major differences between the full sample and the disabled subsamples are found in test scores, both in SAT scores for those who took the test and in the reading and mathematics tests administered by the survey. There are no large differences in either parental education or family income between the disabled and healthy. This is a somewhat surprising finding which runs counter to previous evidence.[5] Other major differences between the disabled and healthy are evident in post-secondary activities. Rather than index each activity by time as well as type, we choose to define activity streams according to first experience with post-secondary education, and then record the duration of particular streams. Specifically, we define four post-secondary alternatives: (1) university education, (2) junior college education; (3) vocational or technical education; and (4) no post-secondary education. Since timing aspects of education are ignored, an individual is defined to have chosen a particular educational stream (i.e., one of the first three above) if the first experience with education is

Table 6.1   Means and Standard Deviations (in parentheses) of Variables

Variable	Full Sample $n = 10430$	School-Reported Disabled $n = 120$	Self-Reported Disabled $n = 461$
Female dummy	.508	.475	.345
SAT-Verbal score (for those with valid SAT scores)	466.345 (333.518)	446.464 (365.075)	451.758 (367.081)
SAT-Quantitative score (for those with valid SAT scores)	499.656 (356.687)	476.107 (389.405)	480.590 (390.103)
No valid SAT dummy	.679	.767	.777
Reading score	52.322 (9.259)	47.908 (10.777)	49.751 (9.792)
Math score	52.397 (9.324)	48.267 (10.489)	49.855 (9.650)
Parent's income (1972; 100's)	132.94 (56.64)	132.86 (61.75)	132.94 (56.58)
Rural dummy (1972)	.066	.075	.100
Large city dummy (1972)	.759	.742	.720
Father—some p-s education dummy	.437	.425	.447
Mother—some p-s education dummy	.358	.383	.377
School-reported disability dummy	.012	1.0	.089
Self-reported disability dummy	.044	.342	1.0
First p-s education at 4-year college or university dummy	.366	.258	.260
First p-s education at junior college dummy	.175	.217	.176
First p-s education at vocational/technical school dummy	.145	.167	.171
No p-s education dummy	.314	.358	.393
Years out before starting p-s education (for those with some p-s education)	.343 (0.774)	.221 (0.468)	.421 (0.953)

of that type. The fourth alternative is a residual category, and also presumed to be an absorbing state.

It is apparent from Table 6.1 that the educational choices of the disabled are different from those of the full sample. In particular, university choices are made less often, and other educational and noneducational choices more often. Whether this is due to disability, or to other variables such as the lower test scores, is the central question that we consider in the first part of our empirical analysis.

Since the focus of our study is on school-reported disabilities, and since the number of individuals in this category is relatively small, the power of any tests attempting to distinguish differential behavior of the disabled and the healthy will be low. Consequently, inferences must be made at lower levels of statistical significance, or else empirical results can be taken to be suggestive only. For example, with regard to low testing power, despite the indication from Table 6.1 that post-secondary educational choices of the school-reported disabled are different, the null hypothesis that the disabled and the healthy have the same choice probabilities can be rejected only at the 70% level, based on a χ^2 test with three degrees of freedom.

The second part of the empirical analysis focuses on the time spent in each defined educational state. Time is accounted by counting one year for each year of full time study, and one-half year for each year of part time study. As mentioned above, educational states are defined as streams, so that cases where subsequent education is of a different type than first post-secondary education are in a sense misclassified. Investigation of these data has shown that instances of such education switching occur relatively infrequently, except for individuals who move from junior colleges to universities. For example, between the first and second year after high school, about 6% of first year enrollments switch type in the second year, and one-third of these switch from junior college to university. The proportion between the second and third years is 10% (of second year enrollments), and two-thirds of these make the junior college to university switch. In subsequent years, about 2% switch type. While the analysis of duration assumes constancy of educational type, this imperfect assumption seems unlikely to seriously affect any main results. It is nevertheless important to remember especially that the junior college alternative in this analysis is for some individuals a combined junior college and university education.

The third part of the empirical analysis examines 1976 earnings for those engaged in full time work in October of that year. Clearly, this presents a potentially serious selectivity bias, since it includes only 60% of the original sample, the remainder being either in school, in part time employment, or unemployed. This selectivity could be particularly serious with regard to the disabled, who are likely to be underrepresented in this subsample, so that findings regarding the effects of a disability should be viewed with this possibility in mind.

The measure of work experience was computed in the same fashion as the duration of education measure, with full time work counting for one year, and part time work for one-half year. Other variables, such as marriage and marriage plans, are strongly related to post-secondary activities, but have been excluded from this analysis since it is likely that they are part of a more complicated structural model.

Estimates

Choice Functions

The model outlined earlier does not point to any specific statistical methodology for the analysis of the educational choice problem, either in terms of parametric families of distributions or required properties of choice rules. The random utility formulation of the problem, however, has been used in conjunction with a polytomous logit representation of choice probabilities, and we follow this general methodology here. Two different logistic models are investigated, corresponding to different assumptions regarding independence of irrelevant alternatives; we find the implications of each to be substantially the same, with the model whose null hypothesis is extreme independence being marginally superior in terms of a comparison of the likelihood functions at their respective maxima.

We assume that, given m alternatives, the probability of choosing the ith alternative, conditional on a variable (or vector of variables) X, is given by

$$(4) \qquad P(A_i) = \exp(X\beta_i) / \sum_{k=1}^{m} \exp(X\beta_k)$$

where the β_k are conformable to X, and where the β_k satisfy the identifying restriction

$$\sum_{k=1}^{m} \beta_k = 0.$$

Incorporating this restriction into (4), the parameter space for the unconstrained problem can be denoted by $\beta = (\beta_1, \beta_2, \cdot \beta_{m-1})$. Then, for the jth observation, define $c(k,j) = 1$ if alternative k is chosen, and $c(k,j) = 0$. otherwise. The log likelihood function for the jth observation then can be written

$$(5) \qquad L_j(X, \beta) = \sum_{k=1}^{m} c(k,j) \log P_j(A_k) \ ,$$

where the probabilities P are given by (4). If follows immediately that given a random sample, the sample log likelihood function is

$$L(\beta) = \sum_{j=1}^{N} \sum_{k=1}^{m} c(k,j) \log P_j(A_k) ,$$

where N is the sample size.[6]

We can use the general method of Jennrich (1969) to transform this maximum likelihood problem into one of nonlinear least squares. Since the probabilities given by (4) are by construction in the open unit interval, and since (5) contains one and only one nonzero term, L_j is negative definite. Furthermore, from (4), it is easy to verify that L_j is a monotonic function of each of the elements of β. Define

$$f_j(X,\beta) = (-L_j)^{1/2}$$

and let $y = 0$. Since L_j is monotonic in β, so is f_j. Now define

$$u_j = y - f_j(X,\beta) ;$$

it is immediately apparent that minimizing $\sum_{j=1}^{N} u_j^2$ is equivalent to maximizing the sample likelihood function.

Table 6.2 shows the results of this method when applied to two different logistic formulations of the choice problem. In the first, reported as columns (a), individuals are presumed to choose among the four defined alternatives when all are in the choice set simultaneously (the extreme model). Most of the effects of socioeconomic variables appear as expected, particularly in the equations defining the probability of university enrollment and no post-secondary education. Higher quantitative ability measures, family income, parents with some post-secondary education, and urban residence are all significant positive contributors to choosing university enrollment, and to a lesser extent, junior college enrollment.

The coefficients indicate that disability has no effect on educational choices which is significant at conventional levels, once other variables are controlled for. At much lower levels of significance, there is some evidence that a disability encourages junior college enrollment and discourages the alternative of no post-secondary education. There may be two interpretations of this finding. One is purely statistical, in that the standard errors associated with the disability coefficients are inflated because disability is a relatively rare event in the sample, and the information passed in the "disabled" observations is swamped by that from the "healthy" observations, so that the power of statistical tests on these coefficients is low.

The second and more straightforward interpretation is that the post-secondary choices of the physically disabled are not systematically different from those of healthy individuals. An intensive examination of the disabled subsample alone seemed to indicate that this lack of systematic effect may stem not from the absence of differences in the behavior of the disabled and healthy, but from the increased difficulty in predicting the choices of the disabled: the logit model applied to the disabled subsample alone was not significantly different than a pure random choice model with no predisposing variables. This lack of systematic behavior was also present even when different types of disabilities, including vision problems, speech and hearing problems, and crippling disabilities, were added to the set of predicting variables.

Columns (b) in Table 6.2 report the parameter estimates of a model which partially relaxes the extreme assumption of the original logit model. The modified model presumes a two-stage decision procedure on the part of individuals, with the probabilities at each stage described by the logistic distribution. The first stage decision is whether or not to engage in some kind of post-secondary schooling, with the second stage determining what type of schooling conditional on the first stage decision. Accordingly, the estimates reported for the "no post-secondary education" alternative are dichotomous logit coefficients, and those reported for the three schooling alternatives are polytomous logit coefficients, again assuming independence among these three alternatives.

The same qualitative picture emerges for all variables, and again there is weak evidence that some schooling alternative is preferred by the disabled, particularly junior college. The two models, of course, do not constitute a nested hypothesis, so that one cannot be tested as a restriction on the other. In any case, their predictive power is nearly the same (with the same number of degrees of freedom), with the log likelihood of the extreme model being -10893.2 and that of the modified model being -10910.5 at their respective maxima.

Hazard Functions

Most economic work has treated education (post-secondary or otherwise) as a homogeneous good, and has focused instead on duration of educational activities. In this section, we estimate the effect of a physical disability on duration for each of the three defined educational alternatives. Since the data contain censored observations (approximately 35% of the individuals ever enrolled in post-secondary education were studying in October, 1976—those not studying in 1976 were presumed to have completed their education), methodologies for analyzing completed spells, such as those suggested by Heckman and Borjas (1980) are inappropriate, and we are forced to draw inferences regarding duration from an analysis of the hazard rate and its dependence on disability and other variables.

The hazard probabilities suffer from the same difficulties of parameterization as the initial choice probabilities, for the reason that they are both

Table 6.2   Post–High School Choices*

Variable	University		Junior College		Vocational-Technical		No P-S Schooling	
	(a)	(b)	(a)	(b)	(a)	(b)	(a)	(b)
Female dummy	-.057 (.086) [-.018]	-.050 (.068)	-.143 (.102) [-.024]	-.122 (.076)	.140 (.112) [.021]	.172 (—)	.060 (—) [.021]	.036 (.026)
SAT-Verbal	.0014 (.001) [.00048]	.0010 (.001)	.0010 (.001) [-.00019]	-.0013 (.001)	.0007 (.002) [.00009]	.0003 (—)	-.0011 (—) [-.00037]	-.0009 (.0005)
SAT-Quantitative	.0021 (.001) [.00064]	.0020 (.001)	-.0016 (.001) [-.00034]	-.0014 (.001)	-.0001 (.002) [-.00007]	-.0006 (—)	-.0004 (—) [-.00024]	-.0008 (.0005)
No SAT dummy	.660 (.436) [.181]	.762 (.362)	-1.309 (.587) [-.258]	-1.069 (.437)	.304 (.703) [.020]	.307 (—)	.345 (—) [.057]	-.036 (.183)
Reading score	.023 (.006) [.008]	.017 (.005)	.006 (.007) [.001]	-.001 (.005)	-.009 (.008) [-.002]	-.016 (—)	-.020 (—) [-.007]	-.012 (.002)
Math score	.043 (.007) [.014]	.030 (.005)	.009 (.007) [.001]	-.003 (.005)	-.017 (.008) [-.003]	-.027 (—)	-.035 (—) [-.012]	-.022 (.002)

Parent's income (100's)	.0020 (.001) [.00068]	.0013 (.001)	.0014 (.001) [.00022]	.0007 (.001)	−.0014 (.001) [−.00022]	−.0020 (—)	−.0020 (—) [−.00068]	−.0012 (.0002)
School-reported disability dummy	−.081 (.426) [−.018]	−.106 (.334)	.229 (.417) [.046]	.185 (.309)	−.024 (.484) [−.001]	−.079 (—)	−.124 (—) [−.029]	−.086 (.113)
Rural dummy (1972)	.025 (.413) [.005]	.011 (.285)	−.202 (.402) [−.037]	−.167 (.262)	.107 (.299) [.014]	.156 (—)	.070 (—) [.018]	.024 (.052)
Large city dummy (1972)	.077 (.211) [.352]	.470 (.146)	.451 (.196) [.076]	.041 (.131)	−.167 (.168) [−.027]	−.511 (—)	−1.261 (—) [−.401]	−.805 (.031)
Father—some p-s education dummy	.280 (.094) [.095]	.174 (.075)	.185 (.111) [.029]	.091 (.083)	−.187 (.127) [−.030]	−.265 (—)	−.278 (—) [−.094]	−.186 (.030)
Mother—some p-s education dummy	.273 (.093) [.095]	.181 (.075)	.057 (.113) [.007]	−.032 (.085)	−.047 (.130) [−.009]	−.149	−.283 (—) [−.093]	−.192 (.031)

*Asymptotic standard errors are in parentheses. Derivatives are in brackets.

determined by the same sequential choice model. Complicating the hazard problem yet further is the notion that education is "lumpy" or has defined units of achievement which may affect the final distribution of educational duration times. The implication is that the hazard rate may not be smooth in the usual sense. For example, in a four-year college program, the hazard rate may be low after three years, and extremely high after four. All of this suggests that it would be hardly defensible to impose any particular parametric scheme either on the hazard rate, or on the completed durations, should they be observed.

We adopt instead Cox's (1972) proportional hazards model which is distribution-free, but which still preserves the parametric notion that different variables may shift some transformation of the duration (or survival) distribution in a parallel fashion. It should be noted again that for purposes of this model activities are defined by first type of post-secondary education, and that exits are defined only by leaving post-secondary education, and not by switching types. Finally, we account for the self-selection problem including as an explanatory variable in the hazards model the estimated log likelihood function of the choice problem for each observation. The extreme model was used, so that the log likelihood function reduces to simply the log of the probability of making the observed choice of alternative. In addition to the log of the probability, the same set of predetermined variables as used in the choice problem were included as explanatory variables. The results are reported in Table 6.3.

The largest effects on the hazard rate are generated by the female dummy variable (women had a higher hazard rate than men), by the location dummies (residents of large cities had a lower rate), and by the parental educational variables, especially for the mother (a lower rate for those whose mothers had some post-secondary education). Test scores have some influence in the expected direction, as does family income for those attending a four-year college or university.

As in the choice problem, the disability effects are ambiguous, and in no case significant at conventional levels. It is interesting to note, however, that junior colleges, which were marginally more attractive to those with a disability, also have lower hazard rates for the disabled, significantly different from zero at the 60% level. These two findings, albeit weak, might be indicative of locational convenience or program flexibility in junior colleges, thereby making this alternative relatively more attractive for longer periods of time. The lower hazard rate also suggests continuation into a four-year college, but the relatively small sample of disabled choosing this alternative prohibits comparison of switching rates into four-year colleges.

The estimated probabilities, included to control for possible self-selection bias, are significant in the university and vocational-technical hazard functions, but in the latter with a positive sign. This implies higher hazard rates for those more likely to choose that alternative. This result may not be unusual if the vocational-technical alternative is predicted to be an educational choice for the unsuccessful, so that high probabilities of choice might be associated with poor prospects for performance. The issue may be one, then, of misspecification of the initial choice probabilities.

Table 6.3   Proportional Hazards Model (Years P-S Schooling)

Variable	University $n = 3817$	Junior College $n = 1827$	Vocational-Technical School $n = 1509$
Female dummy	.147 (.045)	.183 (.062)	.180 (.063)
SAT-Verbal	−.0014 (.0004)	−.0008 (.0008)	−.0003 (.0009)
SAT-Quantitative	.0006 (.0004)	.0002 (.0009)	.0003 (.0009)
No SAT dummy	−.294 (.198)	−.048 (.496)	.454 (.390)
Reading score	−.002 (.004)	−.006 (.004)	−.005 (.004)
Math score	−.010 (.006)	−.021 (.004)	−.101 (.004)
Parent's income (100's)	−.0013 (.0005)	−.0003 (.0006)	.0002 (.0006)
School-reported disability dummy	.132 (.226)	−.226 (.236)	−.061 (.247)
Rural dummy (1972)	.691 (.222)	−.076 (.196)	.175 (.132)
Large city dummy (1972)	−.546 (.184)	−.537 (.154)	−.332 (.091)
Father—some p-s education dummy	−.054 (.053)	−.117 (.065)	.026 (.072)
Mother—some p-s education dummy	−.098 (.051)	−.175 (.063)	−.204 (.070)
Ln. of probability of making the observed choice	−.219 (.113)	−.057 (.154)	.285 (.140)
Censored observations	1,659	562	311
X^2 (13 d.f.)	302.44	159.97	173.42
Average years of p-s education	3.140	2.393	1.553

Standard errors are in parentheses.

Earnings

The ultimate question underlying much of this analysis of educational choices is that of final outcomes, in terms of employment and earnings. A typical empirical finding is that the disabled as adults earn significantly less than the healthy, because of both lower wage rates and fewer hours worked. The evidence for this finding in this case is not so clear cut, as shown by the estimates of a weekly earnings function for those engaged in full time work in October 1976. These estimates are presented in Table 6.4. There is weak evidence for lower earnings, but also evidence that these lower earnings can be partially offset by higher rates of return to education for the disabled. Rates of return average about 3.5% for those who are not disabled, and the point estimates indicate an average incremental rate of return of about 8% for the disabled. This increment, however, was only marginally significant for the university subsample. Moreover, this finding may be an artifact of the selectivity problem mentioned earlier.

To partially correct for such a selectivity problem, the log of the choice probability was included as a regressor in the earnings function, following the similar specification corrections of Heckman (1979) and Rosen and Willis (1979). The estimates, also reported in Table 6.4, indicate no substantial difference between the two specifications, and the correction term appears with a small and insignificant coefficient. It should be noted, however, that this lack of effect may be due not to the absence of selectivity bias, but rather to the source of such bias, which may arise from the hazard functions and not the initial choices. Since the hazard functions are not explicitly parameterized, a correction for this source of bias is not possible.

In addition to the earnings data, preliminary evidence suggests that the disabled have significantly higher unemployment rates. The implication from all of this is that questions of disability and education cannot be fully answered in isolation from early labor force experiences.

Conclusion

While at times it is hard to define common wisdom, our findings in response to the descriptive questions addressed here do not always agree with what one might think is common wisdom. In particular, at conventional levels of statistical significance, we find no systematic differences in the educational choices and progression between the physically disabled and the healthy, once other variables are accounted for. The disabled do not enroll in universities less frequently, nor do they enroll in vocational or technical programs more frequently. At lower levels of significance, we find some preference for education beginning at the junior college level, with longer stays in such programs. We also find weak evidence for lower earnings for the disabled, but also higher rates of return to post-

Table 6.4   Earnings Function[a]
$n = 6219$

Variable	Equation 1		Equation 2	
	Regression Coefficient	t-Ratio	Regression Coefficient	t-Ratio
Female	−.274	−26.31	−.273	−26.30
Reading score	−.0011	−1.50	−.0011	−1.57
Math score	.0039	5.38	.0039	5.36
School-reported disability	−.445	−1.76	−.447	−1.77
Rural	.029	1.36	.029	1.37
Large city	−.0032	−0.23	−.0065	−0.45
University education	.029	5.60	.031	5.73
University education and disability interaction	.083	1.23	.082	1.22
Junior college education	.027	4.11	.025	3.80
Junior college education and disability interaction	.017	0.16	.015	0.14
Vocational-technical education	.036	4.42	.032	3.77
Vocational-technical education and disability interaction	.068	0.90	.068	0.90
Experience	.051	8.90	.050	8.82
Experience and disability interaction	.087	1.27	.087	1.28
Ln. of probability of educational choice	—	—	−.001	−1.20
R^2	.1346		.1348	

[a]Dependent variable is ln (weekly earnings).

secondary education. Of course, our analysis is only partial. We have ignored virtually all timing aspects of the educational process, and we have examined educational choices without regard to finer aspects of educational quality or to explicit costs and benefits of different programs.

Notes

Research for this paper was supported by a grant from the Spencer Foundation to the National Bureau of Economic Research.

1. This multi-period choice problem collapses to a single-period problem in the presence of perfect foresight.

2. The relationship of the conditional expectation to the predetermined variables X can be briefly argued as follows: suppose A_i is chosen in spite of an unfavorable value for X. It follows that A_i must have been chosen on the basis of a very favorable random component, which will be reflected in the conditional expectation. For a more detailed presentation of the selection problem in similar contexts, see Heckman (1979) and Rosen and Willis (1979).

3. See Zacks (1976), pp. 61–93, for a discussion of sufficiency as it relates to conditional distributions.

4. Which it will be, provided the distributions of the underlying e_{i1} are continuous and differentiable.

5. See Edwards and Grossman (1979) and Shakotko (1980).

6. See Dhrymes (1979) for a more complete discussion of the polytomous logit model, and its relation to models of random utility.

References

Cox, D. R. 1972. Regression models and life tables. *Journal of the Royal Statistical Society, Series B* 34: 187–220.

Doob, J. R. 1953. *Stochastic processes.* New York: John Wiley.

Dhrymes, Phoebus. 1979. *Introductory econometrics.* New York: Springer-Verlag.

Edwards, Linda N., and Grossman, Michael. 1979. Adolescent health, family background, and preventive medical care. Working Paper No. 398, National Bureau of Economic Research.

Grossman, Michael. 1972. *The demand for health: a theoretical and empirical investigation.* New York: Columbia University Press for the National Bureau of Economic Research.

Grossman, Michael. 1976. The correlation between health and schooling. In N. E. Terleckyj, ed., *Household Production and Consumption.* New York: Columbia University Press for the National Bureau of Economic Research.

Heckman, James J. 1979. Sample selection bias as a specification error. *Econometrica* 47: 153–62.

Heckman, James J., and Borjas, George. 1980. Does unemployment cause future unemployment? University of Chicago (mimeographed).

Jennrich, R. 1969. Asymptotic properties of nonlinear least squares estimators. *Annals of Mathematical Statistics* 40: 633–43.

Shakotko, Robert A. 1980. Dynamic aspects of children's health, intellectual development, and family economic status. Working Paper No. 451, National Bureau of Economic Research.

Willis, Robert J., and Rosen, Sherwin. 1979. Education and self-selection. *Journal of Political Economy* 87: S7–S36.

Zacks, S. 1976. *The Theory of Statistical Inference.* New York: John Wiley.

7   Employment, Earnings, and Psychiatric Diagnosis

Lee and Alexandra Benham

Why some individuals earn more and why some work more than others are concerns of long standing in economics. In recent years several studies have shown both earnings and labor force participation to be importantly related to health status. With few exceptions, these studies have concentrated almost exclusively on physical health status, giving little direct attention to mental disorders.[1] However, mental disorders affect a substantial proportion of the population: between 10% and 15% of the population have clinically significant psychiatric disorders, and many more suffer from milder disturbances (Woodruff, Goodwin, and Guze 1974, p. 197). This study offers some estimates of the relationships between earnings, employment status, and psychiatric diagnosis.

We are able to undertake this analysis because a remarkable data file has been made available by Lee Robins of the Department of Psychiatry, Washington University, a file originally collected for her classic study of the sociopathic personality, *Deviant Children Grown Up*. It contains detailed sociodemographic and psychiatric information for a sample of individuals born in St. Louis in the 1910s and 1920s, referred to a child guidance clinic during the period 1924–29 or selected as control subjects, and followed up thirty years later. This file permits examination of a wide variety of issues of interest to economists. Integrating mental disorders into a fully articulated model of labor market behavior is not our objective in this, our initial examination of these data. Rather it is to provide descriptive information which links specific psychiatric diagnoses with labor market behavior and to suggest the potential for expanding our

Lee Benham is affiliated with the Division of Health Care Research and the Department of Economics, Washington University. Alexandra Benham is conducting independent research on the consequences of psychiatric disorders. Lee Robins has generously provided the data used in this paper. Financial support for this project was provided by the Division of Health Care Research, Washington University School of Medicine.

understanding of some relationships which have been previously established in the economic literature.

Background

The data file utilized in this paper was originally collected by Lee Robins to study "through a longitudinal investigation the natural history of the psychiatric syndrome variously called sociopathic personality, antisocial reaction, psychopathic personality, and in more venerable days, moral imbecility or constitutional psychopathic inferiority" (Robins 1966, p. 1).

The major part of this sample consists of individuals who were patients at a child guidance clinic, the St. Louis Municipal Psychiatric Clinic, between 1 January 1924 and 30 December 1929, and who were white, were under the age of 18 at the time of referral, and had IQ's of 80 or higher.[2] In Robins' study, 524 individuals, henceforth called clinic patients, met these criteria. Robins also used St. Louis elementary school records to obtain a sample of 100 controls matched by year of birth, by sex, and by average monthly rental in census tract. The controls had to have IQ's of at least 80, to be white, to have attended St. Louis elementary schools for at least two years, and to have no record of school failure, school expulsion, or transfer to a correctional institution while in elementary school. The present analysis utilizes the male subsample of this study population. It consists of 434 males, of whom 365 were clinic patients and 69 were controls.

A substantial amount of information on the clinic patients had been systematically collected by the St. Louis Municipal Psychiatric Clinic in the 1920s, including social history, medical examination, and psychological tests. Robins located the clinic patients approximately thirty years after the referral date and the controls approximately thirty years after their graduation from elementary school. An extensive personal interview was then conducted with all individuals who were located. The interview data were supplemented by information from relatives, police files, school records, army records, credit bureaus, medical and mental hospitals, welfare agencies, and coroner's records, among others. Information was collected on a wide variety of variables, including those conventionally used in economic analysis: employment status, weekly earnings, years of schooling, marital status, and physical health status. In addition, psychiatric diagnoses were made. A major effort was made to collect information for every individual: interviews were undertaken and records were collected from all parts of the country. Of the individuals in the sample, 90% were located or were found to have died; adult records were found for 98%; interviews were obtained for 82% of those not known to have died before age 25. The exhaustiveness of this data collection process is impressive.[3]

Diagnostic Categories

Central to the analysis in this paper are the psychiatric diagnoses used to classify members of the sample. Given the unfamiliarity of these categories to most economists, some discussion of these concepts is warranted.

The notion of psychiatric disease itself is not universally accepted, and considerable confusion and skepticism exist concerning the meaning of particular psychiatric diagnoses. One reason for the skepticism is that in psychiatry, diagnosis usually depends upon what people say in the absence of laboratory tests to confirm the diagnoses.[4] Another reason has been the lack of clearly defined criteria to be used in making differential diagnoses and the absence of replicability.

An approach to these issues which we have found illuminating is that articulated by Woodruff, Goodwin, and Guze in their book, *Psychiatric Diagnosis*. In their view, a disease (including psychiatric disease) is "a cluster of symptoms and/or signs with a more or less predictable course. . . . It is a useful category if precise and if the encompassed phenomena are stable over time" (Woodruff, Goodwin, and Guze 1974, pp. x–xi). This emphasis on classifying by means of patterns of symptoms according to strict criteria and on forecasting future outcomes is an approach followed by an increasing proportion of investigators in psychiatry. The absence of laboratory signs does not preclude diagnostic categories from attaining a high degree of reliability and power to predict the course of the disease over time. The efforts being undertaken in this area by psychiatrists and epidemiologists are impressive and provide a basis for further investigation of a variety of labor market phenomena.[5]

It should be emphasized that psychiatric disorders are of interest to economists not only because scientific standards are being applied in the collection and evaluation of relevant data but also because these diseases have real and significant consequences: "they result in consultation with a physician and are associated with pain, suffering, disability, and death" (Woodruff, Goodwin, and Guze 1974, p. xi). The subsequent analysis here will indicate in summary fashion some of the economic phenomena associated with various psychiatric disorders.

In Robins' study, diagnoses were assigned on the basis of criteria for sociopathy developed by Robins and criteria for other disorders derived from *The Diagnostic and Statistical Manual, Mental Disorders, 1952*, and from various clinical follow-up studies.[6] To assign psychiatric diagnoses to the individuals in the sample, the standard life history for each subject, supplemented by record information, was evaluated independently by two psychiatrists. Diagnoses were based only on information pertaining to the subject's life history after age 18. The subject was assigned a diagnostic category if he met the established criteria at any period in his life after age 18. The diagnoses therefore refer to the occurrence of psychiatric disease in the individuals during a period of approximately twenty-five years (age 18 to age 43, the average age at follow-up).

Criteria for making diagnoses from interviews were established through independent diagnoses by three psychiatrists of the first 150 cases interviewed and subsequent discussion of the reasons for their decisions. For the remaining cases, each of two psychiatrists initially assigned a diagnosis based on the interview alone. After a time lapse of a year or more, two psychiatrists independently reviewed a summary chart of all record information obtained on the individual (e.g., police, credit, housing, military, and mental hospitalization records), the records themselves, the initial diagnosis, and the interview. They then made a final diagnosis, estimated the severity of the illness, and summarized consistency of symptom patterns over time. Cases on which there was disagreement were subsequently reviewed jointly to reach consensus.

Following are the names and brief descriptions of the principal psychiatric disorders coded in this study, and where available, estimates of their lifetime prevalence rates.[7]

WELL: "A subject was called 'no psychiatric disease' only when he did not have at follow-up and had never had more than three symptoms which appeared to be of psychiatric significance (e.g., complaints of tension, emotional lability, vague somatic symptoms without diagnosable medical disease) or even one psychiatric symptom sufficiently disabling to cause him to seek medical help" (Robins 1966, p. 82).

PSYCHOSIS: Included in this diagnostic category are schizophrenia and affective disorders. Schizophrenia is "characterized by fundamental disturbances in reality relationships and concept formations, with affective, behavioral, and intellectual disturbances" (American Psychiatric Association 1952, p. 26). Common features are delusions and hallucinations, strikingly inappropriate affect, unusual motor behavior, and disordered thinking. Affective disorders (depressive and manic-depressive) are defined by a "primary, severe, disorder of mood, with resultant disturbance of thought and behavior" (American Psychiatric Association 1952, p. 24). Organic brain syndrome, characterized by "diffuse impairment of brain tissue function" and entailing impairment of orientation, memory, all intellectual functions, judgment, and affect, was also coded in this category (American Psychiatric Association 1952, p. 14). Schizophrenia is estimated to affect 1–2% of the population. Estimates of the prevalence of affective disorders vary widely; some studies estimate 5%

of men and 9% of women are likely to have primary affective disorders at some time.

SOCIOPATHY: "The term sociopathic personality is used in this study to mean a syndrome characterized by *a gross, repetitive failure to conform to societal norms in many areas of life, in the absence of thought disturbance suggesting psychosis.* . . . The criteria for the diagnosis of sociopathic personality were developed before designing the interview. For each of 19 areas of the subject's life in which he might fail to conform to societal norms, specific criteria for 'failure to conform' were set up. It was decided, *a priori*, that these criteria must be met in at least five life areas before a diagnosis of sociopathic personality could be *considered*. But a diagnosis of sociopathic personality was not made mandatory, no matter how many of the criteria had been fulfilled.

"The symptom areas used to diagnose sociopathic personality were: work history, marital history, drug use, alcohol use, arrests, belligerency, sexual behavior, suicide attempts, impulsiveness, truancy combined with other school problems, financial dependency, performance in the Armed Forces, vagrancy, somatic complaints, pathological lying, [failure to maintain] social relationships, use of aliases, lack of guilt, and 'wild' behavior in late adolescence. All but one of these, truancy, referred only to behavior after age 18. . . . The median number of areas in which subjects given a final diagnosis of sociopathic personality met the criteria for disturbed behavior was 11. Only 6% had symptoms only in the minimum five areas" (Robins 1966, pp. 79–80). Estimates of the prevalence of sociopathy in the population vary widely. Indirect estimates suggest that it is common.

ALCOHOLISM: "This study defined alcoholics as persons with 'well-established addiction to alcohol *without recognizable underlying disorder.*' Sociopaths, schizophrenics, and other psychotics who were addicted to alcohol were excluded from this category. Subjects were *not* excluded, however, if they simultaneously had neurotic symptoms and were addicted to alcohol" (Robins 1966, p. 244). The lifelong expectancy rate for alcoholism among men is about 3–5%; for women, about .1–1%.

NEUROSIS: "The chief characteristic of these disorders is 'anxiety'. . . . In contrast to those with psychoses, patients with psychoneurotic disorders do not exhibit gross distortion or falsification of external reality (delusions, hallucinations, illusions) and they do not present gross disorganization of the personality. Longitudinal (lifelong) studies of individuals with such disorders usually present evidence of periodic or constant maladjustment of varying degree from early life. Special stress may bring about acute symptomatic expression of such disorders" (American Psychiatric Association 1952, p. 31). Symptoms associated with anxiety neurosis include dizzy spells, dyspnea, palpitations, chest pain, anxiety attacks, anxiety in crowds, nervousness, and weak feelings. Approximately 5% of the adult population is affected by anxiety neurosis.

UNDIAGNOSED BUT SICK: "Undiagnosed but psychiatrically ill" was assigned when the individual appeared to be psychiatrically ill but it was not possible to make a specific diagnosis (Robins 1966, p. 76).

NO ESTIMATE: "No estimate as to whether well or sick" was assigned when no decision could be reached as to whether the individual was psychiatrically ill or well. Most of the individuals receiving this diagnosis were not personally interviewed at follow-up, e.g., were among the missing or dead. (Robins 1966, pp. 76–77).

Empirical Estimates

Some relationships between psychiatric status and earnings, employment status, and the principal economic variables used to explain them are explored below, using calculations of means and simple multivariate equations. No attempt is made in this paper to impose a fully specified model on the data.

Table 7.1 shows cross-tabulations of employment status and earnings by psychiatric diagnosis. It is worth emphasizing that individuals were assigned a diagnostic category if they *ever* fulfilled the criteria for the diagnosis after age 18. If the disease was in remission at the time of follow-up, they are still included under the diagnosis. These results thus are likely to understate the effects for those whose disease was active at the time of follow-up. Several of the differences are substantial, and diagnoses associated with low wage rates are also associated with low employment rates. It is of some interest that those diagnosed as well have neither the highest earnings nor the highest rate of employment: that distinction belongs to the neurotics.

Column 5 of Table 7.1 shows educational attainment, a variable which is almost universally included in earnings functions. A vast theoretical and empirical literature exists on the relationship between educational attainment and earnings. Why some individuals obtain more education than others has been much less frequently explored, but several studies indicate a strong familial pattern both for educational attainment and for earnings level (Taubman 1976; Jencks 1979). Education varies with psychiatric diagnosis in this sample. Since each of the psychiatric diseases coded here tends to be more prevalent among first-degree relatives of persons diagnosed as having that disease, these results suggest one of the mechanisms which may underlie familial patterns of educational attainment and of economic success.[8]

Marital status is of interest in this context because of the well-established relationship between marital status and labor force participa-

Table 7.1   Earnings, Employment, IQ, and Education by Psychiatric Diagnosis

Psychiatric Diagnosis	Weekly Earnings, in Dollars[a]			Employed Full Time		Employed Full or Part Time or in Armed Services		IQ Category[b]			Years of Schooling		
	Mean	SD	N[c]	%	N[c]	%	N[c]	Mean	SD	N[c]	Mean	SD	N[c]
Entire sample	116.44	56.52	283	78	361	84	361	2.35	1.24	413	9.82	3.16	358
Well	118.97	51.09	94	90	110	95	110	2.49	1.23	99	11.10	3.07	110
Psychosis	82.61	60.23	23	57	37	62	37	2.00	1.10	41	8.27	2.98	37
Sociopathy	102.91	47.73	48	56	68	66	68	2.17	1.17	81	8.22	2.45	68
Alcoholism	99.29	52.79	26	79	29	86	29	2.13	1.09	31	8.45	2.05	29
Neurosis	144.50	58.94	44	96	46	98	46	2.90	1.39	42	12.03	3.11	46
No diagnosis, but sick	121.66	57.75	41	84	56	88	56	2.21	1.15	71	9.12	2.62	55
No estimate	143.21	75.93	7	73	15	87	15	2.50	1.41	48	10.08	3.51	13
Severe psychiatric disease, ever	103.81	53.17	101	66	137	72	137	2.18	1.16	146	8.56	2.71	136

[a]For persons with known positive earnings.
[b]IQ categories: 1 = 80–89 IQ
                2 = 90–99 IQ
                3 = 100–109 IQ
                4 = 110–119 IQ
                5 = 120 + IQ.

[c]Number of nonmissing observations for this category.

tion, and between marital status and health. Marital status is the single most important variable in "explaining" labor force participation of mature men.[9] A substantial literature exists on the economics of the family, but persuasive evidence is sparse on the reasons why the labor force participation of unmarried men is low and why they are less healthy.[10] In Table 7.2 the differences in marital status by psychiatric diagnosis are large.

The question naturally arises as to whether the result observed for sociopaths simply reflects the inclusion of marital instability among the criteria used in their classification. Those who were classified as sociopaths in the sample we investigated had on average 10.0 antisocial criteria, of which one at most could have been marital status. (Individuals classified as well had on average 1.1 antisocial criteria.) Thus, sociopaths engaged in a wide variety of antisocial acts, and their classification would not have been significantly changed if marital status had been excluded as a diagnostic criterion. Furthermore, as noted below, the onset of antisocial behavior almost invariably predates the age of marriage. These results suggest one of the reasons for the low labor force participation among those not married: psychiatric disorders are highly correlated with reduced market activity and with worse marital circumstances.

The principal variable used in relating health status to economic behavior in most economic studies has been the individual's response to questions of the form, "Is your health excellent, good, fair, or poor?" The subjects in Robins' study were classified at the time of follow-up as in good, fair, or poor self-reported general health status (if still alive and located). The distribution of persons across these three categories by psychiatric diagnosis is shown in Table 7.3. Persons who were in poor mental health were on average in poorer physical health and had higher death rates.[11]

Table 7.2   Marital Status by Psychiatric Diagnosis

Psychiatric Diagnosis	Married and Together	Separated, Widowed, Divorced	Always Single	N[a]
Entire sample	72%	15%	13%	400
Well	90	5	5	110
Psychosis	44	12	44	41
Sociopathy	53	39	8	72
Alcoholism	65	23	13	31
Neurosis	80	11	9	46
No diagnosis, but sick	77	14	9	66
No estimate	76	6	18	34
Severe psychiatric disease, ever	58	25	17	141

[a]Number of nonmissing observations for this category.

Table 7.3   Current Health Status by Psychiatric Diagnosis

Psychiatric Diagnosis	Alive and Health Good	Alive and Health Fair	Alive and Health Poor	Dead	Not Located for Follow-up	N[a]
Entire sample	62%	9%	2%	10%	16%	434
Well	89	3	1	7	0	110
Psychosis	55	14	7	5	19	42
Sociopathy	50	12	4	16	18	82
Alcoholism	71	6	0	19	3	31
Neurosis	78	20	0	2	0	46
No diagnosis, but sick	50	14	4	12	20	74
No estimate	24	0	0	12	63	49
Severe psychiatric disease, ever	61	15	5	11	9	148

[a]Total number of observations for this category.

Table 7.4 estimates some multivariate relationships with weekly earnings for employed individuals as the dependent variable. The sample is restricted to those who were alive at the time of follow-up and were employed, with known education, marital status, and earnings. Among these persons, neurotics earned approximately 23% more than those classified as well, and psychotics earned approximately 43% less. The impact of psychiatric diagnosis is altered only slightly when measures of physical health status are introduced.

The marital status variable has the expected positive association with earnings, although this association is somewhat diminished when psychiatric diagnosis is included. Neurosis and psychosis continue to have a significant independent effect in this specification. If anything in Table 7.4 is a surprise, it is the absence of statistically significant differences for the sociopaths, the alcoholics, and the undiagnosed but sick, as compared to the well.

The coefficient of the variable "years of schooling" approximates the rate of return to education, here estimated as 5.8%. The inclusion of variables for experience does not alter the education coefficient, and the experience variables themselves are statistically insignificant. The coefficients of neurosis and psychosis are diminished somewhat when education is included.

The child guidance clinic patients were not a random sample of the population of boys in St. Louis in the 1920s. A large proportion of the clinic patients were having some trouble in school at the time of referral to the clinic, and the overall level of school achievement and attainment for this group was low. That fact alone would lead us to expect low earnings for this group. What is more interesting is the question of the

Table 7.4   LN Weekly Earnings as a Function of Psychiatric Diagnosis and Other Variables[a]

Independent Variables	Regressions					
	1	2	3	4	5	6
Psychiatric Diagnosis[b]						
Psychosis	−.430	−.396	−.310		−.353	−.390
	(3.8)	(3.4)	(2.9)		(3.0)	(3.4)
Sociopathy	−.033	−.004	.144		.014	−.017
	(.4)	(.05)	(1.7)		(.2)	(.2)
Alcoholism	−.112	−.101	.047		−.076	−.087
	(1.1)	(1.0)	(.5)		(.7)	(.8)
Neurosis	.226	.256	.177		.271	.240
	(2.9)	(3.2)	(2.4)		(3.4)	(3.0)
No diagnosis, but sick	.063	.071	.135		.085	.075
	(.7)	(.8)	(1.7)		(1.0)	(.9)
No estimate	.145	.139	.290		.224	.229
	(.7)	(.7)	(1.6)		(1.1)	(1.1)
Other Variables						
Physical health fair[c]		−.170	−.131		−.176	
		(2.0)	(1.7)		(2.1)	
Physical health poor[c]		.181	.236		.151	
		(.8)	(1.2)		(.7)	
Married with spouse present				.143	.116	.115
				(1.9)	(1.5)	(1.5)
Years of schooling			.058			
			(6.7)			
Constant	4.693	4.698	4.062	4.583	4.590	4.585
	(103.9)	(104.5)	(39.5)	(68.1)	(55.2)	(55.0)
R^2	.12	.14	.28	.02	.15	.13

[a]OLS regressions for the subsample of 244 males who were still alive at follow-up, were employed full or part time or were serving in the armed forces, and had known positive earnings, known education, and known marital status. t-statistics appear in parentheses.
[b]The excluded dummy variable for this set is "well".
[c]The excluded dummy variable for this set is "physical health good".

rates of return to schooling for these clinic patients. As discussed earlier, controls were matched with the clinic patients by a variety of characteristics, but the controls differed in the important respect that no information suggested they engaged in antisocial behavior in elementary school. It is of interest to note that (in specifications not shown here) the rates of return to education do not differ significantly between the clinic patients and the controls, and there is no significant interaction between control status and education.

In Table 7.5 measures of IQ are included in the regressions. IQ has a strong independent impact on earnings, and when it is included, the estimated rate of return to education falls to 4.5%. The impact on earnings of neurosis and psychosis remains significant.

Table 7.6 shows some regression estimates for employment status. In this case, the sample is composed of all individuals who were alive at the time of follow-up with known employment status, education, and marital status. Individuals were counted as employed if working full or part time or serving in the army. The results indicate that psychotics and sociopaths were significantly less likely to be employed. As expected, individuals in poor physical health were also significantly less likely to be employed, but including physical health status in the specifications alters the psychiatric coefficients only trivially.

It will be noted that the variables given most theoretical attention, wages and income, are not included in these employment equations directly. These are ignored for two reasons. First, the literature seems fairly consistent in indicating the relative unimportance of these effects for men of this age; hence it appears unlikely that conventionally measured income and substitution effects would alter the partial estimates of psychiatric diagnosis. Second, we do not have meaningful income and wage rates for those not employed. Education can be interpreted in part as a proxy for lifetime wealth.

Many studies have found marital status to be significantly related to employment status. In this sample, unmarried men had an employment rate of 70% whereas those married had an employment rate of 94%. When psychiatric status and marital status are considered simultaneously, the effects of both on employment are diminished. Part of the relationship between marital status and labor force participation heretofore observed may be bound up with psychiatric disorder. This does not answer the question of the extent to which marriage is a cause or an effect, but for some disorders, such as antisocial personality, the symptoms usually begin prior to the age of marriage. Indeed, in Robins' study, there were no cases of men who were diagnosed as adult sociopaths who did not display sociopathic tendencies prior to age 16. In the case of psychotics, many never married. Certainly for those cases it cannot be argued that marital breakup precipitated psychiatric disorder.

The psychiatric diagnoses discussed above are one way to chara
the mental health of individuals. Many studies have used rate
sion to mental hospitals to examine the relationship b
health and socioeconomic status or other characte
While the rate of admission to mental hospitals is
it is a much more commonly available one. Fo
not including an examination of the de
number of times an individual has h
proxy for health status.

Table 7.5   **LN Weekly Earnings as a Function of Psychiatric Diagnosis, IQ, and Other Variables[a]**

Independent Variables	Regressions		
	1	2	3
Psychiatric Diagnosis[b]			
Psychosis	−.347	−.301	−.252
	(3.2)	(2.9)	(2.4)
Sociopathy	.012	.126	.146
	(.2)	(1.5)	(1.8)
Alcoholism	−.065	.049	.081
	(.7)	(.5)	(.8)
Neurosis	.172	.142	.156
	(2.3)	(1.9)	(2.2)
No diagnosis, but sick	.087	.144	.160
	(1.1)	(1.8)	(2.0)
No estimate	.169	.280	.382
	(.9)	(1.6)	(2.1)
Other Variables			
IQ 90–99[c]	.170	.105	.101
	(2.4)	(1.5)	(1.5)
IQ 100–109[c]	.222	.111	.104
	(2.9)	(1.4)	(1.4)
IQ 110–119[c]	.370	.238	.239
	(3.9)	(2.5)	(2.5)
IQ 120 or over[c]	.533	.294	.299
	(5.1)	(2.6)	(2.7)
missi⋅	.446	.354	.351
	(3.7)	(3.0)	(2.8)
			.141
			(2.1)
		.045	.046
		(4.7)	(4.8)
	4.476	4.062	3.923
	(70.2)	(37.8)	(31.1)
	.24	.31	.32

ͺales who were still alive at follow-up, were
ᵗhe armed forces, and had known positive
ᵗatus. *t*-statistics appear in parentheses.
⁏
‑89.''

Table 7.6 **Employment in the Labor Force as a Function of Psychiatric Diagnosis and Other Variables[a]**

Independent Variables	Regressions				
	1	2	3	4	5
Psychiatric Diagnosis[b]					
Psychosis	−.293	−.273	−.182	−.271	−.164
	(4.8)	(4.4)	(2.9)	(4.3)	(2.6)
Sociopathy	−.304	−.297	−.236	−.278	−.214
	(6.1)	(5.9)	(4.7)	(5.3)	(4.1)
Alcoholism	−.012	−.018	.030	.011	.050
	(.2)	(.3)	(.5)	(.2)	(.8)
Neurosis	.007	−.005	.016	−.003	.006
	(.1)	(.1)	(.3)	(.1)	(.1)
No diagnosis, but sick	−.032	−.031	.0004	−.015	.014
	(.6)	(.6)	(.008)	(.3)	(.3)
No estimate	−.082	−.083	.004	−.069	.016
	(.8)	(.8)	(.04)	(.7)	(.2)
Other Variables					
Physical health fair[c]			.053	.041	.046
			(1.0)	(.8)	(.9)
Physical health poor[c]			−.331	−.362	−.348
			(3.3)	(3.7)	(3.5)
Married with spouse present				.181	.181
				(4.5)	(4.5)
Years of schooling				.009	.008
				(1.6)	(1.5)
Constant	.971	.972	.805	.868	.713
	(32.9)	(33.4)	(17.1)	(12.3)	(9.1)
R^2	.16	.20	.24	.17	.25

[a]OLS regressions for the subsample of 314 males who were still alive at follow-up and had known employment status, known education, and known marital status. Individuals who were employed full or part time or who were serving in the armed forces are counted here as employed in the labor force; the remainder are counted as unemployed. t-statistics appear in parentheses.

OLS estimates are reported here for ease of interpretation. Logit estimates (when transformed) give results very similar to those shown: the same set of variables is significant, and in only one case (physical health poor) does the transformed coefficient of a significant variable differ more than .02.

[b]The excluded dummy variable for this set is "well".

[c]The excluded dummy variable for this set is "physical health good".

Table 7.7 shows patterns of hospitalization by psychiatric diagnosis. There are differences in the use of medical hospital services by diagnosis, but these are relatively small compared to the differences in the use of mental hospital services. Individuals diagnosed as psychotic or sociopathic used on average substantially more mental hospital services than those diagnosed as well.[12] Psychotics make up a high proportion of the long term patients in mental hospitals, so the large number of years spent in mental hospitals by this group is not surprising.[13]

From Table 7.8 it can be seen that the mean characteristics of individuals who were in the labor market full time differed substantially from the mean characteristics of those who were not. Among the characteristics of interest in this table are the variables related to medical and mental hospitalization. Medical hospitalization appears to be similar for all groups except those not located for follow-up, for which the number of nonmissing observations is small. This is in contrast to mental hospitalizations. For those males fully employed, there was only one mental hospital admission for every five individuals over their lives up to the time of the follow-up. The mean stay per admission was ten weeks. Simple calculations indicate that for those males not fully employed, which includes those who were institutionalized at the time they were surveyed, the mean number of admissions per individual was 1.08 and the mean stay per admission was 1.26 years. Compared to those who were fully employed, those not fully employed had over five times as many admissions and six times as long a stay per admission in mental hospitals. The impact of psychiatric disease in this sample is heavily concentrated among the unemployed and those out of the labor force.

Conclusion

Our objective in this paper has been to illustrate the strong association between psychiatric diagnoses, earnings, and employment status. Part of our motivation for studying the effects of mental disorders is an interest in the question of why some individuals have very low earnings. We have not attempted here to specify the direction of causality or the nature of the structural relationships among the variables, but one of our ultimate objectives is to see how well we can predict who will be in the lower tail of the permanent income distribution.

One would expect health status to play a major role in determining who ends up on the bottom of the income distribution. What is particularly intriguing about mental disorders in this context is that some disorders, including antisocial personality, are substantially related to earnings and employment status (and mortality) and have a relatively early age of onset. This pattern of early onset of symptoms and strong association with education, marital status, employment status, and earnings suggests

Table 7.7 Hospitalization for Physical and Psychiatric Illnesses by Psychiatric Diagnosis

Psychiatric Diagnosis	Total Number of Medical Hospital Admissions			Total Years of Medical Hospitalization			Total Number of Mental Hospital Admissions			Total Years of Mental Hospitalization		
	Mean	SD	N[a]	Mean	SD	N[a]	Mean	SD	N[a]	Mean	SD	N[a]
Entire sample	2.47	2.60	346	0.14	0.30	315	0.43	1.57	418	0.49	2.80	434
Well	1.97	2.37	109	0.08	0.24	108	0.01	0.10	109	0.00	0.01	110
Psychosis	2.39	2.27	36	0.21	0.31	29	2.62	3.33	42	3.63	7.16	42
Sociopathy	2.88	2.57	64	0.27	0.48	58	0.54	1.52	80	0.66	3.15	82
Alcoholism	2.36	1.82	25	0.07	0.10	22	0.73	2.13	30	0.07	0.29	31
Neurosis	2.57	2.39	46	0.12	0.25	45	0.02	0.15	46	0.04	0.24	46
No diagnosis, but sick	3.20	3.55	56	0.11	0.19	45	0.04	0.26	74	0.01	0.08	74
No estimate	1.50	1.79	10	0.06	0.08	8	0.00	0.00	37	0.00	0.00	49
Severe psychiatric disease, ever	2.82	2.51	130	0.20	0.38	115	1.00	2.20	146	1.34	4.62	148

[a]Number of nonmissing observations for this category.

Table 7.8   Earnings, Education, and Hospitalization Levels for
                   Subsamples of the Study Population

Subsample (N)	Weekly Earnings, in Dollars[a]			Years of Schooling			Total Number of Medical Hospital Admissions		
	Mean	SD	N[b]	Mean	SD	N[b]	Mean	SD	N[b]
Alive and employed full time with known education and marital status (235)	122.19	56.78	235	10.29	3.22	235	2.48	2.54	231
Alive with known employment status, education, and marital status (314)	117.79	56.08	264	9.93	3.20	314	2.50	2.61	308
Dead (45)	94.58	57.56	12	9.37	2.76	39	2.15	2.46	33
Missing (not located for follow-up) (70)	108.33	75.62	6	6.60	1.08	5	2.50	3.70	4

[a]For persons with known positive earnings.
[b]Number of nonmissing observations for this category.

that mental disorders may provide more than a small clue to understanding and predicting who will be very poor.[14] It is also likely that familial patterns of mental disorders will show up as a significant factor in explaining familial patterns of earnings. Research in this area is likely to be of value in increasing the precision of forecasts about market participation and earnings of individuals.

Notes

1. Bartel and Taubman (1979) have examined the relationship between mental disorders and earnings and labor market participation. In that study, all mental disorders are combined into one category. The aggregate impact of mental disorders has been examined by Cooper and Rice (1976), and the economic cost of alcoholism has been studied by Berry and Boland (1977). For several decades psychiatric epidemiologists and sociologists have explored the relationship between socioeconomic status and mental disorders and have found that most psychiatric disorders are disproportionately concentrated among lower socioeconomic groups. There is a continuing exchange over the direction of causality. For an early example of research in this area see Faris and Dunham (1939). For a list of recent references to this literature, see Wheaton (1978).

2. Only 20% of all cases seen by the clinic over this period fulfilled all these criteria. The major loss was due to the IQ restriction: 55 to 65% of all referrals had IQ's below 80.

3. For a description of the original interview used by the St. Louis Municipal Psychiatric Clinic and the follow-up interview, see Appendices B and C in Robins (1966).

4. "Historically, once etiology is known, a disease stops being 'psychiatric.' Vitamins were discovered, whereupon vitamin-deficiency psychiatric disorders no longer were

Total Years of Medical Hospitalization			Total Number of Mental Hospital Admissions			Total Years of Mental Hospitalization		
Mean	SD	N[b]	Mean	SD	N[b]	Mean	SD	N[b]
0.12	0.26	217	0.20	1.01	233	0.04	0.29	235
0.14	0.31	286	0.42	1.68	31	0.37	2.05	314
0.11	0.17	26	0.36	0.87	44	0.83	4.12	45
0.48	0.68	2	0.50	1.43	58	0.82	4.37	70

treated by psychiatrists. The spirochete was found, then penicillin, and neurosyphilis, once a major psychiatric disorder, became one more infection treated by non-psychiatrists" (Woodruff, Goodwin, and Guze 1974, p. xi).

5. A substantial amount of recent research in psychiatry has been directed toward developing better predictors of the onset of mental disorders and more complete knowledge of their natural histories. A major effort is ongoing at Washington University to refine instruments for psychiatric diagnosis. The Diagnostic Interview Schedule, based on the format of the Renard Diagnostic Interview (Department of Psychiatry, Washington University) is currently in use in studies sponsored by the Division of Biometry and Epidemiology of the National Institute of Mental Health to assess the prevalence and incidence rates of specific psychiatric disorders in the general population. This instrument can be administered by individuals not specifically trained in clinical psychiatry and is computer scorable.

The techniques used in the Robins study were earlier versions of the current set of criteria and techniques, but Robins has indicated in private conversation that there is no reason to believe a significant shift in diagnostic classification of individuals would take place if the more recent criteria were applied.

6. See especially Wheeler et al. (1950).

7. Where estimates are available, the prevalence rates for the general population are subject to wide confidence intervals, and many can be considered only rough approximations. But even conservative estimates indicate that many individuals are affected. Prevalence rates are from Woodruff, Goodwin, and Guze (1974).

8. See Woodruff, Goodwin, and Guze (1974) for discussion and references concerning the familial patterns of each of these diseases.

9. "Marital status is the single most powerful predictor of labor force participation for prime age males" (Bowen and Finegan 1969, p. 40).

10. Economists are generally reluctant to examine variables such as marital status seriously even when they have a quantitatively important relationship with the behavior being examined, if a satisfactory theoretical explanation does not exist a priori. Whatever the merits of this methodology, it has at least one unintended benefit. The quantitative

estimates associated with these "uninteresting" variables are much less likely to be subject to investigator bias than those coefficients of theoretical interest.

11. Only individuals who died after age 25 were included in the sample of 434. The death rate before the age of 25 was approximately 4% for clinic patients and 1% for controls (Robins 1966, p. 32).

12. Alcoholics had low average utilization, but recall that in this study alcoholism as a diagnosis was possible only for individuals who were not diagnosed as sociopathic or psychotic.

13. Most of the time period examined here (between the 1920s and 1960) predated the development of the drugs which have dramatically shortened the length of stay in mental hospitals for many patients.

14. As noted earlier, a substantial literature outside economics exists on the relationship between mental disorders and socioeconomic status.

References

American Psychiatric Association, Committee on Nomenclature and Statistics. 1952. *Diagnostic and statistical manual, mental disorders, 1952.* Washington: American Psychiatric Association.

Bartel, Ann, and Taubman, Paul. 1979. Health and labor market success: the role of various diseases. *The Review of Economics and Statistics* 61: 1–8.

Berry, Ralph E., Jr., and Boland, James P. 1977. *The economic cost of alcohol abuse.* New York: The Free Press.

Bowen, W.G., and Finegan, T.A. 1969. *The economics of labor force participation.* Princeton: Princeton University Press.

Cooper, Barbara S., and Rice, Dorothy P. 1976. The economic cost of illness revisited. *Social Security Bulletin* 39: 21–36.

Faris, R.E.L., and Dunham, H.W. 1939. *Mental disorders in urban areas: an ecological study of schizophrenia and other psychoses.* Chicago: University of Chicago Press.

Jencks, Christopher. 1979. *Who gets ahead? The determinants of economic success in America.* New York: Basic Books.

Robins, Lee N. 1966. *Deviant children grown up: a sociological and psychiatric study of sociopathic personality.* Baltimore: Williams and Wilkins Company.

Taubman, Paul. 1976. The determinants of earnings: genetics, family and other environments; a study of white males. *American Economic Review* 66: 858–70.

Wheaton, Blair. 1978. The sociogenesis of psychological disorder: reexamining the causal issues with longitudinal data. *American Sociological Review* 43: 383–403.

Wheeler, E.O.; White, P.D.; Reed, E.W.; and Cohen, M.E. 1950. Neurocirculatory asthenia (anxiety neurosis, effort syndrome, neurasthenia). *Journal of the American Medical Association* 142: 878–88.

Woodruff, Robert A., Jr.; Goodwin, Donald W.; and Guze, Samuel B. 1974. *Psychiatric diagnosis.* New York: Oxford University Press.

8 Children's Health Problems: Implications for Parental Labor Supply and Earnings

David S. Salkever

A considerable amount of empirical research has been carried out on the economic impact of adults' health problems (e.g., Bartel and Taubman 1979; Luft 1975; Grossman and Benham 1974). A principal objective of the research has been to estimate the effects of these problems on the labor supply and earnings of illness victims. Policymakers and analysts have also expressed interest in these estimates as inputs to the process of allocating health sector resources among prevention and treatment programs for various diseases (Fuchs 1966; Fein 1958; Klarman 1965; Rice, Feldman, and White, 1976). By contrast, very few econometric studies have examined the economic impact of health problems on other family members. In particular, little is currently known about impacts on the spouses of illness victims or the parents of children with health problems. As a result, consideration of these impacts in policy analyses have been based on conjecture or, more frequently, ignored altogether.

The present study focuses on the effect of chronic health problems and disabilities among children on parental labor supply and earnings. The severity of these problems, along with the long-term expense and difficulty of coping with them, raises the possibility of substantial impact on the psychological, physical, and economic health of the child's family. While relatively few children report such problems, a dramatic increase

David S. Salkever is with the School of Hygiene and Public Health at the Johns Hopkins University. Helpful comments on the preliminary work were received from Mark Rosenzweig, Michael Grossman, Victor Fuchs, and other conference participants. Extremely capable research and programming assistance was provided by Alison Jones, Michele Alperin, and Bruce Lubich. Thanks are also due to Valerie Knell for preparing the several versions of the manuscript. Financial assistance from Maternal and Child Health Research Grant MC–R–240426, Bureau of Community Health Services, U.S. Dept. of Health and Human Services, is gratefully acknowledged. The author is solely responsible for any opinions expressed in the paper as well as for any errors of omission or commission.

has occurred over the past decade. According to National Center for Health Statistics data (Table 8.1), the number of children with activity limitations due to chronic conditions nearly doubled from 1967 to 1978. The reasons for this increase are not presently known, but it seems likely that a variety of factors are involved, including more sophisticated medical therapies which increase survival rates for children born with physical impairments and the growing emphasis on "mainstreaming" and deinstitutionalization in public educational and social services programs.[1]

Most previous research on economic impacts of children's health problems consists of descriptive evidence based upon interviews of small samples of families. Several of these studies indicate pronounced negative effects on maternal market work. Meyerowitz and Kaplan (1967) interviewed 111 families in Texas with children suffering from cystic fibrosis and found that while 54% of the mothers were employed prior to diagnosis of their children's problem, only 26% were employed after the diagnosis was made. Similarly, Barsch's (1967) data from interviews with 177 families of handicapped children in Milwaukee showed a maternal employment rate of only 25%. (This is comparable to the rate during the 1960s for all married women with children under 6 and considerably below the overall rate for mothers.) Barsch's data also indicate higher maternal employment rates for families with mongoloid children and deaf children than for three other handicapping conditions studied (cerebral palsy, other neurologic impairments, and blindness). Moreover, Barsch reported that the majority of the working mothers worked only part time. Recent research shows higher maternal employment rates, however. Both the McCubbin et al. (1979) study of 100 families of children with cystic fibrosis and the study by Breslau et al. (1980) of 370 families with handicapped children report about one-half of all mothers

Table 8.1   Numbers (Percentage) of Noninstitutionalized Children (0–17 years) with Limitations in Activity Due to Chronic Conditions, Selected Years

	Activity Limitation	Limitation in Major Activity
1967	1,418,000 (2.1)	712,000 (1.1)
1972	1,921,000 (3.0)	1,037,000 (1.6)
1978	2,309,000 (3.9)	1,178,000 (2.0)

Source: U.S. National Center for Health Statistics, *Vital and Health Statistics: Data From the National Health Survey*, Series 10, Nos. 52, 85, and 130 (Washington: U.S. Dept. of HEW).

with either full or part time employment. McCollum's (1971) Connecticut study of 54 families of children with cystic fibrosis found that 41% of the mothers were employed. Reported evidence on other labor market effects is even more scanty. McCollum reported that 62% of the fathers in her sample took on overtime work or second jobs to help pay the cost of medical treatments. In contrast, the study by Sultz et al. (1972) of 390 families in New York State found only a small minority of families reporting employment changes to obtain additional income.

The only prior econometric research is in two preliminary studies by Salkever (1980, forthcoming). The first of these utilized 1972 data from the Panel Study of Income Dynamics to estimate child disability effects on maternal work probability and hours of work. Results for two-parent families indicated little effect on the probability that a mother worked at all during the year but a fairly strong negative effect on annual hours of work. Regressions for one-parent families showed negative effects on work probability but no effect on hours of working mothers. No significant effects were found for nonwhite two-parent families. The second study, based on 1972 Health Interview Survey data, reported that in white two-parent families mothers of disabled children were significantly less likely to report working as a usual activity or that they had worked at all during the two weeks preceding the interview; however, no significant child disability effects were observed for mothers in nonwhite or one-parent families.

The present study expands upon this preliminary research in several ways. In addition to estimating child disability effects on maternal labor supply, it also examines effects on paternal labor supply and on earnings per hour and earnings for both parents. Moreover, it utilizes a much larger data base on households with disabled children than any previous study and it differentiates among types of functional limitations and disabilities caused by health problems.

Theoretical Considerations

The relationship between children's disabilities and parental labor supply can be described within the framework of a simple household production model.[2] In particular, let us assume that the family seeks to maximize a utility function $U(H, X)$ whose arguments are the levels of child health (H) and other goods (X).[3] Child health production is described by the function $G(M, C_1, C_2; H_0)$ where M is purchased medical inputs, C_1 and C_2 are maternal and paternal child health production time and H_0 is the child's health endowment. Other goods are produced according to the function $X(Q, P_1, P_2)$ where Q is purchased nonmedical goods and services, and the P_i's are parental time inputs. Letting L_i denote parental market work time and T_i denote total time available, the parental time constraints are $T_i = C_i + P_i + L_i (i = 1, 2)$. The family's binding expenditure constraint is $Q + \Pi M = Y + w_1 L_1 + w_2 L_2$ where Y is unearned income, the w_i's are parental wage rates, Π is the price of M, and Q is the numeraire good.

The family's optimal levels of X and H can be depicted as the tangency of an indifference curve and an opportunity locus as shown at Points A and B in Figure 8.1. The opportunity locus is derived by maximizing X for a given level of H (or vice versa) subject to the time, budget, and production function constraints. If either production function displays nonconstant returns to scale, the opportunity locus will be nonlinear. When the child's health endowment is reduced from H_0^1 to H_0^2 because of a chronic health problem, the opportunity locus shifts leftward from $X^1 H^1$ to $X^2 H^2$. If this decline in health endowment also increases (decreases) the marginal products of M, C_1, and C_2, the slope of the opportunity locus will become less (more) negative.

Further restrictions on the model are necessary if we are to determine whether parental labor supplies (the L_i's) increase or decrease in response to a decline in H_0. Consider the simple case where the health

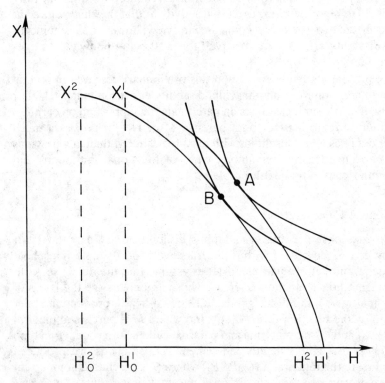

Fig. 8.1   Family consumption decisions with differing child health endowments.

production relationship takes the form $H = G(M, C_1, C_2) + H_0$ and $G(\cdot)$ and $X(\cdot)$ are characterized by constant returns to scale. Because these assumptions imply constancy of optimal factor input ratios and optimal input-output ratios (for given values of Π, w_1 and w_2), we can write the family's opportunity locus as

$$(1) \qquad (w_1 + \theta w_2 + \beta) \; \frac{X}{\gamma} + (w_1 + \rho w_2 + \alpha \Pi) \; \frac{(H - H_0)}{\delta}$$

$$= Y + w_1 T_1 + w_2 T_2 \; ,$$

where θ, β, ρ and α are the optimal values of the input ratios P_2/P_1, Q/P_1, C_2/C_1, and M/C_1, and where γ and δ are the optimal values of the input-output ratios $X(\cdot)/P_1$ and $G(\cdot)/C_1$. Similarly, the parental time constraints become

$$(2a) \qquad L_1 + \frac{X}{\gamma} + \frac{(H - H_0)}{\delta} = T_1$$

$$(2b) \qquad L_2 + \frac{\theta X}{\gamma} + \rho \frac{(H - H_0)}{\delta} = T_2.$$

Allowing L_1, X, H, and H_0 to vary and taking differentials in equations (1) and (2a), we can show that when H_0 declines, maternal labor supply (L_1) will also decline if (1) $dH_0 - dH < 0$ and (2) $(w_1 + \rho w_2 + \alpha \Pi) < (w_1 + \theta w_2 + \beta)$. The first of these two conditions follows from the reasonable assumption that X is a normal good (i.e., $dX/dH_0 > 0$). The second condition implies that maternal time costs comprise a larger fraction of total costs in producing child health than in producing other goods. The analogous result holds for the response of paternal labor supply (L_2) to a decline in H_0. It also follows, in this simplified model, that the labor supply response to children's health problems will be more negative for mothers than for fathers provided that the production of child health is relatively more maternal-time intensive (i.e., $\theta > \rho$).[4] Finally, it is clear that these same conclusions hold if the model is generalized to allow for the possibility of a proportionate increase in the marginal productivity of all child health inputs (i.e., a decrease in δ) as H_0 declines.[5]

While this simple model describes impacts of children's health problems in terms of income effects and changes in the productivity of child health inputs, a number of other possible effects must be recognized. For example, one might expect these problems to influence parental wage rates for several reasons. Since wage rates are related to work experience, labor supply effects in any time period will impact on wages in subsequent time periods. Moreover, parents may spend some nonworking time in the accumulation of human capital. Pursuing educational programs to acquire or improve marketable skills and migration to take advantage of better job opportunities are examples of this phenomenon.

Here again effects of child health problems on the amount of time spent in these pursuits implies corresponding effects on observed wage rates. Finally, even if one abstracts from any intertemporal effects, it may be more reasonable to regard individuals' market opportunities as described by a continuum of jobs offering differing combinations of wages and required time and effort rather than by a single fixed wage rate. In this situation, both wages and hours of work are determined by parental labor supply decisions, and thus both may be influenced by child health problems.

Further generalizations of the standard labor supply model point to further possible avenues of influence for child health problems. In recent work, Cogan (1977) has focused attention on the fixed money and time costs of working and presented empirical estimates relating these costs to maternal child care responsibilities. One might reasonably presume that children's health problems increase these costs and thereby impact on parental labor supply decisions. Based on Cogan's analysis, one would expect these increased fixed costs to reduce the probability that a mother works; the effect on hours of work of working mothers is ambiguous, since higher fixed money costs imply longer hours of work while higher fixed time costs imply shorter hours. An additional factor, brought out in Heckman's (1974, 1977) treatment of the relationship between labor supply and the availability of nonparental child care, is variable costs of work (i.e., costs which vary with the mother's hours of work). If these costs are constant per hour of work, they are equivalent to a reduction in the mother's hourly wage. They could also rise more than proportionately with hours of work. For example, if mothers of school age children work full time, they may face after-school child care costs which would not be incurred if they only worked part time. In either case, one might conjecture that upward shifts in the level of these variable costs due to children's health problems will reduce maternal labor supply. The possibility of direct preference effects should also be noted. In the model sketched above, utility depended only on the attained levels of X and H. However, in view of the evidence that children's physical health problems are associated with increased stress or psychological problems of parents (Breslau et al. 1980; Cummings et al. 1966; Cummings 1976), it may be more realistic to assume that parental time spent at home also has a direct effect on utility (apart from its effect on the level of X and H) and that this effect will depend upon child health endowments.

Empirical Models and Estimation Techniques

The foregoing discussion suggests the following empirical representation of child health problem effects on parental labor supply and wages:

(3a) $$L_1 = F_1(Z_1, w_1, w_2, Y, H_0, u_1)$$

(3b) $L_2 = F_2(Z_1, w_1, w_2, Y, H_0, u_2)$

(4a) $w_1 = F_3(Z_1, Z_2, A, Y, H_0, u_3)$

(4b) $w_2 = F_4(Z_1, Z_2, A, Y, H_0, u_4)$

where Z_1 denotes parental and family characteristics which affect preferences and productivity in home production of X and H, Z_2 denotes parental characteristics which affect market productivity, A denotes area labor market conditions which affect offered wage rates, and the u_i's are random disturbance terms. Note that in the wife's wage equation (4a), the inclusion of Z_1, Y, H_0, and the elements of Z_2 and A which pertain to the husband's market productivity and market opportunities is intended to capture the influence of these variables on the wife's accumulation of human capital. A similar rationale applies to the specification of the husband's wage equation (4b).[6]

In our empirical analyses, the work hours equations (3a and b) were estimated in reduced form (obtained by replacing w_1 and w_2 by the right sides of equations (4a and b). In addition, earnings relationships, which can be represented by multiplying the wage equations by the corresponding reduced-form hours equations, were also estimated. Estimation of the work hours, wage, and earnings regressions for wives involved two steps: estimation of a probit maternal work probability regression and estimation of hours, wages, and earnings regressions based on data for working wives with Heckman's (1977) selectivity variable (computed from the probit regression) included to correct for sample censoring. This procedure is preferable to the alternative of using Tobit regression since it is consistent with both the standard labor supply model and the fixed-cost model recently developed by Cogan (1977).

Since the household equilibrium conditions are different for families with working wives and those with nonworking wives, husband's hours, wage, and earnings regressions were estimated separately for those two groups of households (again with the inclusion of selectivity variables).[7] All hours, wage, and earnings regressions for both husbands and wives were estimated with ordinary least squares.[8]

Two different sets of regression estimates were used to measure the effects of the variables relating to children's health problems. The first set was based on a simple additive model in which it was assumed that the coefficients for all other variables were the same for families that reported children's health problems and for families without such problems. Data from both types of families were used to estimate these regressions and no interactions between the child health problem variables and other variables were included. The second set, which was used to examine interactions between children's health problems and other family characteristics, involved two stages. First, earnings and maternal work probability regressions were estimated from data on families with no child health problems. The estimated coefficients from these regressions were used to compute predicted dependent variable values for families with children's health problems, and deviations of actual from predicted values for these families. Then, these deviations were used as dependent variables in regressions estimated from data for these same families.

Data Base And Definition Of Variables

The data base for our analysis was the Survey of Income and Education (SIE). This survey was administered to 151,170 households throughout the United States during the period April–June 1976. The interviews included detailed questions about labor market activity and income (similar to those used in the Current Population Survey) as well as a large number of questions dealing with sociodemographic characteristics, housing, health insurance, and disabilities of household members.[9]

Because the prevalence rates for children's disabilities are rather low (see Table 8.1), the large sample size of the SIE was particularly important for the purposes of this study. Information was available on approximately 4,000 households containing children aged 3 to 17 with reported disabilities. (Disability data for children under 3 was not reported in the SIE.) This data base is roughly four times larger than that employed in any of the previous studies cited above.

The study sample for our analysis was constructed in several steps. First, all SIE households were divided into two groups: those containing children with reported health problems and those containing no children with reported health problems. Second, a 1-in-10 random sample of the second group of households was selected. Third, from the households with reported child health problems and the random sample of other households we selected out all white, two-parent, single-family households with no married childen, children over 18, other relatives living with them, or reported maternal health problems. This process yielded a study sample of 5,885 families composed of 2,685 families containing children with reported health problems (referred to as "disabled families") and 3,200 families with no such children (referred to as "nondisabled families").

Characteristics of these families are described in Table 8.2, which presents definitions and mean values for all independent and dependent variables used in our regressions. The independent variables are of four types: family characteristics, location variables, area labor market conditions, and variables pertaining to children's health problems. Family characteristics include number and ages of children (KIDOT2 through KIDNUM in Table 8.2), age and education of both parents, husband's health status (HEALTHLM and DUMHUSLM), a proxy for unearned

Table 8.2   **Variable Definitions and Mean Values**

Independent Variables		Mean Values	
Name	Definition	Disabled Families (*n*-2685)	Nondisabled Families (*n*-3200)
KID0T2	Number of children 0–2 years.	.163	.387
KID3T4	Number of children 3–4 years.	.219	.250
KID5T9	Number of children 5–9 years.	.921	.651
KIDNUM	Number of children	2.859	2.136
WIFEAGE	Wife's age (years)	35.233	32.884
WFAGESQR	WIFEAGE^2	1287.100	1147.047
WFEDUC	Wife's years of education	12.117	12.623
WFEDSQR	WFEDUC^2		
HUSBAGE	Husband's age (years)	38.447	35.618
HSAGESQR	HUSBAGE^2	1537.125	1350.477
HSEDUC	Husband's years of education	12.435	13.151
HUSEDSQR	HSEDUC^2		
HEALTHLM	= 1, if husband has any reported health problem	.129	.066
DUMHUSLM	= 1, if husband needs any help in daily activities	.009	.004
CASHDUM	= 1, if family assets in savings accounts, savings bonds, checking accounts, and cash total more than $5000	.228	.249
DFARMINC	= 1, if family has income or losses from farming	.063	.061
DUMVET	= 1, if husband is veteran of armed forces	.535	.487
DUMALIEN	= 1, if husband immigrated to U.S. since 1970	.004	.008
DUMSPAN	= 1, if husband is of Spanish origin	.033	.039
NE	= 1, if in New England	.156	.137
MA	= 1, if in Mid-Atlantic region	.076	.079
ENC	= 1, if in East North Central region	.134	.144
WNC	= 1, if in West North Central region	.147	.149
SA	= 1, if in South Atlantic region	.088	.097
ESC	= 1, if in East South Central region	.036	.034

Table 8.2 (continued)

Independent Variables		Mean Values	
Name	Definition	Disabled Families (*n*-2685)	Nondisabled Families (*n*-3200)
WSC	= 1, if in West South Central region	.066	.059
M	= 1, if in Mountain region	.193	.197
BIGSMSA	= 1, if residence is in one of the 20 largest SMSA's	.143	.142
MEDSMSA	= 1, if residence is in one of the 78 next largest SMSA's	.211	.202
OTHMETRO	= 1, if identified in SIE as in other SMSA's	.098	.095
OTHNONM	= 1, if identified in SIE as not in an SMSA	.235	.262
HUSBWAGE	Area wage for husband	5.675	5.832
HSUNEMRT	Area unemployment rate for husband	.048	.047
WIFEWAGE	Area wage for wife	3.453	3.592
WFUNEMRT	Area unemployment rate for wife	.068	.068
DUMDIS	= 1, if family has a child with a health problem	1.0	0
WORK[a]	Number of children limited in schoolwork (but not attendance) by health problems	0.671	0
CANTABS[a]	Number of children limited in schoolwork and unable to attend regular school or frequently absent because of health problems	0.045	0
PLAY[a]	Number of children with health problems but not limited in schoolwork or attendance	0.383	0
USMOB	Number of children usually or occasionally needing assistance in getting around outside the home	0.045	0
USHELP	Number of children usually or occasionally needing assistance in daily activities	0.070	0
DIS3T4	Number of children aged 3–4 with health problems	.072	0

Table 8.2 (continued)

Independent Variables		Mean Values	
Name	Definition	Disabled Families (n-2685)	Nondisabled Families (n-3200)
DIS5T9	Number of children aged 5–9 with health problems	.389	0
DIS10T13	Number of children aged 10–13 with health problems	.360	0
DIS14T17	Number of children aged 14–17 with health problems	.296	0
Dependent Variables			
Name	Definition		
ANNHRS1	Husband's hours worked in 1975	2128.874	2147.030
ANNHRS2	Wife's hours worked in 1975	651.578	690.071
DUMWFWK	= 1, if $ANNHRS_2 > 0$	.542	.548
WIFEEARN	Wife's earnings in 1975	1927.674	2244.432
HUSBEARN	Husband's earnings in 1975	12,130.397	12,284.951
WWAGE	Wife's earnings per hour in 1975	3.250	3.684
HWAGE	Husband's earnings per hour in 1975	6.502	6.356

[a]This variable is based on data for disabled children aged 5–17.

income or wealth (CASHDUM), a farm residence dummy (DFAR-MINC), and other background characteristics of the husband (DUM-VET, DUMALIEN, DUMSPAN). These variables are included to account for variations in husbands' and wives' market and nonmarket productivity and preferences. Locational variables indicate region of residence (NE through M with the West being the omitted region) and metropolitan or nonmetropolitan status (BIGSMSA through OTHNONM).[10] Area labor market conditions are described by race-sex specific unemployment rates (HSUNEMRT and WFUNEMRT) and race-sex-education specific wage rates (HUSBWAGE and WIFE-WAGE) calculated from data on all SIE respondents. In most cases these variables are defined for the metropolitan area in which the family resides, for all metropolitan areas within the state of residence (except SMSA's specifically identified in the SIE), or for the nonmetropolitan areas of the state of residence for non-SMSA families. In a minority of cases, the entire state or even larger geographical aggregates had to be used because more specific areas were not identified or because the numbers of individuals in particular race-sex-education groups were small.

Variables pertaining to children's health problems are of four types. DUMDIS indicates the presence of a child with any reported chronic health problems.[11] The variables PLAY, WORK, and CANTABS relate to what Nagi and Luken (1975) have termed "role disabilities." In particular, these variables indicate whether children's health problems limit their ability to function in a regular school setting.[12] Functional limitations in mobility and in activities of daily living (eating, dressing, personal hygiene) are indicated by the variables USMOB and USHELP. DIS3T4, DIS5T9, DIS10T13 and DIS14T17 differentiate among families by the age of the disabled children.

The last segment of Table 8.2 reports mean values for our seven dependent variables. Note that the mean values for the wage variables only apply to persons reporting nonzero hours and earnings. Also note that the wage and earnings variables are defined to include self-employment and farm income as well as salary and wage income. The first two types of income probably include some returns to capital, but it is not possible to break this out with the SIE data.

With regard to differences between disabled and nondisabled families, Table 8.2 shows that the disabled families have more children above the age of 4, more children in total, and parents who are about 2.5 years older on average. These differences are to be expected since prevalence rates increase with age and the probability of having at least one disabled child increases with the number of children in the family. (Moreover, since health problem data were not reported for children under 3, families with only children under 3 could not be defined here as disabled families.) Parents in nondisabled families have slightly higher levels of education and considerably lower rates of paternal health problems.

Differences in mean values for the dependent variables are rather small but do show a consistent pattern. Maternal annual hours of work, earnings, and earnings per hour are clearly lower for disabled families, but the fraction of mothers who worked at all is virtually identical for the two groups. Paternal earnings and annual hours are only slightly lower in disabled families, while paternal earnings per hour are slightly higher.

Empirical Results for the Simple Additive Model

For each of our dependent variables, at least four different regressions employing different sets of child health variables were estimated. Each regression was first estimated with all other independent variables (besides the child health variables) included. They were then reestimated deleting independent variables (other than the child health variables) with verylow t-statistics.[13] All regressions except those on DUMWFWK also included a selectivity variable.[14] The resulting coefficients for the child health variables are shown in Tables 8.3 and 8.4.[15]

Looking first at the maternal work status regressions in Table 8.3, we observe in regression A that the coefficient for DUMDIS is small and insignificant, indicating that on average children's health problems do not deter mothers from working.[16] However, the results for regressions B–D suggest that this finding is not consistent across all age groups and types of disabilities. The significant or nearly significant negative coefficients for WORK, CANTABS, and USMOB imply that health problems which limit the ability to function in school and which limit mobility do in fact reduce maternal work probabilities. Moreover, the magnitude of the estimated effects is sometimes fairly large. For example the coefficient for CANTABS in regression D (-0.2304) implies that for a mother who would otherwise have a 0.5 probability of working, the presence of a child whose health problem interferes with school attendance reduces this probability to 0.421. In contrast, the strongly positive coefficients of DIS3T4 and DIS14T17 suggest that children's health problems have less of a deterrent effect in families with very young or older disabled children.

The maternal work hours regressions in Table 8.3 generally show more significant negative effects on children's health problems, particularly when the disabled child needs assistance in mobility. Variations in impact by age of the disabled child are similar to those for the work status regressions, although the positive effects for children aged 3 to 4 is somewhat weaker and the effects for children aged 5 to 9 and 10 to 13 are more strongly negative. It is also surprising that the coefficients of CANTABS are much less significant than the coefficients of WORK and similar to the latter in magnitude. Comparing the results for regressions B through E, one observes some instability in the results for WORK, CANTABS, DIS10T13, and DIS14T17 stemming from collinearity of the health problem variables.

Negative health problem effects on maternal wages are also rather pronounced. The significant coefficient of -0.1 for DUMDIS implies a 9.5% reduction in maternal wages due to the presence of a disabled child.[17] Results for CANTABS imply even larger reductions for mothers of children limited in their ability to attend school. Coefficients of WORK are also significantly negative, but only when DIS5T9 and DIS10T13 are not included in the regression. Finally, it is interesting to note that coefficients of DIS3T4, DIS5T9, DIS10T13, and DIS14T17 indicate increasingly negative effects as the child's age increases. Presumably, this pattern of results reflects the cumulation over time of impacts on labor market experience and investment in human capital.

Table 8.3   Estimated Effects of Children's Health Variables: Maternal Labor Supply and Earnings

Dependent Variable		DUMDIS	PLAY	WORK	CANTABS	USHELP	USMOB	DIS3T4	DIS5T9	DIS10T13	DIS14T17
Maternal work status	A	−0.036 (0.37)									
	B		0.0461 (1.06)	−0.0583 (1.60)	−0.1958 (1.68)	0.1076 (0.90)	−0.2685 (1.83)	0.1262 (1.62)			
	C			−0.0832 (1.62)	−0.2462 (2.02)	0.1176 (0.98)	−0.2766 (1.88)	0.1236 (1.23)	0.0168 (0.28)	−0.0115 (0.20)	0.1131 (2.01)
	D			−0.0757 (2.12)	−0.2304 (2.01)		−0.1906 (1.57)	0.1248 (1.25)			0.1109 (2.15)
Annual work hours, working wives	A	−101.84 (3.28)									
	B		10.66 (0.27)	−123.34 (3.06)	−120.78 (0.91)	2.77 (0.03)	−529.07 (2.93)	51.56 (0.50)			
	C			−79.58 (1.46)	−144.52 (0.98)	40.65 (0.35)	−581.67 (3.19)	50.28 (0.49)	−55.86 (1.05)	−159.66 (3.36)	180.12 (2.85)
	D			−152.94 (3.44)	−196.48 (1.38)		−561.07 (4.03)	54.24 (0.52)		232.78 (3.82)	
	E			−97.01 (1.77)	−103.18 (0.77)		−522.37 (4.11)		−16.57 (0.30)	−80.82 (1.64)	78.15 (1.66)

	1	2	3	4	5	6	7	8	9	10
Logarithm of wages, working wives										
A	-0.1000 (3.53)									
B		-0.0724 (2.14)	-0.0746 (2.48)	-0.2977 (3.07)	0.0184 (0.02)	-0.0291 (0.22)	-0.0279 (0.35)			
C			-0.0123 (0.30)	-0.2251 (2.24)	-0.0144 (0.14)	0.0379 (0.29)	-0.0263 (0.32)	-0.0373 (0.78)	-0.0729 (1.65)	-0.0929 (2.18)
D			-0.0533 (1.81)	-0.2628 (2.71)		0.0309 (0.30)	-0.0225 (0.28)			-0.0668 (1.71)
F				-0.1971 (2.04)				-0.0500 (1.35)	-0.0864 (2.41)	-0.0929 (2.44)
Logarithm of earnings, working wives										
A	-0.2265 (4.37)									
B		-0.1237 (1.98)	-0.1752 (3.04)	-0.0302 (1.68)	-0.0811 (0.05)	-0.3250 (1.32)	-0.0787 (0.51)			
C			-0.0175 (0.23)	-0.1702 (0.90)	-0.0729 (0.40)	-0.3481 (1.41)	-0.0847 (0.55)	-0.1070 (1.20)	-0.2834 (3.59)	-0.0221 (0.27)
D			-0.1556 (2.71)	-0.2887 (1.59)		-0.3973 (2.09)	-0.0798 (0.52)			
G			-0.0970 (1.62)	-0.2588 (1.45)		-0.4511 (2.40)			-0.2047 (2.98)	0.0809 (1.05)

t-statistics in parentheses.

Negative health problem effects on earnings of working mothers are particularly strong, since they are the combined result of the negative wage and hours effects noted earlier. The DUMDIS coefficient of − 0.227 implies a 20% earnings reduction for mothers in disabled families. Again there is evidence from the results for WORK, CANTABS, and USMOB that school-related role disabilities and mobility limitations are particularly important, although collinearity with the age-related variables is also apparent. Coefficients of the age-related variables are most negative for the age groups 5 to 9 and, particularly, 10 to 13. Possible reasons for this pattern of results are discussed later in this paper.

Estimated effects on labor supply, wages, and earnings of fathers are reported in Table 8.4. Relatively few of the coefficients reported there approach statistical significance. In the work hours regressions, limitations in schoolwork and attendance, daily activities, and mobility tend to have negative effects, but the only significant coefficients are for CANTABS with husbands of working wives. Among the estimated wage effects, only the negative coefficients of CANTABS and DIS3T4 in the regressions for husbands of nonworking wives are significant. In the earnings regressions for husbands of nonworking wives, significantly positive coefficients are observed for DIS5T9, DIS14T17, and PLAY while the coefficients of DIS3T4 and the variables for school-related and functional limitations tend to be negative. On the whole, the results in Table 8.4 suggest that the presence of children with such limitations tends to reduce paternal labor supply and earnings while the presence of a chronically ill child without such limitations tends to have a more positive impact as the age of the child increases. It is also interesting that the results for DUMDIS show consistently more negative effects for husbands of working wives than for husbands of nonworking wives, although they are clearly not significant.

Estimated Interaction Effects

An analysis of interaction effects of children's health problems was undertaken for two reasons. First, it provided alternative estimates of the impacts shown in Tables 8.3 and 8.4 that did not involve the strict assumptions of the simple additive model. Second, it permitted us to explore the possibility that health problem impacts vary with parental and family characteristics. While our interest in this possibility was primarily exploratory, there were two hypotheses deriving from the results of previous research (Salkever, forthcoming) which we wished to test. One was that negative health problem effects on maternal labor supply would be smaller for families with young children and/or large numbers of

Table 8.4   **Estimated Effects of Children's Health Variables: Paternal Labor Supply and Earnings**

Dependent Variable		DUMDIS	PLAY	WORK	CANTABS	USHELP	USMOB	DIS3T4	DIS5T9	DIS10T13	DIS14T17
Annual work hours, husbands of working wives	A	−25.90 (0.90)									
	B		22.15 (0.65)	−25.78 (0.85)	−165.70 (1.66)	34.51 (0.33)	−133.23 (0.98)	−45.62 (0.55)			
	C			−54.81 (1.30)	−189.10 (1.83)	27.01 (0.26)	−124.82 (0.91)	−44.70 (0.54)	38.79 (0.79)	29.81 (0.66)	8.71 (0.20)
	D			−27.88 (0.94)	−165.61 (1.66)		−103.71 (0.97)	−48.10 (0.58)			−5.65 (0.14)
	H			−31.23 (1.08)	−177.62 (1.81)						
Annual work hours, husbands of nonworking wives	A	15.63 (0.46)									
	B		64.23 (1.49)	31.98 (0.95)	−28.91 (0.27)	−114.14 (1.11)	−108.12 (0.90)	−4.69 (0.06)			
	C			−27.17 (0.56)	−96.02 (0.98)	−118.60 (1.14)	−110.31 (0.92)	−7.69 (0.09)	82.97 (1.60)	21.27 (0.39)	80.03 (1.31)
	D			9.71 (0.30)	−80.81 (0.74)		−159.76 (1.53)	−12.42 (0.14)			57.12 (1.03)
	I		55.43 (1.32)			−106.75 (1.05)	−109.97 (0.93)				

Table 8.4 (continued)

Dependent Variable		DUMDIS	PLAY	WORK	CANTABS	USHELP	USMOB	DIS3T4	DIS5T9	DIS10T13	DIS14T17
Logarithm of wages, husbands of working wives	A	−0.017 (0.53)									
	B		0.036 (0.96)	−0.023 (0.69)	0.054 (0.50)	0.001 (0.01)	0.026 (0.17)	−0.043 (0.47)			0.070 (1.47)
	C			−0.044 (0.95)	0.016 (0.14)	0.016 (0.14)	0.016 (0.11)	−0.045 (0.49)	−0.011 (0.20)	0.024 (0.49)	
	D			−0.038 (1.16)	0.025 (0.23)		0.023 (0.19)	−0.046 (0.50)			0.064 (1.46)
Logarithm of wages, husbands of nonworking wives	A	0.015 (0.54)									
	B		0.033 (0.93)	−0.0002 (0.01)	−0.195 (2.13)	0.006 (0.08)	0.040 (0.42)	−0.184 (2.70)			
	C			−0.033 (0.83)	−0.231 (2.38)	0.009 (0.011)	0.043 (0.45)	−0.183 (2.69)	0.023 (0.54)	0.043 (0.97)	
	D			−0.007 (0.28)	−0.205 (2.23)		0.050 (0.58)	−0.187 (2.76)			0.038 (0.77)
	K		0.033 (0.98)		−0.182 (2.10)			−0.185 (2.72)			0.019 (0.42)

Logarithm of earnings, husbands of working wives

	C1	C2	C3	C4	C5	C6	C7	C8	C9	C10
A	−0.028 (0.82)									
B		0.030 (0.77)	−0.035 (0.99)	−0.081 (0.70)	−0.020 (0.17)	0.029 (0.18)	0.002 (0.02)			
C			−0.053 (1.09)	−0.114 (0.95)	−0.008 (0.06)	0.021 (0.13)	0.001 (0.01)	−0.007 (0.12)	0.019 (0.38)	0.059 (1.19)
D			−0.049 (1.40)	−0.109 (0.93)		0.009 (0.07)	−0.0003 (0.004)			0.055 (1.19)

Logarithm of earnings, husbands of nonworking wives

	C1	C2	C3	C4	C5	C6	C7	C8	C9	C10
A	0.029 (0.96)									
B		0.090 (2.36)	0.006 (0.21)	−0.016 (0.16)	−0.058 (0.64)	−0.128 (1.22)	−0.138 (1.86)			
C			−0.079 (1.82)	−0.113 (1.06)	−0.057 (0.63)	−0.127 (1.21)	−0.139 (1.87)	0.094 (2.05)	0.061 (1.26)	0.115 (2.13)
D			−0.019 (0.67)	−0.069 (0.68)		−0.138 (1.49)	−0.148 (2.00)			0.074 (1.54)
J			−0.080 (1.87)	−0.123 (1.17)		−0.158 (1.69)	−0.140 (1.89)	0.092 (2.00)	0.059 (1.19)	0.122 (2.33)

t-statistics in parentheses.

children. The other was that these negative health problem effects would be stronger for lower income families.

Interaction effects were examined by regressing child health variables and other parental and family characteristics on the differences between actual and predicted dependent variable values for disabled families. (The predictions were derived from regressions for nondisabled families.) Five sets of parental and family characteristics variables were included in the analysis: parental education (HSED, WFED), the variables describing the number and ages of children in the family (KID0T2, KID3T4, KID5T9, KIDNUM), the large SMSA location dummies (BIGSMSA, MEDSMSA), other characteristics associated with the family's economic status (HEALTHLM, DFARMINC, DUMSPAN, and CASHDUM), and selectivity variables (obtained from maternal work status regressions for nondisabled families). The large SMSA dummies were included on the presumptions that families in urbanized areas had access to more supportive services and that the availability of these services would influence parental labor market behavior.[18]

The analysis of interactions began by including all the child health variables (except PLAY and DUMDIS) and all the parental and family characteristics variables just mentioned in preliminary regressions. Variables in the latter set with the lowest estimated t-statistics were then deleted from the interaction regressions shown in Table 8.5. (DFARMINC was insignificant in all cases and does not appear in the table.) Looking first at the maternal work status findings, we note several similarities to the additive model findings. First, the reported mean dependent variable value of -0.01 indicates little average impact on maternal work status; the fraction of mothers in disabled families who worked (0.542) was only .01 below the predicted fraction based on the maternal work status regression for nondisabled families. Second, significantly negative effects on maternal work probabilities are again observed for WORK, CANTABS, and USMOB, while DIS14T17 is significantly positive. The positive coefficients for KID0T2, KID3T4, and KID5T9 are in accord with our expectations, although only KID0T2 is significant. Results for HEALTHLM, DUMSPAN and CASHDUM are consistent with the income-interaction result from our previous study, but the findings for WFED do not fit this pattern.

The results for health problem variables in the maternal earnings regressions are also somewhat similar to the additive model results. The mean dependent variable value of -0.195 is close to the value of -0.2265 for the corresponding DUMDIS coefficient in Table 8.3. Also, the coefficient of DIS10T13 is again significantly negative. However, the strongly negative effects of WORK, CANTABS, and USMOB in the additive model are greatly diminished in the interaction analysis. Evidence on the hypothesized interactions with economic status and with numbers and ages of children is mixed. While the coefficients for KID-NUM, WFED, HEALTHLM, and DUMPSPAN are consistent with the results of our previous study, the significantly negative coefficients of KID5T9 and HSED contradict these results.

Results for earnings of husbands of working wives show no significant interactions except the strongly positive effect of the SMSA location dummies. For husbands of nonworking wives, the strong negative effects of school-related disabilities and mobility limitations are consistent with the estimates of the additive model. It is difficult to interpret other significant or nearly significant coefficients because their signs are not consistent with one another; while MEDSMSA and KID0T2 are positive, BIGSMSA and KIDNUM are negative. Finally, it is interesting to note that while the mean dependent variable values for both groups of husbands are more negative than the corresponding DUMDIS coefficients in Table 8.4, comparison between the two groups again suggests a more negative effect of health problems for husbands of working wives.

Summary and Discussion

Our empirical results provide rather consistent evidence that children's chronic health problems have a more pronounced negative effect on labor supply and earnings for mothers than for fathers. A possible explanation for this finding, suggested by our simple theoretical model, is that the production of child health is relatively more maternal-time intensive. In addition, we have found that on average the reduction of maternal labor supply and earnings is due primarily to shorter hours of work and lower wage rates for mothers of chronically ill children rather than to reductions in the probability that these mothers work at all. This finding, which is consistent with results from our previous studies, could possibly indicate that health problems impact on maternal labor supply primarily through effects on the variable costs of maternal work. For example, if the costs of nonparental after-school care for school-age children with disabilities are greater than the corresponding costs for their nondisabled counterparts, net wages (i.e., wages minus variable costs of working per hour) for their mothers will fall more sharply as hours of work increase beyond the length of the school day.

With regard to the labor supply and earnings impacts of differing types of disabilities, our estimates generally show that these impacts are more negative for school-related disabilities and mobility limitations than for limitation in activities of daily living or playing with other children. In particular, the additive model results show strong negative impacts of the former types of disabilities in most of the maternal regressions, in the work hours regressions for husbands of working wives and in the wage and earnings regressions for husbands of nonworking wives. In the in-

Table 8.5   Interaction Analysis for Maternal Work Status and Parental Earnings

Independent Variables	Maternal Work Status		Dependent Variables — Ln (Earnings) Working Wives		Ln (Earnings) Husbands of Working Wives	Ln (Earnings) Husbands of Non-Working Wives	
	(1)	(2)	(3)	(4)	(5)	(6)	(7)
WORK	-0.027 (1.42)	-0.032 (1.93)	0.032 (0.42)		-0.029 (0.53)	-0.076 (1.81)	-0.081 (2.24)
CANTABS	-0.086 (1.87)	-0.087 (1.96)	-0.050 (0.27)		-0.077 (0.58)	-0.140 (1.36)	-0.144 (1.45)
USMOB	-0.091 (1.69)	-0.068 (1.52)	-0.179 (0.75)	-0.273 (1.47)	0.057 (0.32)	-0.178 (1.76)	-0.204 (2.27)
USHELP	0.0345 (0.76)		-0.126 (0.68)		-0.032 (0.23)	-0.048 (0.55)	
DIS3T4	0.018 (0.36)		0.048 (0.27)		0.132 (1.02)	-0.138 (1.60)	-0.138 (1.76)
DIS5T9	-0.012 (0.35)		0.082 (0.60)		0.037 (0.40)	0.063 (0.97)	0.064 (1.56)
DIS10T13	-0.011 (0.38)		-0.168 (1.35)	-0.183 (2.50)	0.049 (0.56)	-0.013 (0.20)	
DIS14T17	0.044 (1.47)	0.051 (2.41)	-0.004 (0.32)		0.043 (0.52)	0.015 (0.22)	
HSED			-0.027 (1.70)				

WFED	−0.007 (1.57)	−0.007 (1.54)	0.045 (2.24)	0.046 (2.29)		−0.118 (2.11)	−0.116 (2.09)
HEALTHLM	−0.081 (2.86)	−0.082 (2.94)	0.130 (1.16)	0.132 (1.18)		0.116 (2.24)	0.117 (2.26)
BIGSMSA					0.155 (1.90)		
MEDSMSA	0.058 (2.55)	0.058 (2.55)			0.242 (3.55)		
DUMSPAN	−0.086 (1.63)	−0.087 (1.63)	−0.255 (1.20)	−0.254 (1.19)	−0.156 (1.03)		
CASHDUM	0.057 (2.48)	0.057 (2.47)					
KID0T2	0.037 (1.57)	0.039 (1.66)				0.081 (1.60)	0.080 (1.59)
KID3T4	0.033 (1.28)	0.040 (1.85)					
KID5T9	0.020 (1.45)	0.019 (1.58)	−0.125 (1.82)	−0.089 (1.79)			
KIDNUM			0.067 (1.91)	0.060 (1.88)		−0.043 (2.51)	−0.042 (2.56)
SELECTIVITY						0.348 (3.41)	0.354 (3.51)
R^2	0.018	0.018	0.015	0.014		0.052	0.051
Mean dependent variable value		−0.010	−0.195		−0.100	−0.067	−0.067

t-statistics in parentheses.

teraction analysis, similar effects of school-related and mobility limitations are obtained for maternal work status and earnings of husbands of nonworking wives, but negative effects on earnings of working mothers and earnings of working wives' husbands are weaker.

Variations in health problem impact with the age of the disabled child are strongest in the maternal regressions with the additive model. Effects on maternal work probabilities, work hours, and earnings are most negative for the 5 to 9 and 10 to 13 age groups while the negative maternal wage effects increase with age. The additive model results for fathers shows a weak tendency for hours, wage, and earnings effects to become more positive with age. In the interaction regressions, the patterns of age effects on maternal work status and parental earnings are less clear.

Finally, the interaction analysis tends to confirm our previous findings that negative effects of children's health problems on maternal work status are stronger in lower income families and families with fewer young children. However, analogous results for parental earnings are rather mixed.

A number of factors could be invoked to explain the age-related variations in health problem impact reported here. The greater reduction in maternal labor supply for disabled children in the 5 to 13 age group suggests that while mothers of healthy children can cut back substantially on child care responsibilities as their children reach school age, mothers of disabled children are much less able to substitute educational services for their own time inputs.[19] Similarly, while healthy children start assuming more responsibility in caring for themselves as they enter the 10 to 13 age group, mothers of disabled children may be reluctant to rely on self-care until their children are somewhat older.

Differences in the types of reported health problems may also be relevant. Although the distribution of problem types reported in the SIE is, in general, similar across age groups, it is noteworthy that hearing and speech limitations are more than twice as prevalent for the 5 to 13 age groups than for the 14 to 17 age groups. (In contrast, among the other reported types of problems, only back impairments and arthritic or rheumatic problems clearly increase in prevalence with age.)[20] If parental time inputs (for home therapy, regular visits to health professionals, etc.) are in fact typically greater for hearing and speech limitations and other problems more frequently reported in the 5 to 13 age groups, a more negative effect on maternal labor supply would be expected.[21]

It is also possible that age differences in health problem impacts may be due, at least in part, to unmeasured parental characteristics. For example, if mothers with a very strong labor force attachment prior to childbearing are more likely to have children with health problems because they devote less time to prenatal care, or because they subsequently devote less time to child health maintenance and illness prevention activities, a positive bias in our disability coefficients would result. If this bias is strongest for mothers of young children, the more positive coefficients for DIS3T4 reported here would occur.

More generally, a variety of biases could result from unmeasured parental characteristics in a cross-sectional study such as this one. Although mothers with reported chronic health problems were excluded from the study, some variation in maternal health levels is probably still present in the data. If so, any positive association between maternal and child health levels will presumably cause a negative bias in the disability coefficients of the maternal labor supply and earnings regressions. Similarly, the probability of having a disabled child is positively related to the number of children, so that unmeasured parental preferences for large families (which presumably are negatively related to maternal preferences for market work) will cause a similar negative bias.[22] Moreover, families with disabled children are only so classified in our study if they have not chosen to institutionalize these children. While this raises the possibility of a systematic selection bias, the effect of such a bias oh our estimates is difficult to predict a priori.

These various threats to the validity of our cross-sectional findings could be greatly diminished by using panel data and examining changes in parental labor supply and earnings after the onset of children's chronic health problems. However, because the prevalence rates for these problems are low, the sample size for a prospective panel study would have to be extremely large to yield enough households with such problems. As an alternative, panel data could be collected retrospectively on a large number of households with disabled children, but one might question whether this retrospective approach yields sufficiently reliable data.

Conclusion

The major conclusion emerging from this analysis is that children's chronic health problems have substantial economic impacts, particularly in the form of reduced maternal earnings. A conservative estimate of the annual magnitude of this earnings reduction can be derived by assuming no effect on maternal work probability, using the 20% negative effect implied by the maternal earnings coefficient for DUMDIS in Table 8.3, and using a mean maternal earnings figure for nondisabled families of $4,100. (Using the data in Table 8.2, the exact figure is $2244.43/0.548 = $4,095.68.) This yields a per family annual reduction of $820 (in 1975 dollars). Assuming that half of the more than two million mothers with disabled children work, and thus experience this earnings reduction, we estimate that the total annual reduction is roughly $1 billion (in 1975 dollars). Of course, our estimates may overstate the earnings reduction for types of families excluded in our study (e.g., nonwhites, single-parent families, families where mothers have chronic health problems). However, this is probably offset by omitting the negative effects on maternal work probability and paternal earnings which were found to be significant for certain types of health problems.

Our finding that this economic impact depends on the extent to which health problems limit children's abilities to participate in educational activities is also of interest from a policy research standpoint. These limitations, which were reported by more than 60% of the children with health problems in the SIE, result from the interaction of physiological or psychological abnormalities and impairments with the structure and characteristics of available educational programs. Following the passage in 1975 of P.L. 94–142 (The Education for All Handicapped Act), increasing amounts of resources have been devoted to special education programs and to making regular programs more accessible to handicapped children. It has been suggested that the major economic benefits of these expenditures will occur in future years as more handicapped children become productive, tax-paying adults. Our own analysis raises the possibility of more immediate benefits in the form of increased parental productivity and earnings, and suggests that evaluation researchers should attempt to determine the extent, if any, of such benefits.

While the present study has focused on parental labor supply and earnings, it is likely that children's chronic health problems have a variety of other effects on parental behavior and time allocation. In particular, effects on child-spacing and family size, which have been ignored in the present study, may themselves have important secondary effects on parental labor supply and earnings.[23] Children's health problems may also affect other aspects of parental time allocation, such as the total amount of time spent in housework and child care.[24] Moreover, the distribution of this time among children in the household may also be affected; by causing parents to spend less time with healthy siblings, children's health problems may have deleterious effects on intellectual development or even the future health of these siblings.[25] Still other interesting areas for future research include possible impacts on family stability and parental mental and physical health,[26] and more detailed analysis of specific categories of chronic diseases. We hope that sufficiently large and detailed data sets will become available in the future to permit investigation of these issues.

Notes

1. Another possible explanation is aging of the population of children, since prevalence of chronic health problems increases with age; however, Bureau of the Census estimates for 1967 and 1979 show that the median age of the under-18 population increased by only about

one year during that time span. Alternatively, one might argue that the prevalence increase is mostly due to increased reporting of chronic conditions. As visits to physicians have increased, more chronic illnesses among children have been diagnosed; this has probably increased the percentage of children reporting disabilities in the household surveys conducted by the National Center for Health Statistics. However, the increase in prevalence shown in Table 8.1 for the 1967–72 period should contain only a minimal upward bias since per capita physician visits for children were virtually unchanged over this period, according to National Center for Health Statistics data. Moreover, the increases in prevalence of major activity limitations probably are not strongly influenced by this upward bias since we would expect that few of these limitations went unreported even in 1967.

2. Several other economic analyses of child health have used similar models. See, for example, Edwards and Grossman (1977a).

3. H could be interpreted as the average level of child health for all children in the family or as the health level for one particular child (with health levels for other children included in the composite good X). We do not explicitly consider the possibility of intrafamily variations in child health levels.

4. If one makes the more extreme assumption that paternal time inputs into child health production are zero (Inman 1976), then $\rho = 0$ and it follows from equation 2b that if X is a normal good, the occurrence of child health problems will increase paternal labor supply.

5. Another interesting property of this simple model is that the reduction in parental earnings in response to a child health problem (i.e., $w_1 dL_1 + w_2 dL_2$) must be less than the welfare cost to the family of this problem as measured by the relevant copensating income variation $(w_1 + \rho w_2 + \alpha \Pi) dH_0 / \delta$. (We assume δ is constant.) This offers some justification for viewing empirical estimates of earnings reductions (i.e., so-called "indirect costs of illness") as lower bounds on the relevant welfare cost figures. (We are indebted to Michael Grossman for suggesting this point.)

6. A recent study of maternal labor supply using a similar wage equation is Nakamura et al. (1979). While that study only includes selected elements of Z_1 in the wage equation because of this effect on work experience (i.e., labor supply in prior periods), this approach logically implies the more inclusive specification used here.

7. Of course, the selectivity variables are defined differently for the two groups. For husbands of working wives (and for working wives), the variable is the ratio of the probability density (calculated from the maternal work status regression) to the estimated probability of working. For husbands of nonworking wives, it is the ratio of the probability density to the estimated probability of not working.

8. Since heteroscedasticity is to be expected on a priori grounds in censored samples, the OLS estimates of t-statistics for the regression coefficients may be biased away from zero. However, the results cited in n. 15 suggest that in fact the extent of this bias may be small.

9. For more detailed information on the methods and content of the SIE, see U.S. Department of Commerce (1978).

10. OTHMETRO and OTHNONM can only be nonzero for residents of Massachusetts, Connecticut, New York, Pennsylvania, Ohio, Indiana, Illinois, Michigan, Wisconsin, Minnesota, Iowa, Virginia, North Carolina, Georgia, Florida, Tennessee, Alabama, Louisiana, Texas, Colorado, New Mexico, Arizona, and Oregon.

11. All health problems reported in the survey are chronic or long-term. Short-term problems (e.g., broken bones) are not indicated in the data.

12. The SIE questions on which these variables are based first determined whether each child aged 5 to 17 had a physical, emotional, or mental condition which limited or interfered with regular school work. If they did have such a condition, a question was then asked about limitations in ability to attend school. If they did not, a question was asked about physical, emotional, or mental conditions which limited the child's ability to take part in sports, games, or similar activities. If the response to this last question was negative, the child was not considered to have a health problem. For children aged 3 to 4 only this last question

about limitations in play was asked. Also, the reader should note that classification of emotional and mental conditions as health problems in the SIE is consistent with recent epidemiological work emphasizing that this type of problem (termed "the new morbidity") is an important portion of the total spectrum of child health problems (Haggerty et al. 1975, pp. 94–113; Starfield et al. 1980).

13. This deletion had little effect on the estimated coefficients for the child health variables.

14. In most cases, the selectivity variables were computed from maternal work status regressions using the same selection of child health variables. For example, in Table 8.3 maternal wage regression D used a selectivity variable calculated from maternal work status regression D. For the regressions labeled E through K in Tables 8.3 and 8.4 maternal work status regression C was used to calculate the selectivity variables.

15. Complete results for all these regressions are available from the author. It should also be noted that the residuals from several of the hours and earnings regressions reported here were examined for evidence of heteroscedasticity. More specifically, since the censored sample model implies that the residual variance will be a function of the value for the selectivity variable (Cogan 1977; Nakamura et al. 1979), we grouped the observations in each regression into ten roughly equal groups ordered by this value. We then calculated the mean square residual for each of the ten groups. These mean figures were generally close to one another (with the largest being no more than roughly 1.5 times the smallest) except in the husband's earnings regressions. Moreover, variation in the mean squares among the groups did not seem to be systematically related to the value of the selectivity variable. Thus, it seems safe to conclude that sample censoring is not an important source of heteroscedasticity in the data.

16. Coefficients are regarded as significant if their t-statistics exceed 1.645, which indicates significance at the 0.1 level in a two-tailed test.

17. Since the dependent variables in the wage regressions are natural logarithms, the percentage reductions referred to in the text are calculated as $(1-e^{bx})$, where b is the estimated coefficient and x is the variable under discussion.

18. All regressions for nondisabled families used for predictions and all regressions on disabled families reported here were estimated by OLS. Selectivity variables used in these regressions were based on a probit maternal work status regression for nondisabled families.

19. Regression results for the variables KID0T2, KID3T4, KID5T9, and KIDNUM are consistent with this explanation. In the maternal work status, hours, and earnings regressions, coefficients for the first two of these variables are always large and significantly negative, while coefficients of the latter two indicate less negative effects which are sometimes insignificant.

20. Other types of health problems reported in the SIE are mental retardation, visual impairments, other musculoskeletal problems (besides back problems), digestive disorders, respiratory disorders, emotional and nervous disorders, and heart disease. Note, however, that 40% of the reported problems did not fall into any of the categories mentioned here or in the text. Data on the nature of these problems was not available.

21. The SIE data also indicate that the reported health problems for this age group were more likely to involve limitations in schoolwork. In particular, the percentages of children with schoolwork limitations (including those with attendance limitations) were 73.7, 64.6, and 40.6 for the age groups 5 to 9, 10 to 13, and 14 to 17 respectively. These figures are not surprising in view of collinearity between WORK, CANTABS, DIS5T9, and DIS10T13 already noted.

22. A related criticism, based on the analysis of Rosenzweig and Wolpin (1980), is that it might be more appropriate to view parental labor supply and child-bearing decisions over the life-cycle as jointly determined. From this perspective, independent variables relating to fertility (such the number and ages of children), which are typically included in standard

labor supply analyses, are viewed as endogenous and estimated labor supply equations containing these independent variables are *conditional* labor supply functions. Furthermore, estimates of these functions may be biased by unobservable preference variations among households. If, in the present analysis, these fertility-related independent variables are simply excluded, the possibility of bias still remains since unobserved preference variations are related to family size and thus to the probability of having a disabled child. If, however, the disability variable could be defined in a manner unrelated to fertility, estimated child disability effects free of this bias would be obtained. For example, one might define a disability dummy equal to 1 if the family's firstborn child was disabled at birth (or shortly thereafter) and use this in labor supply regressions which excluded fertility-related variables. As an approximation to this procedure, we reestimated regressions A and B for maternal work status and parental earnings, excluding disabled families where the oldest child was not disabled and excluding nondisabled families with no children over 2 years of age. The results for both specifications A and B are similar to the findings in Tables 8.3 and 8.4. The DUMDIS coefficients are small and clearly insignificant except in the maternal earnings regression where a highly significant coefficient of -0.1822 is obtained. The coefficients of WORK, CANTABS, and USMOB in the maternal work status regression are all negative with t-statistics greater than 1; however they are smaller in magnitude than those in Table 8.3 and only the WORK coefficient is clearly significant. The positive coefficient of PLAY is also significant. In maternal earnings regressions B, the coefficients for WORK, CANTABS, and USMOB are not significant, while the negative coefficients for DIS3T4, USHELP, and PLAY became larger and highly significant. In summary, regardless of the weight one gives to the Rosenzweig-Wolpin critique of the standard labor supply model, it does not appear to have important implications for our major empirical results.

23. Note, however, that the estimation method described in n. 22 does capture these secondary effects.

24. We are currently examining this possibility with 1976 data from the Panel Study of Income Dynamics.

25. For indirect evidence that parental time inputs influence children's intellectual development, see Edwards and Grossman (1977*a*). Empirical evidence on the interrelationships of children's health and intellectual development over time is presented in Shakotko et al. (1980) and Edwards and Grossman (1977*b*).

26. Further research in the project described by Breslau et al. (1980) is examining some of these impacts.

References

Barsch, Ray, 1968. *The parent of the handicapped child.* Springfield, Illinois: Charles C. Thomas, p. 62.

Bartel, Ann, and Taubman, Paul. 1979. Health and labor market success: the role of various diseases. *Review of Economics and Statistics* 61: 1–8.

Breslau, Naomi; Staruch, Kathleen; and Gortmaker, Steven. 1980. The burden of caring for the disabled child. Paper presented at the Annual Meeting of the American Sociological Association, New York, August 1980.

Cogan, John. 1977. Labor supply with time and money costs of participation. R–2044. Santa Monica, Cal.: The Rand Corporation.

Cummings, S.T. 1976. The impact of the child's deficiency on the father: a study of fathers of mentally retarded and of chronically ill children. *American Journal of Orthopsychiatry* 46: 246–55.

Cummings, S.T.; Bayley, Helen C.; and Rie, Robert E. 1966. Effects of the child's deficiency on the mother: a study of mothers of mentally retarded, chronically ill, and neurotic children. *American Journal of Orthopsychiatry* 36: 595–608.

Edwards, Linda, and Grossman, Michael. 1977a. An economic analysis of children's health and intellectual development. Working Paper No. 180, National Bureau of Economic Research.

———. 1977b. The relationship between children's health and intellectual development. Working Paper No. 213, National Bureau of Economic Research.

Fein, Rashi. 1958. *Economics of mental illness*. New York: Basic Books, pp. 108–39.

Fuchs, Victor R. 1966. The contribution of health services to the American economy. *Milbank Memorial Fund Quarterly* 44: 65–101.

Grossman, Michael, and Benham, Lee. 1974. Health, hours, and wages. In Mark Perlman, ed., *The economics of health and medical care*. New York: Halsted Press.

Haggerty, Robert J.; Roghman, Klaus J.; and Pless, Ivan B. 1975. *Child health and the community*. New York: John Wiley, pp. 94–113.

Heckman, James. 1977. Sample selection bias as a specification error. Working Paper No. 172, National Bureau of Economic Research.

———. 1974. Effects of child care programs on women's work effort. *Journal of Political Economy* 82: 491–519.

Inman, Robert P. 1976. The family provision of children's health: an economic analysis. In Richard N. Rosett, ed., *The role of health insurance in the health services sector*. New York: National Bureau of Economic Research.

Klarman, Herbert E. 1965. *The economics of health*. New York: Columbia University Press, pp. 162–73.

Luft, Harold. 1975. The impact of poor health on earnings. *Review of Economics and Statistics* 57: 43–57.

McCollum Audrey. 1971. Cystic fibrosis: economic impact on the family *American Journal of Public Health* 61: 1335–40.

McCubbin, Hamilton; Patterson, Joan; McCubbin, Marilyn; Wilson, Lance; and Warnick, Warren. 1979. Parental coping and family environment: critical factors in the home management and health status of children with cystic fibrosis. Paper presented at the annual meeting of the American Public Health Association, New York, November 1979.

Meyerowitz, Joseph, and Kaplan, Howard. 1967. Familial responses to stress: the case of cystic fibrosis. *Social Science and Medicine* 1: 249–66.

Nagi, Saad Z., and Luken, Paul C. 1975. Childhood disability: a social epidemiology. Unpublished paper. Mershon Center, The Ohio State University.

Nakamura, Masao; Nakamura, Alice; and Cullen, Dallas. 1979. Job opportunities, the offered wage, and the labor supply of married women. *The American Economic Review* 69: 787–805.

Rice, Dorothy P.; Feldman, Jacob J.; and White, Kerr L. 1976. The current burden of illness in the United States. An occasional paper of the Institute of Medicine. Washington: National Academy of Sciences.

Rosenzweig, Mark R., and Wolpin, Kenneth I. 1980. Life-cycle labor supply and fertility: causal inferences from household models. *Journal of Political Economy* 88: 328–48.

Salkever, David S. Forthcoming. Childen's health problems and maternal work status. *Journal of Human Resources.*

———. 1980. Effects of children's health on maternal hours of work: a preliminary analysis. *Southern Economic Journal* 47: 156–66.

Shakotko, Robert A.; Edwards, Linda N.; and Grossman, Michael. 1980. An exploration of the dynamic relationship between health and cognitive development in adolescence. Working Paper No. 454, National Bureau of Economic Research.

Starfield, Barbara; Gross, Edward; Wood, Maurice; Pantell, Robert; Allen, Constance; Gordon, I. Bruce; Moffatt, Patricia; Drachman, Robert; and Katz, Harvey. 1980. Psychosocial and psychosomatic diagnoses in primary care of children. *Pediatrics* 66: 159–67.

Sultz, Harry; Schlesinger, Edward; Mosher, William; and Feldman, Joseph. 1972. *Long-term childhood illness.* Pittsburgh: University of Pittsburgh Press, pp. 101-106.

U.S. Department of Commerce. 1978. Bureau of the Census. *Microdata from the Survey of Income and Education.* Data Access Description No. 42.

3 Health and Public Policy

9   The Choice of Health Policies with Heterogeneous Populations

Donald S. Shepard and Richard J. Zeckhauser

Introduction

The Problem

Expending resources to secure health benefits is engaging in a game of chance. We might observe that, on average, a 65-year-old patient with an inguinal hernia and known medical characteristics who chooses an elective herniorrhaphy has about a 90% chance of completely successful surgery—surviving the operation without recurrence of the hernia—and a 10% chance of failure (0.3% chance of death, and 9.7% chance of recurrence) (Neuhauser 1977). In decision theory, we are used to considering such problems as if they were analogous to playing a roulette wheel, the outcome determined by the fall of a ball.

Many medical interventions, we shall argue here, do not fit this paradigm. It is not an entirely random process that determines which individuals have successful operations. The successes may tend to be different, in ways that may or may not be observable, from the 10% that have poor outcomes. That is, the population is heterogeneous.

Heterogeneous or mixed populations are ones in which the probability of loss from the population varies among members, in its initial value, in

Donald S. Shepard is adjunct research associate, Kennedy School of Government; economist, Veterans Administration Outpatient Clinic; and lecturer, Harvard School of Public Health. Richard J. Zeckhauser is professor of Political Economy, Kennedy School of Government. Research was supported by grant number SOC 77–16602 from the National Science Foundation to the Kennedy School of Government, by the Health Services Research and Development Service of the Veterans Administration, and by the Institute for Research on Poverty, University of Wisconsin.

Kenneth Arrow, Victor Fuchs, other participants in the NBER Conference on Economic Aspects of Health, Benjamin Barnes, and Nancy Jackson gave us helpful comments. Michael Riddiough, Claudia Sanders, and John Bell kindly shared their data from the study of the pneumococcal pneumonia vaccine by the Office of Technology Assessment.

its evolution over time, or in its response to an intervention. In a health context, the population is people who have not yet suffered some sickness, complication, or death; the loss is the onset of that condition. Variations along such dimensions as age and sex are well known; hence we traditionally standardize mortality statistics with respect to such variables. Medical characteristics, such as smoking or general medical history, may also be employed as classifying variables. Here our concern is not only such directly recorded variables, but others that may go unnoticed or that are even inherently unobservable.

The benefits of medical procedures often vary according to the patient's characteristics. With herniorrhaphy, for example, an occupation requiring heavy lifting and straining, obesity, use of steroid drugs which discourage healing (perhaps to treat asthma), or chronic lung disease (which may cause coughing) would all reduce the chances of successful surgery. Where explanatory variables can be readily observed and classified, we are likely to standardize on them. Thus, for example, we might express surgical mortality as corrected by such variables as age, urgency of operation (elective or emergency), and the patient's general health. Frequently, however, the explanatory variables are either unmonitorable, unrecognized, or sufficiently difficult to classify that they go unmentioned. Although surgeons attempt to ascertain the risk of heart attack during or after general surgery through medical history and routine tests, they typically forego the greater predictive accuracy that could be achieved through invasive cardiac tests such as coronary angiography, because the value of the information would not justify the risks.

Individuals differ, then, in their chances of contracting an illness, failing to respond to treatment, or dying. This paper is concerned with the policy implications of that heterogeneity in the population, with the ultimate purpose of helping officials who must decide where to direct health interventions. Understanding the effects of population heterogeneity will permit more accurate assessment of the benefits and costs of various possible interventions, thus contributing to better policy.

The salient characteristics of heterogeneity differ depending whether the characteristics that predict an individual's probability of loss are observed and are used as a basis for prediction. If so, we say that the population embodies "observed heterogeneity." Accurate assessments then require that we trace the way each of the several observed risk groups evolves over time. That is, we predict the expected health benefits each risk group receives from alternative interventions, and the expected resources the interventions will require each year. Policy choices involve not only these epidemiological and modeling considerations, but ethical and economic issues entailed in setting priorities for offering health programs to different categories of individuals.

By "latent heterogeneity" we denote the situation in which different subgroups of the population are at different levels of risk, but the differentiating factors are not used as a basis for prediction. They may be unobservable, unobserved, or observed and ignored because they are not known to be relevant. With latent heterogeneity, the economic and ethical issues related to setting priorities within the population are obviated; distinctions simply are not made among individuals. However, important and generally unrecognized statistical questions arise that must be attended to if accurate assessments of benefits and costs are to be made.

Observed Heterogeneity

In cases of observed heterogeneity, we assume that the benefits and costs returning to members of the different risk groups can be determined by established methods. The policy task is to establish priorities for the risk groups in receiving interventions. This is essentially a problem in public expenditure theory, where the objective is to maximize the difference between benefits and costs, or in the constrained resource case, to maximized benefits subject to some resource limit. Complications arise in three areas: (1) a metric must be established for health benefits; (2) in addition to their immediate costs, medical interventions have implications for future costs which may be paid from other pockets; (3) determining the order in which different groups shall be offered medical interventions on the basis of predicted benefits and costs has significant ethical implications. These issues are explored later.

Latent Heterogeneity

Even though a human population appears homogeneous, there will be differentials in risk among its members that persist over time; i.e., there will be latent heterogeneity. Most interventions directed towards heterogeneous populations will offer differential benefits to the members of that population at various risk levels. Hence, they will change the mix among the surviving population. Even when the nature of the different risk groups is unclear, recognizing the fact of latent heterogeneity will make it possible to predict the effects of interventions more accurately.

Evidence

The existence of heterogeneity in a population's risk levels can be diagnosed by observing losses from the population over time and comparing that pattern with a theoretical norm that assumes homogeneous risk. As the simplest case, suppose we could confidently assume that loss rates for each individual were constant over time; heterogeneity would then reveal itself by a decline in loss rates over time as the high-risk members were eliminated from the population. This sort of population heterogeneity could explain why students' failure rates decline over successive years in colleges, or why rates of recidivism decline after longer periods of abstention from alcohol or smoking. (See Shepard 1977.)

With smoking, for example, it is frequently alleged that the first few weeks of forbearance are the most difficult. Surely there is another phenomenon at work. Some individuals, for whatever reasons, are more likely to return to smoking in any given period. Persons with a high probability of recidivism tend to be eliminated from the "not smoking" population early. That effect tends to reduce recidivism in the population over time.

In earlier analyses (Shepard and Zeckhauser 1977, 1980a) we have looked at the relapse problem in relation to hernia recurrence. The annual rate of recurrence drops from 30/1,000 person-years during the first year after the initial hernia repair, to 9.1/1,000 during years one through five, to 3.4/1,000 for years five to ten. Heterogeneity with respect to per period probability of recurrence offers a straightforward explanation for this observed pattern: each individual remains at the same level of risk indefinitely, but a larger proportion of the recurrence-prone individuals are removed early. The alternative explanation is that the recurrence rate for each recipient of the operation falls over time. Physicians whom we consulted told us, however, that it was highly unlikely that the observed patterns reflected a strengthening of tissues over time. Wounds gain maximum strength in a few weeks, not a few years. A further piece of evidence supports the hypothesis that there is patient-to-patient heterogeneity in recurrence rates. The probability that a patient undergoing herniorrhaphy ever experiences a first recurrence is about 10%; the probability that he suffers a second recurrence, given that he had a first recurrence, is 35% (Neuhauser 1977). The higher rate for second recurrences is consistent with the fact that persons with a first recurrence are primarily those with above-average recurrence probabilities.

Even if individuals' loss rates do not remain constant over time, we will still be able to detect heterogeneity, as long as loss rates conform to some predictable patterns. Consider, for instance, a group of people who have stopped smoking. We assume that there is substantial heterogeneity in the initial relapse rates back into smoking, and that each individual's loss rate increases exponentially over time. It may nevertheless turn out that, for the population as a whole, observed relapse rates decline over time. The selection factor that applies to the population as a whole overcomes the increasing risk factor that applies to each individual separately. Consider now an individual whose initial relapse rate is unknown. His risk of relapsing appears to decline over time, as he remains in the population, whereas actually it is increasing. The source of the paradox is that the individual is simultaneously undergoing two effects. By surviving he reveals (with increasing confidence) that he is a better risk than the initial population average. Whatever his true risk level, however, that risk is increasing on a period-by-period basis.[1]

Possible Biases in Assessment and Interpretation

Latent heterogeneity must be considered when choosing interventions or when interpreting data derived from experiments, e.g., the differential survival of those given a new drug in a randomized controlled trial.

Without proper attention to latent heterogeneity, we will misestimate the long-term benefits and costs of medical interventions. We want to state at the outset that our problem is not the familiar bias due to confounding of treatment differences with patient differences. We are assuming that outcomes with and without interventions are compared for populations that are *initially* identical. The bias that we discuss arises because an intervention selectively eliminates certain members of the mixed population from further follow-up, so that after a time, the makeup of the population differs from what it would have been without the intervention.

Latent heterogeneity usually biases inferences about the effects of an intervention. One type of inference, termed a population projection, estimates the effect of a treatment on a population from its effect on homogeneous risk groups. Projections that ignore heterogeneity will generally make the intervention appear better than it really is. A second type of inference estimates the effect of the intervention on each individual, or homogeneous risk group, from its observed effect on the population. Generally, the effect on each individual will be stronger than the observed effect on the population. *Heterogeneity generally attenuates the effect on the population compared to the effect on the individual.*

Predicting the Benefits of an Intervention on a Population with Latent Heterogeneity

Analytic models enable us to predict the gains when interventions reduce loss rates in heterogeneous populations. The recommended procedure, which we shall refer to as a "standardized assessment," begins by classifying the population into homogeneous strata. Within each stratum, the time-specific (which implies age-specific when age is of consequence) loss rates are computed with and without the intervention. For each stratum, an output measure of interest is computed, such as mortality, life expectancy, or duration of freedom from a disease. The overall outcome measure for the population is computed by averaging the measures for each stratum weighted according to initial prevalences.

This paper compares the standardized assessment procedure with the most widely used methodology for evaluating interventions, which we shall refer to as a "traditional assessment." A traditional assessment starts with the pattern of losses under baseline conditions varying with both age and time, derived from some observed data or a statistical model. (If no adjustment is made for age and time, a procedure we term a "naive assessment," then greater biases may result [Shepard and Zeckhauser 1980*a*].) The active intervention is assumed to change age- and time-specific loss rates. The traditional assessment, in contrast to the recommended procedure, assumes (usually implicitly) that the presence of the intervention does not alter the population mix at any point in time. Output measures are computed using mortality rates that are adjusted to allow for the direct effect of the intervention, but take no account of the intervention's effect in changing the mix in the population.

Recent trends in U.S. mortality (discussed later) and a number of other illustrations suggest that interventions change the mixture of risk groups in the population, most often increasing the proportion of high-risk persons. For example, a simulation has shown that the continued availability of a mobile coronary care unit would increase the percentage of surviving males over age 30 who had had heart attacks from 12% to 15% (Zeckhauser and Shepard 1976). This group is at substantially higher risk for future coronary events.

When carrying out the recommended standardized assessment, a critical problem is to stratify the population appropriately. Stratification variables might include lifestyle characteristics, such as smoking and drinking habits, single medical variables, or multivariate risk scores. In some instances, socioeconomic factors may be employed as proxies for underlying causal fctors. Many factors that influence mortality risk may be unobserved; some may never be observed, though their presence can be inferred through experiment.

The important point is that stratification should proceed far enough that the individuals within a risk category are relatively homogeneous. The reward for painful efforts at classification is an assessment procedure that avoids the systematic bias inherent in traditional assessments.

Formal Concepts for Assessing Interventions

Consider a mixed population whose risk categories are indexed by j, with the initial prevalence of each being r_j. Interventions are indexed over i; $i = 1$ represents the baseline intervention. If we let $\mu_{ij}(x)$ denote the instantaneous hazard rate, survival at age x will be

$$(1) \qquad \ell_{ij}(x) = \exp[- \int_o^x \mu_{ij}(t)\,dt] \ ,$$

where $\ell_{ij} = 1$ at $x = 0$. The mixed population's survival at age x, denoted by $\ell_{i.}(x)$, is a weighted average of $\ell_{ij}(x)$,

$$\ell_{i.}(x) = \sum_j r_j \ell_{ij}(x) \ .$$

The *prevalence*, or proportion, of survivors of risk category j under intervention i at age $x, r_{ij}(x)$, is

$$(2) \qquad r_{ij}(x) = r_j \, \frac{\ell_{ij}(x)}{\ell_{i.}(x)} \ .$$

The overall hazard rate under intervention i at age $x, m_i(x)$, is a weighted average by prevalence of the hazard rates for the individual risk groups:

$$(3) \qquad m_i(x) = \sum_j r_{ij}(x) \, \mu_{ij}(x).$$

Biases Inherent in Traditional Assessments

In a traditional assessment, the prevalence of risk category j at age x is taken to be its baseline value, $r_{ij}(x)$. Bias arises when the population is subjected to an active treatment, $i = 2$ for illustration. Risk is estimated to be

$$m_2'(x) = \sum_j r_{1j}(x) \, \mu_{2j}(x) \ ,$$

where comparison with (3) reveals that the unbiased estimate replaces r_{1j} with r_{2j}.

Our interest is in the difference between the (incorrectly weighted) traditional assessment and the standardized assessment. This difference, $\Delta m(x)$ at age x, is defined by

$$\Delta m = m_2(x) - m_2' \, (x)$$

where a positive difference indicates that the traditional assessment overstates the benefit of the intervention in reducing mortality.

In an earlier analysis (Shepard and Zeckhauser 1980*a*) we identified this bias. Here we shall prove some of its properties.[2] Let us define comparative survival gain as

$$(4) \qquad g_j(x) = \frac{\ell_{2j}}{\ell_2} - \frac{\ell_{1j}}{\ell_1}.$$

Thus, g_j measures the gain in survival to group j relative to overall survival gain in treatment. The group that gains the most has the highest value for g_j. We prove below that the bias of the traditional assessment depends on which risk group gains relatively most in survival.

Theorem 1

Let $m_2'(x)$ be mortality calculated by the traditional assessment and $m_2(x)$ be mortality standardized for appropriate risk indicators. Let μ_{ij} be mortality rates and g_j be the relative survival gain as defined above. Then $\Delta m(x) \equiv m_2(x) - m_2'(x) = $ covariance (μ_{2j}, g_j).

Proof

First we establish the chain of equations in (5) by substituting from the definitions of $r_{ij}(x)$ in (2) and of g_j in (4):

$$(5) \qquad r_{2j} - r_{1j} = r_j(0) \left[\frac{\ell_{2j}}{\ell_{2.}} - \frac{\ell_{1j}}{\ell_{1.}} \right] = r_j(0) g_j(x) .$$

To simplify notation, we have shortened $r_{1j}(0)$ and $r_{2j}(0)$ (which are identical) to $r_j(0)$ or r_j. Next we sum both sides of (5) over j, obtaining

$$\sum_j r_{2j} - \sum_j r_{1j} = \sum_j r_j(0) g_j(x).$$

The left side is $1 - 1 = 0$ and the right side is the mean of the g_j, weighted by $r_j(0)$. Thus the weighted mean of g_j is zero. Now multiply both sides of (5) by μ_{2j} and sum over j:

$$(6) \qquad \sum_j \mu_{2j}(r_{2j} - r_{1j}) = \sum_j r_j(0) \mu_{2j}(x) g_j(x).$$

Recalling the definitions of $m_2(x)$ and $m_2'(x)$, the left side in (6) is $\Delta m(x)$. The right side is the weighted cross product of $\mu_{2j}(x)$ and $g_j(x)$.

Recalling that the weighted mean of $g_j(x)$ is zero, we can subtract the product of the means of $g_j(x)$ and $\mu_{2j}(x)$ (termed g *and* $\mu_{2.}$, respectively) from the right side, yielding

$$
\begin{aligned}
(7) \qquad \Delta m(x) &= \sum_j r_j(0) \mu_{2j}(x) g_j(x) - \mu_{2.}(x) g_.(x) \\
&= \text{covariance}\,(\mu_{2j}(x), g_j(x)) .
\end{aligned}
$$

Q.E.D.

This theorem represents our central result with respect to bias. For example, if the absolute benefit of the intervention is greater for high-risk individuals, then the greater values of g_j will be associated with the larger values of $\mu(x)$. This implies that the covariance is positive. The bias will be positive as well. From this it follows: *Traditional assessment methods will overstate the benefits of interventions that offer a greater reduction in force of mortality for high-risk than for low-risk individuals.*

The expression for $\Delta m(x)$ reveals that the magnitude of the bias depends on time, x. At time zero, there is no bias, for selective mortality has not yet affected the composition of the population. After a long period of time virtually all survivors with or without the intervention will be low-risk individuals; the bias is small. In the intermediate run the bias is greatest. Traditional assessments implicitly underestimate the number of high-risk individuals for intermediate times. In a numerical example involving a hypothetical intervention to reduce the risk of dropping out of medical treatment for hypertension, we found that the maximum bias occurred at 3.5 years after the start of the intervention. At that point, loss rates were underestimated by 31% in a traditional assessment (Shepard and Zeckhauser 1980a).

A common complaint in recent years has been that our dramatically increased national expenditures on health care and other health promoting activities have not done much to lengthen life expectancy. (See, for example, Fuchs 1974.) But perhaps they have, at least for an individual at any particular risk level. The problem may be that heterogeneity masks such effects by producing a weaker overall population of survivors.

How then should an individual feel about health care? Suppose that health improvements had reduced age-specific mortality for all initial risk levels regardless of age by $X\%$ from 1940 to 1980. (The preventive fraction is $X\%$.) If an individual knows his prior risk level, he can calculate his current risk level as $X\%$ less. If he does not know his prior risk level, then he must compare the age-specific mortality rates for men of his age today and 40 years ago. This comparison will generally show an expected decline in age-specific mortality that is less than $X\%$. The reason is that an individual alive now at an intermediate age, say age 60, has a higher probability of being a high-risk individual than an unselected individual of the same age 40 years ago.

To illustrate numerically, assume as above, that there were two equal sized risk groups, with forces of mortality of 5% (indexed by $j = 1$) and 10% ($j = 2$) per year. A vaccine would cut both of these rates in half (X equals 50%). If a person survived for 10 years *without* the vaccine, the chance that he was a high-risk ($j = 2$) person is $r_{12}(10)$, or 38%, from equations (1) and (2). If he survived for 10 years *with* the vaccine, his chance of being a high-risk person is higher, $r_{22}(10)$, or 44%. Though each individual has improved his chances of survival, the population as a whole contains a larger proportion of high-risk people than before the vaccine.

Bias for Common Epidemiological Models

Most of the examples we have encountered in our study of heterogeneity suggest that traditional assessments will overstate the benefits of interventions. However, this is an empirical rather than a logical proposition. If the covariance between benefit and risk were negative, the bias would be in the opposite direction. To discover an example of negative covariance—what we believe to be the unusual case—simply look for an intervention that offers its greatest benefits to healthier individuals. Programs that benefit employed persons might meet this criterion, since those who are employed are likely to be healthier than the population overall. Presumably, the health benefits to the population at large of workplace health and safety programs are understated. If we restricted our attention to benefits to employed persons and considered other sources of heterogeneity within the employed group, the covariance would probably turn positive again. For example, among employed individuals, those in the least healthy jobs might gain most from an occupational health program.

Two of the most widely used models of mortality both illustrate a positive bias. They are the multiplicative and logistic models. The multiplicative model assumes that the effects of an intervention are independent of other determinants of risk. The intervention merely applies a constant multiple, a, to whatever level of instantaneous risk previously held. The term for this multiple in epidemiology is the risk ratio. Thus

$$\mu_{2j}(x) = a\,\mu_{1j}(x) \qquad \text{where } 0 < a < 1.$$

Frequently the multiplicative model is written with $\mu_{ij}(x)$ as an increasing function of age (such as the Gompertz function), which enables it to reproduce realistic mortality experience from around age 30 onwards.

The logistic model applies a constant factor to the odds of death in a discrete time interval. It has been widely applied in cardiovascular epidemiology. The logistic model requires that for an interval of time Δx starting at time x,

$$q_{2j} = 1/[1 + \exp(b_j + \alpha)] \ ,$$

where b_j is defined so that

$$q_{1j} = 1/[1 + \exp(b_j)] \ .$$

Here q_{ij} is the probability of death in the interval and $\alpha > 0$.

For each of these two widely applied models of risk, the covariance defined in Theorem 1 is positive. Traditional assessments of interventions will overstate their benefits. (See Appendix A for theorems and proofs.)

Conditions When Latent Heterogeneity is Important

Explicit attention to latent heterogeneity has been shown to eliminate a source of bias in predicting the effects of population interventions, but it also increases the complexity of an analysis. In circumstances where the gain in precision is small, the additional complexity may not be worthwhile. As the source of bias in traditional assessments is the changing mixture of risk groups due to an intervention, the magnitude of bias depends on the extent of selection. The selection effect will be substantial if the baseline mortality rate or loss rate is high, the difference in loss rates between risk groups is large, and the intervention has a powerful effect on losses. A high loss rate means that a substantial portion (roughly at least 20%) experiences the event under consideration within the time period at issue. A large difference in loss rates means that the high-risk group has at least twice the risk of the low-risk group; and a powerful intervention is one that cuts the risk of losses by, say, 30% or more.

More formally, manipulating results obtained by Shepard (1977, p. 154) shows that the proportional bias in mortality, $\Delta m(x)/[m_2(x) - m_1(x)]$, is approximated to first order by the product of the following factors:

1) the number of years over which the intervention is considered;
2) the average loss rate over that period in the baseline intervention;
3) the square of the coefficient of variation in initial loss rates among risk groups in the baseline intervention.

In an example developed elsewhere (Shepard and Zeckhauser 1980a), cigarette smoking was an important source of latent heterogeneity in the analysis of the benefits of controlling blood pressure in a hypertensive male from age 50 onward. Suppose we wished to know the intervention's effect at age 75, that is, after twenty-five years. In the baseline intervention, the cohort with a diastolic blood pressure of 110 mm Hg faces a mortality pattern that rises exponentially (at rate of 0.08 per year) from an initial level at age 50 of 20/1,000 per year. Thus the average mortality over the period is .064 per year. Since smokers consuming a pack or more a day have about twice the risk of "others" (nonsmokers and light smokers), the coefficient of variation is 0.33. The approximation gives a proportional error of 17% (25 × 0.064 × 0.33,[2] expressed as a percentage), close to the directly calculated bias of 16% (Shepard and Zeckhauser 1980a, p. 428).

When death is the loss being modeled, then latent heterogeneity is important only where mortality risks are substantial. This condition occurs when advanced age is combined with a chronic condition of moderate importance, as in the example of moderate hypertension above, or where a medical condition imposes extremely high risk, as with survivors of a recent heat attack in our later discussion of sulfinpyrazone. For events other than death, the annual loss rates are much higher. Examples include dropping out of a treatment program, relapsing in a behavior such as abstinence from smoking, or the recurrence of a medical problem such as a hernia. Here the bias within a few years can be substantial. (See Shepard and Zeckhauser 1980a, p. 423.)

Latent Heterogeneity and the Bias in Future Health Cost Estimates

Since the difference between the traditional and standardized assessment lies only in the evolution of risk groups over time, the two procedures will give identical estimates of short-run costs. Heterogeneity, however, is likely to be of significance in assessing the long-run costs of survivors. Let us assume, as we have previously, that the high-risk individuals receive differentially greater benefits. Usually we would also expect them to have the highest expected annual costs should they survive. However, this factor alone is not sufficient to prove the direction of bias in lifetime costs. High-risk individuals are likely to live a shorter time. Hence their costs (even discounted costs) might actually be lesss.

Our policy concern is not with expected lifetime costs themselves, but rather with costs per unit of benefit. We should normally expect high-risk individuals to be at a disadvantage in costs per unit of benefit. If they are, and if the intervention benefits the high-risk group more, then the use of a traditional assessment will be too favorable to an intervention. We shall return to this subject in our discussion of cost-effectiveness.

Drawing Inferences about an Intervention from Population Data

In the preceding section, we assumed that the effect of an intervention on a homogeneous risk group was known, and we established procedures for predicting its effect on a mixed population. In the two examples of this section, we work in the opposite direction. We assume that we have observed the longitudinal effects of an intervention on a population. We want to infer the effects on individuals (or homogeneous risk groups) to understand better the structural effect of the intervention. We also want to be able to extrapolate from observed data to effects for different forms of the intervention, or to time periods beyond those for which we have direct data.

Our first example traces age-specific mortality reductions over the past forty years. The intervention is a general improvement in health conditions (medicine, environment, and standard of living). We believe the observed patterns are suggestive of a heterogeneous population, with higher risk groups receiving greater benefits from mortality reduction.

Sulfinpyrazone (brand name Anturane) is examined second. It is a highly controversial drug for which a major new use has recently been investigated: preventing death in the months after a heart attack. The authors of a randomized study reported that while the drug appeared to be effective initially, it apparently offered no protection beyond six months (Auturane 1980). That inference is not valid, as we shall demonstrate, if those who have died in the absence of the drug are at higher risk after six months than those who would have survived without it.

A method for drawing appropriate inferences in such situations is of general importance. Frequently, when mortality curves of populations under different treatments coincide after a period of time, it is thought that the treatment no longer has any effect. Our models provide a different interpretation. Two opposite effects, one of selection, the other of differential risk, may be canceling each other.

Inferring the Presence of Heterogeneity:
Changes Over Time in U.S. Mortality

Figure 9.1 shows the decline in age-specific death rates by decade for adult white males in the United States from 1930 to 1970. (The age range of 25 through 84 was selected because simple exponential [Gompertz] mortality models can be applied over that range.) It is striking that the reduction in mortality rates around age 70 is only a fourth as large as around age 30. The higher the age group (except for 75–84), the smaller is

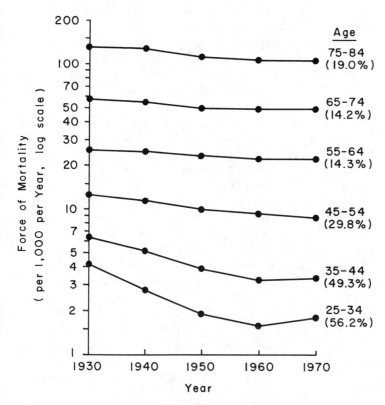

Fig. 9.1   Age-specific mortality rates for white males in the U.S., 1930–70 (with percentage declines in parentheses). Source: see table 9.A.1

the reduction in mortality. Percentage gains in life expectancy follow a similar pattern. Life expectancy at birth has increased from 59.1 to 68.2 years over this period, a gain of 9.1 years or 15%. At age 40, however, the gain in remaining life expectancy is only 2.8 years or 10%. For other sex and color groups, a similar pattern can be reported.

What factors might be responsible for this pattern of gains? Improved nutrition, sanitation, and medical care have undoubtedly figured prominently. Improvements in medical technology in this interval, particularly the introduction of sulfa and antibiotic drugs, may have been of greatest benefit to children and young adults. Yet these drugs have also been important in the treatment of diseases that affect the aged, like bacterial pneumonia. For example, the annual death rate between ages 70 and 75 from pneumonia, influenza, and respiratory disease has fallen by 70% from 1930 to 1960, from 4.6 to 1.4 per 10,000.

We offer an explanation for these data that emerges from our earlier discussion: the population consists of persons at different risk levels, and improvements in medicine, nutrition, and sanitation have interacted with the risk factors that were operating. Suppose that the population consists of persons who fall into one of two classes, "constitutionally weak" or "normal." The weak are especially prone to disease and remain at high risk until they succumb. They have only a small chance of surviving to middle age. The medical and environmental changes since 1930 benefited the normal to some extent, but were of greater benefit to the weak. At earlier ages, we see a substantial decline in death rates because weak persons are being saved. At more advanced ages, we now have a greater proportion of weak persons among the survivors. This structural change partially offsets (though it does not overcome) the fact that the prognosis for each weak and each normal person at every age level has improved; the improvement results in a modest reduction in mortality rates at advanced ages.

Since this hypothetical constitutional weakness may be an unobservable risk factor, our explanation is unlikely to be proved conclusively. Nevertheless, a simple simulation shows that our explanation yields results generally consistent with the data. Our model, described in Appendix B, fits the data markedly better than the competitive best polynomial model with the same number of parameters. Although we do not wish to claim that mortality improvements favoring high-risk persons were the sole factor responsible for the pattern of decline in age-specific mortality rates, it is encouraging that our model generates results consistent with the observed pattern.

We have reported previously (Shepard and Zeckhauser 1980a) that the hypothesis of constitutional weakness can also explain the crossover effect in remaining life expectancy. A national or racial group whose life expectancy at birth is lower (e.g., nonwhites compared to whites) may expeience more powerful selection; this phenomenon can explain why the remaining life expectancy in the United States for nonwhites exceeds that for whites of the same sex beyond about age 70, while whites have a greater life expectancy at birth.

Deducing the Benefits of an Intervention—The Sulfinpyrazone Example

The best way to get a long-term estimate of the benefits of an intervention is to employ a randomized controlled trial. If the size of the population is large, the experiment is well-controlled, the experimental group is perfectly representative of the population to which the actual program will be offered, and the intervention is to be used precisely as tested in the trial, no additional modeling is required. We need merely examine the magnitude of the benefit conferred in the randomized trial.

In many situations, however, we wish to extrapolate from results of a randomized trial to other situations, so we must resort to modeling. *The*

New England Journal of Medicine reported the performance of sulfin-pyrazone (Anturane), a drug designed to offer protection against cardiac deaths to post–heart attack patients (Auturane 1980). Participants in a randomized trial were followed for 24 months. The data in the original article show that sulfinpyrazone offers considerable protection over months 1 through 6. The annualized mortality rate was 5.0% with the active drug as opposed to 10.3% with the placebo. During months 7 through 24, however, there was virtually no difference between the two groups in annualized mortality (4.1% with the drug versus 3.7% with the placebo).

The article concluded that sulfinpyrazone offered protection for six months, but not beyond. The implied clinical recommendation was that physicians should prescribe the drug for a six-month period but no more.[3] Unfortunately, there has been no controlled trial that compares only six months of use of the drug with longer use. All experience to date under a trial is with continued use or no use (placebo). The intervention that appears to be recommended by the data is only a minor modification (as to duration) from the protocol actually followed in the trial. Yet, as we shall see, any assessment of what would happen to a population that stopped taking the drug after six months is at best a careful speculation. The policy implications of this trial depend critically on inferring the benefits to an individual particpant.

We offer a contrary interpretation of the small differential after six months, based on the heterogeneous population concept. (See Shepard and Zeckhauser 1980*b* for a brief informal argument.) Participants within each treatment group vary in their probability of cardiac death. Suppose, as seems plausible, given experience with other interventions, that sulfin-pyrazone was most helpful to those whose mortality rate would have been highest. Then, the drug-treated group surviving at seven months would have a larger proportion of high-risk patients than would the group receiving the placebo. If that is true, then the equal experience of treatment and control groups beyond six months would illustrate a continuing positive benefit from drug treatment.

We have modeled this situation using techniques equivalent to those employed for the U.S. mortality example as described above. With two risk groups we achieved an excellent fit, fitting annualized mortality rates to less than a tenth of a percentage point for both placebo and sulfinpyra-zone groups for months 1 through 6 and 7 through 24. (See Table 9.1.) The high-risk group, which comprises 4.4% of the population at the outset, has a risk of 0.814% per *day*, which is reduced by 75% with sulfinpyrazone. The low-risk group has a mortality of 3.41% per *year*, which is reduced 32% by the drug.[4]

The important point is that the model assumes that the benefit of sulfinpyrazone treatment persists through the entire twenty-four months. Its continuing effectiveness is masked in the aggregate mortality rates

Table 9.1   Annualized Percentage Mortality Rate

Months in Study	Placebo		Sulfinpyrazone	
	Actual	Model	Actual	Model
Up to 6	10.3	10.3	5.0	5.0
7 through 24	4.1	4.1	3.7	3.7

because it is offset by the increased proportion of high-risk survivors in the treatment group. As shown in Table 9.2, which is derived from our model, the proportion of high-risk subjects in the sulfinpyrazone group surviving at six months is three times as great as in the placebo group.

If the world corresponded exactly to our model—though we have too little data to make any claims along this line—discontinuing treatment after six months would lead to an increase in the annualized cardiac mortality rate of the sulfinpyrazone group from 3.7% to 5.5%. In sum, the evidence is consistent with the hypothesis that selection within a heterogeneous population prevented sulfinpyrazone from having superior mortality experience after six months, despite the fact that it was offering continuing benefit.

A controlled trial randomizing for stopping versus continuing therapy beyond six months could test the hypothesis that the selection effect over months 1 through 6 had masked the beneficial impact of the intervention in months 7 through 24. Leaving aside sampling questions, suppose the controlled trial found that patients on continued therapy did better than those discontinuing at six months. Such a finding would provide further information from which to infer the structure of different risk groups, but still might not provide sufficient information to identify uniquely a complex model. The finding would, however, answer the policy-relevant question concerning continued administration of the drug.

Policy Choice with Observed Heterogeneity

With latent heterogeneity, the intellectual challenge is to infer the composition of a population and predict the way it will respond to an intervention. With observed heterogeneity, the problem is one of resource allocation: which individuals should receive which interventions?

Table 9.2   Percentage of Survivors in High-Risk Group

Months After Entry	Placebo	Sulfinpyrazone
0	4.40	4.40
6	1.05	3.11
24	0.01	1.08

Discrimination can be made on the basis of standard demographic variables such as age and sex, medical characteristics such as blood pressure, individuals' preferences, or any other variable that is observable and that helps predict how an individual will respond to an intervention. (Since it will seldom be possible to classify the population into truly homogeneous risk groups, the methods outlined in our discussion of latent heterogeneity will have to be employed to predict how the identifiable subpopulations will respond to an intervention.)

To set priorities for interventions, it is not sufficient merely to estimate benefits; costs must be considered as well. With costs, as with benefits, heterogeneity may play a significant role. Simple extrapolations that do not allow for heterogeneity will provide biased assessments of costs. Recent work on the high-cost users of medical care suggests that expenditures are highly skewed; a small percentage of individuals accounts for a very high percentage of costs (Zook and Moore 1980). For example, the most costly 12% of hospital patients in a year account for more expenditures than the remaining 88%. This suggests that heterogeneity is not only important conceptually when addressing the cost question, but is likely to be of policy consequence. (See Zook, Moore, and Zeckhauser 1981.)

The major question we shall address first is: How should we set priorities for an intervention when we can estimate the benefits and costs it will generate for different members of the population?

Efficient Resource Allocation: The Cost-Effectiveness Paradigm

For simplicity, we shall consider the case in which there is only one intervention that is an alternative to the status quo. We assume that the objective is to maximize total health benefits obtained by all persons treated within a fixed total cost (in present value terms) to the medical care system. The policy must therefore establish priorities among different classes of individuals for receiving the intervention. The policy may also have to determine how much money to spend, which in effect is the question of how far to proceed down the priority list.

In the usual case, health interventions will offer positive net health effects but incur positive net costs. The policymaker then confronts a classic public expenditure problem. To maximize total benefits subject to a budget, he should follow the cost-efectiveness criterion. Cost-effectiveness (CE) is defined as the ratio (Shepard and Thompson 1979):

$$CE = \frac{\text{Net costs paid from the constrained budget}}{\text{Net health benefits}}$$

Net health effects may be expressed in any metric common to all the alternative programs being compared. Two metrics which have proved particularly useful are years of life (improvements in life expectancy) and quality-adjusted life years, QALYs. QALYs generalize the concept of life expectancy to adjust for quality of life, applying different weights according to functional status. (QALY totals may also be adjusted for timing, discounting future years of life. It should be understood that the discounting process is controversial, particularly with noneconomists.)

Net costs of a health intervention are the sum of three costs: (1) the costs of the intervention itself, including treatment of any resulting side effects; (2) the medical costs or savings for the condition at which the intervention is aimed, called related treatment costs; and (3) general induced medical costs for other conditions, as a result of longer life.[5] In the example of the pneumococcal pneumonia vaccine, which we develop later, the intervention cost is that of giving a vaccination. The related treatment savings are the avoided costs of hospitalizations for cases of pneumonia prevented by the vaccination. The general medical costs are the costs incurred during added years of life by persons who would otherwise have succumbed to pneumonia.

The inclusion of long-term treatment costs on a parallel basis might prove controversial. Do we really mean to imply that policy should be formulated with an eye to how much society will have to spend in the future, if an intervention succeeds in saving a life? The uncomfortable conclusion may be yes. If it is cost-effectiveness we seek in medical care, then not immunizing those with expensive chronic diseases might be the preferred policy, even though the immunization might yield them more expected QALYs than it would those who were healthy. The disadvantaged would be denied precisely because their disadvantage will persist in the future.

Suppose the existing pattern of health expenditures has been optimized so that at the margin of expenditure on each individual, each individual receives the same number of QALYs for the last unit of expenditure. The problem when considering a new potential intervention is that preserving an individual carries along his average QALYs and dollar expenditures, not his marginal quantities. If the newly contemplated activity itself entails an expense, we will direct it first to individuals who offer us large inframarginal surpluses.

A related question is how we should account for the nonmedical costs of keeping a person alive, his tax contribution, his drain on social services, etc. Should he survive, his own utility from the resources he expends on himself would be captured in his QALY stream. Conventional cost-effectiveness analyses in health consider medical care as the only constrained resource (see Shepard and Thompson 1979). A more comprehensive analysis would tally non-medical costs. Under this perspective, if a person saved by a health intervention provides (drains) net resources for the rest of society, the QALYs they generate to (cost) others should be added to the individual's QALY stream to get the net benefits to all from his survival.

Consider the extreme case of perfect observability in which each internally homogeneous category could be considered separately for an intervention. If we seek maximum benefits for our budget, we should simply compute the cost-effectiveness value separately for each category. For a category k, we would compute expected costs with and without the treatment; the difference would yield net costs. Then we would do the same with benefits. The cost-effectiveness of applying the treatment to individuals in this category would be

$$(8) \qquad CE_k = \frac{\text{Net costs}_k}{\text{Net health benefits}_k} .$$

Those categories with the most favorable (i.e., lowest) ratio should be accorded the highest priority to receive the intervention.

Dealing with Latent Heterogeneity within Categories

Realistically, it will be impossible to classify the population finely enough to eliminate all within-category heterogeneity. In most of the examples mentioned above, the presence of some important variables could be inferred only by observing responses to interventions. In other instances, physical evidence only becomes available too late to use for predictions. For example, autopsies of soldiers killed in Vietnam showed that 45% of these young men already had some evidence of atherosclerosis, and 5% had severe atherosclerosis (McNamara et al. 1971). The ability to classify individuals on this risk factor prospectively could greatly help us in our ability to intervene to moderate or prevent coronary heart disease. Unfortunately, there is presently no practical mass screen for monitoring of atherosclerosis. Its differential presence, among even young men, is a source of heterogeneity in risk.

To conduct an assessment when latent heterogeneity remains within categories, we must take the same approach to the population within each category as we did earlier to overall latent heterogeneous populations to make predictions and draw inferences. Within each category we start by identifying the prevalence for each (unobservable) group, r_j, and its associated costs and health benefits. Then we compute a standardized assessment for each of the costs and benefits for the entire category. Finally, the cost-effectiveness ratio is computed as average net costs divided by average net health benefits. Thus, we have

$$CE = \frac{\text{average net costs}}{\text{average health benefits}} = \frac{\sum_j r_j \cdot \text{net costs}_j}{\sum_j r_j \cdot \text{QALYs}_j} .$$

(Note that we do not compute a weighted average of the cost-effectiveness ratios for the different groups.)

Although there may be within-category heterogeneity, the procedure yields only a single cost-effectiveness ratio that tells us the marginal return of offering it to all or none within the category. Nevertheless, although different groups within a category cannot be made the basis for policy, it is important to identify them in order to make an accurate assessment of both benefits and costs.

Earlier in this paper we addressed the probable bias with health benefits. We shall also want an accurate assessment of costs, for our real concern is the bias in cost-effectiveness ratios if a traditional assessment if employed. If those who differentially survive because of the intervention in general cost more per QALY (what we might think of as the normal case), then there will be a downward bias—the intervention will be regarded too favorably—and vice versa. A weighted average of cost-effectiveness ratios for the different risk groups summarizes the bias. It is important to note, however, that the weights are not the relative prevalences of the different groups, but rather the relative total QALYs each group offers; that is, CE_k is weighted by $r_k \cdot QALYs_k$. This procedure is equivalent to dividing average costs (weighted by prevalences) by average health benefits (similarly weighted).

Constraint on Expected Costs

Let us put our cost-effectiveness approach into practice. Consider an extreme example of an intervention that reduces an individual's immediate mortality, but has no effect on his morbidity or subsequent mortality. To which risk category should it be offered first? To answer this question we shall have to have four pieces of information:

1) the change in probability of survival for each risk category, call it δ_j;
2) future discounted QALYs within that category for a survivor, $QALYS_j$;
3) future discounted costs for an individual in that category, $COSTS_j$; and
4) the intervention costs (including costs of side effects).

If the goal is to maximize total health benefits within a budgetary constraint on total health care costs, then cost-effectiveness ratio CE_j for ordering risk groups is a special case of (8):

$$CE_j = \frac{\delta_j \times COSTS_j + INTERVENTION\ COST}{\delta_j \times QALYS_j}$$

The interventions should be offered to all risk groups for which CE lies below some established cutoff, the shadow price of QALYS given the budget.

Constraint on the Level of Intervention

In some circumstances resources other than dollars may be constrained. Particularly under present regulatory conditions, hospital days, number of operations, and physician time could each be a constrained resource. Under such conditions, it is no longer appropriate to employ traditional cost-effectiveness ratios comparing dollar cost and health effectiveness. Say the constraint is on the number of procedures undertaken, where δ_j, the decrease in current mortality, is the only health effect. In this case it is appropriate to multiply the δ_js by the net benefits that are offered in each group. (Note they are not multiplied by cost-effectiveness ratios.) Such net benefits are appropriately computed using a shadow price on QALYS, λ. Thus,

(9)   EXPECTED NET BENEFITS$_j$ (in dollar terms) =
          $(\lambda \text{ QALYS}_j - \text{COSTS}_j) \times \delta_j$.

The expected net benefits criterion in (9) would alter priorities indicated by traditional cost-effectiveness ratios in either direction—that is, toward the high-risk or the low-risk group. Suppose an intervention reduced mortality in the high-risk category by 10%, and in the low-risk category by only 5%. Each QALY is assigned a shadow price of 1. As depicted in Table 9.3, with the number of persons who can be offered the intervention constrained, it is appropriate to give the intervention first to the high-risk category in Example A and to the low-risk category in Example B, as the asterisks show.

An analyst who was entranced with the traditional CE ratio approach might mistakenly employ expression (8) to establish priorities. Consider a situation where the intervention cost was low. The analyst would assign the intervention first to the low-risk category in A and to the high-risk category in B, exactly the opposite of the correct assignment defined by (9). Priorities depend upon which resource is constrained.

The same principles apply if interventions reduce morbidity, hence present treatment costs. The formulas are only a trifle more complicated.

Ethical Issues

Throughout history, the cornerstone of the medical ethic has been to provide for each individual the medical care that offers him the most favorable prospects. Although the rising costs of medical care have been a subject of concern since the Commission on the Cost of Medical Care of the 1930s, public policy has rarely explicitly confronted the trade-off between health and resources. Even within current cost containment efforts, such as Certificate of Need and PSROs, the stated goal has been to foster efficiency without a sacrifice in health, rather than to save resources through the purchase of less health. Nevertheless, the notion that health might be too expensive at the margin in some circumstances appears to have been the implicit justification for many programs designed to contain medical expenditures.

Table 9.3   Policy Choice with Constraints on the Level of Intervention

	Example A			Example B		
	Survivors QALYS	Costs	Expected Net Benefits	Survivors QALYS	Costs	Expected Net Benefits
High-risk	10	2	.8*	10	9	.1
Low-risk	11	1	.5	11	7	.2*

*Higher priority risk group.

The Central Ethical Problem

Once factors other than the promotion of health status enter policy decisions, as they do if resource costs are considered at all, a central ethical problem arises. Some policies beneficial to health will be accepted, and others will not. Some may be accepted for certain classes of individuals, but not others. Society, in effect, will refuse to spend resources to provide particular health benefits for particular individuals.

On that ethical basis can such a refusal be made? Are we justified in weighing resource costs to society as a whole against health benefits to an individual, and if so, on what basis should we do the weighing? In this paper we have approached a number of problems of this sort using the tools of cost-effectiveness. But we have not justified that approach, nor have we explored its implications.

Let us take as a premise that policy priorities must be set, and that some interventions that offer some health benefits will have to be forgone. We see three bases on which a set of policies could be justified. First, if there were some widely accepted mechanism for calibrating and valuing health benefits in dollar terms, we could merely apply it and choose the set of policies that maximized expected total societal benefits. (This is the approach of benefit-cost analysis.) An appropriate mechanism for such valuations does not now exist, however, and is not likely to in the near future.

A second basis for discrimination would emerge if all members of a society agreed to a set of policies for health promotion (and for financing those policies), weighing in their own minds the associated benefits and costs. Such agreement is unlikely to be forthcoming, however, for reasons linked to the theme of the paper. Heterogeneity in the population, if observable, will hurt us if consensus is our goal. The candidate for a heart-bypass operation would certainly like to have that procedure covered by health insurance, but most of society might think the benefits not worth the resources entailed; the 60-year-old bachelor might not support an immunization campaign against childhood diseases, whereas young mothers would be staunch partisans.

A third approach might be possible if we could get around the disagreement problem that arises because each individual judges from his own position. Suppose we could return all individuals to a hypothetical original position, where no one knew who he would end up to be, and each attached equal probability to the possibility that he would be each member of society. We could ask a representative citizen at this position what mixture of policies he would prefer. Presumably he would seek to maximize his overall expected welfare, taking both health and resource costs into account. In effect, before he is conceived, before his genetic and environmental factors become set, we would ask an individual to lay out a health protection plan for his whole life, not knowing whether he would be born with a birth defect, contract cancer, live in a polluted city, or work as a truck driver. He would be free to choose how much money would be devoted to medical care in any circumstance, but would know that he would have to pay for that care—through taxes, insurance, or out-of-pocket. His program would include items that offered high benefits relative to their costs. In essence, he would be using some form of cost-effectiveness analysis to maximize his expected utility, not knowing his future identity. As a real life approximation to an original position, we might think of a committee of young faculty members at a university trying to draw up to a health plan for the junior faculty. They would not know who would be paralyzed in an auto accident, who would have a baby with spina bifida, who would want to spend many weekly hours with a psychiatrist.

Whatever ethical sustenance one secured from an original position argument, and however far back that original position extended, one should not expect that such policies would be widely accepted once the world played out its lotteries, i.e., once heterogeneity revealed itself, identifying who was healthy, whose health was threatened, and who was sick with which disease. A program designed on cost-effectiveness principles might lead to a highly unequal ex post result. Even though we could point out that the set of outcomes merely reflected the gambles that a disinterested individual would have been willing to take, we should still expect the actual losers to be grumblers. Consider an individual whose unfavorable health prognosis made it undesirable to spend more resources to increase his chance for short-run survival. He could justifiably complain that his welfare is being disregarded.

Our thought experiment started by placing the individual in a contingent claims market for resources, the states of the world to depend on his health. The discomforting reality is that following the efficiency dictate of securing an equal marginal return from all expenditures, he might find it optimal to transfer more resources towards high-health rather than low-health states. If so, once lotteries are played out, arguments about ex post inequity will arise. With contingent claims markets for money, in contrast to health, the individual will almost invariably wish to allocate his major transfers to situations where he would otherwise have low income. The ethical problem of transfering more to the better as opposed the worse off does not arise. So too, it would be more convenient if the nature of the health production process were such that expected utility maximization required allocating resources in a pattern inversely proportional to health status. Any lack of negative covariance between health state and the return to expenditure generates automatic dissatisfaction.

In practice, we should expect society to respond to such dissatisfaction and the accompanying charges of inequity. Through its political processes, society would attempt to devote additional resources to poor-outcome states even though the return to those resources was below what could be secured in high-outcome states. Moreover, in contrast to the framework we laid out above, we would expect that policy-makers would play down the importance of anticipated future expenditures for medical care in the decision process. That is, even though we might have accepted the lottery before the fact, we would smooth out dissatisfaction afterwards through an inefficient overallocation to poor-outcome states. Natural redistributional proclivities would reinforce any tendencies in this direction.

Social Acceptability of Categories

A number of the categories that are most useful in making medical predictions, notably sex and race, have become lightning rods for debate in a variety of policy areas. We can foresee circumstances where strong political pressures, clothed in ethical trappings, would be brought to bear requiring or prohibiting that medical priorities be set or not be set on the basis of such categorizations.

It is not beyond belief that there may be social pressures to stop classifying data or basing medical predictions on these highly charged variables. This is particularly likely if such predictions may ultimately influence policy choices, hence the expenditure of public funds. Forces for knowledge suppression will be more difficult to counteract if, as seems likely, the classifying variables, though correlating with risk, are either not causal or cannot be shown to be causal.

Appropriate Output Measure

Even if we accept cost-effectiveness analysis unquestioningly, and can avoid conflicts on appropriate risk categories, we still do not escape ethical dilemmas. What output measures should be employed as we assess the benefits of interventions?

An alternative quite different in spirit from the original position approach might suggest that the QALY, or some other indicator that could be calibrated appropriately, is a basic unit of accounting. Not to maximize QALYs would be to throw away a resource that society valued. Thus, we should be coverting the outputs of health policies into QALYs, just as we often convert alternative energy supplies into barrels of oil when making energy policy decisions. A major difficulty with a universal unit approach is that QALYs are not readily transferable from individual to individual. As we choose among health policies, we are basically shuttling QALYs from one individual to another. Securing maximum total QALYs and then dividing up the pie is not a possibility.

A second difficulty relates to appropriate ways for tallying QALYs within an individual. Apart from discounting considerations, should individuals be (or are they) risk averse on the total health received over a period of years? The QALY measure merely adds across years, perhaps with discounting.[6] Utility functions for longevity and health status can contain risk aversion, but they are more difficult to interpret (see Pliskin, Shepard, and Weinstein 1980). But risk aversion may raise other ethical questions. We might find ourselves denying additional years of health to individuals who had already lived a long time, to provide lesser sums of comparable years to individuals who were younger. Would that be appropriate? We have no resolution for these problems; we merely wish to suggest that intriguing ethical issues persist.

Process

If the resources involved were small, as they may be with any single intervention, then we could afford the luxury of avoiding triage decisions. However, the costs of life preservation across all areas of our modern technological society are becoming so great that protecting ourselves against unpleasant aspects of our value system may be too costly. When the point is reached at which self-delusion is no longer worthwhile, if it has not been already, we believe that a policy of expected QALY optimization per dollar of expenditure will garner strong intellectual support.

It would have been more comfortable for us to avoid this issue, as most cost-effectiveness analyses have in the past. Given the vibrant societal debate about cost-effectiveness and risk-benefit analyses, ducking did not seem desirable.[7] If the Secretary of Health and Human Resources has to decide whether to provide federal funds for heart transplantation, as Secretary Patricia Harris did, we should be willing to discuss the principles that underlie such decisions. Often we can avoid the most discomforting aspects of life-versus-resource decisions. If we can remove the resources before we know who would receive them, then in effect we can capitalize on an original position type of self-interest on the part of citizens who concur. Thus, we can close down hospital beds or limit CAT scanners. (Here is not the place to judge the effectiveness of such programs for ultimate resource savings.) However, if individuals had a good idea of who the beneficiaries of those resources might be, prior limitations might be more difficult. Thus, we would have a harder time eliminating a machine that benefited an identified group, such as asthma patients, than a CAT scanner that offered the same total benefits per year at the same cost. As Schelling (1968) has eloquently stated, an identified life is often valued more highly than a statistical life.

Voluntary versus Involuntary Behavior

One final element may be relevant to our ethical analysis. When we devise our optimal portfolio of policies, we consider whether an individual is denied some interventions to improve his health because of actions over which he had no control. If a choice must be made, most citizens would prefer to grant an intervention to an individual who incurred a respiratory disease because he lived in a polluted area than to one who contracted the disease by smoking. Our society seems to believe that individuals should suffer the consequences of their sins, but not of variables over which they have no control.

In practice, the determination of what behaviors are voluntary is quite complex. Consider smoking. Can we be confident that there is not a strong genetic predisposition towards smoking, at least for some individuals? And would we really say that smoking is voluntary if environmental factors beyond an individual's control, such as smoking parents, strongly predicted smoking behavior? From an economic standpoint perhaps the best way to judge the voluntariness of any behavior would be to determine how much an individual engaging in it would have to be paid to reduce or give it up. Alternative numeraires would convey different impressions. To get a numeraire other than dollars, we could look at a smoker's hourly wage, and determine how many minutes of work he would do for a cigarette. (Because smoking is habit forming, we might also inquire about willingness-to-pay before a person has taken up the practice. Voluntariness may depend on the time that a behavior is examined.)

Denying or offering a health program based on an individual's behavior will have the side effect of changing incentives. Thus, denying an intervention to a smoker will in effect raise the price of smoking, which could have an effect on behavior if the elasticity of demand for smoking were high. In examining the effects of a pattern of interventions, we must look not only at what they accomplish vis-a-vis the status quo, but also how they change the status quo by affecting individual's behaviors.[8]

We already tax smoking. Denying some medical interventions would represent a further tax.[9] From the standpoint of efficiency, we want to make sure that the total tax equals the social cost of smoking, which depends largely on the subsidized health care services smokers receive.

Age is obviously a variable beyond an individual's control, and on that basis many would find it morally objectionable as a basis for assigning priority to medical benefits. Our view, however, is that it may be one of the less objectionable variables, assuming that society is designing a fairly stable set of interventions over time. Each individual has his opportunity to be young, when he may be given priority for some interventions, and old, when he may be denied them. (The reciprocal argument applies, of course; with the pneumonia vaccine the intervention is provided first to the old.) Providing less in the way of medical resources to the old is not unlike providing them less in the way of educational resources. Those resources simply provide more value when the individual is young.

Summary

In medicine there is a well established tradition of basing predictions on factors such as age, sex, and race. This tradition, however, is accompanied by the ethic that the regimen that is medically best for the patient should be prescribed. This tradition may be challenged if constraints on resources force us to forego some medically beneficial, albeit cost-ineffective treatments. Attention to medical expenditures is now forcing us to set priorities.

Any apparatus that selects one health-promoting policy over another raises profound ethical questions. Common analytic tools for making such choices, such as cost-effectiveness analysis, though often innocuous in appearance, carry strong moral overtones. Such techniques are often justified in policy debate on the grounds that they are the only logical or rational method of choice. Whatever the validity of that argument, it alone is unlikely to be sufficient to carry the day in the highly contentious policy arena. Direct ethical support is needed as well, and could perhaps be elicited by an original position argument—that is, by persuading individuals that they themselves would choose a cost-effectiveness approach were their own distinctive characteristics and interests still undetermined.

The Choice of Health Policies

Given an understanding of the concept of heterogeneity, how should we design policy interventions? We illustrate the relevance of our concepts by considering a pneumonia vaccination program. We then summarize what strike us as the more important policy implications of our analysis.

Pneumococcal Pneumonia Vaccine: An Illustration of Heterogeneity

The pneumonia vaccine example illustrates several concepts. (1) Medical research can generally identify numerous risk factors for elevated incidence and/or case fatality from a disease (observed heterogeneity); for some factors, the effects can be quantified; other risk factors can only be assessed qualitatively. (2) The cost-effectiveness framework can be applied to observed classes for which quantitative data are available to establish priorities among them for an intervention. (3) Within standard categories of observed heterogeneity (such as age), there is substantial latent heterogeneity which biases traditional assessments of benefits. (4) Assessments that control for observed heterogeneity, but not for unobserved characteristics, estimate the benefits and cost-effectiveness of an intervention too favorably.

Pneumococcal Pneumonia Vaccine

"Pneumovax" is a vaccine designed to prevent the fourteen most common valences of pneumococcal pneumonia; it was licensed by the Food and Drug Administration in 1977. A cost-effectiveness analysis of the vaccine by the Office of Technology Assessment (OTA 1979; Willems et al. 1980) provides much of the foundation for this example. By conservative estimates pneumococcal pneumonia is responsible for between 5,000 and 17,000 deaths per hear in the United States (Willems et al. 1980).

Age is an observable risk factor with marked influence on both the incidence and case fatality rate. The largest set of population-based data that illustrate its importance comes from Massachusetts for 1921 through 1930, during which time lobar pneumonia was a reportable disease (Heffron 1979, pp. 300–305). Age patterns for lobar pneumonia can serve as a reasonable indicator for all pneumococcal pneumonia.[10] Using Heffron's (1979, p. 299) assumption that reported cases were about half of total cases, we infer that the attack rate per year in the Massachusetts data rose steadily with age in adults, from 13 per 1,000 persons aged 20–29 to 80 per 1,000 persons aged 80 and above. Data from this pre-antibiotic era reveal that the case fatality rate also rose with age. The combined effect of both factors is that the age-specific death rate due to lobar pneumonia in persons aged 80 and above was twenty-six times as high as that for persons aged 20–29. Recent data confirms that similar patterns still hold for the antibiotic era. Incidence rises with age (beyond the teens) (Oseasohn et al. 1978), as does case fatality (Sullivan et al. 1972; Austrian and Gold 1964).

A number of other observable characteristics have been found to be associated with differences in the age-specific death rate from pneumonia (and presumably pneumococcal pneumonia in particular). These include sex (males are higher), race (nonwhites are higher), overcrowded housing (Heffron 1979, p. 316), probably alcoholism (Heffron 1979, p. 158), fatigue, acute infections such as influenza, and chronic diseases such as infections of the respiratory tract and cancer (Heffron 1979, p. 335). Austrian and Gold (1964) and Mufson (1974) found that case fatality rates from bacteremic pneumococcal pneumonia were above average in persons with chronic lung disease, chronic heart disease, chronic renal failure, diabetes mellitus, and other metabolic disorders. In view of such associations, the approved indications for administering Pneumovax include "persons having severe chronic physical conditions such as chronic heart disease, chronic bronchopulmonary disease, chronic renal failure, diabetes mellitus or other chronic metabolic disorders; persons in chronic care facilities; persons convalescing from severe disease." (OTA 1979, p. 54).

Application of Observed Heterogeneity: Disaggregating by Age

Using vital statistics data, the OTA (1979) study computed the expected health gain from vaccination against pneumococcal pneumonia as a function of age in terms of dicounted quality-adjusted life years. Averting death in a younger person generally confers a larger remaining life expectancy than in an older person. Nevertheless, for pneumococcal pneumonia vaccination, the increase in discounted QALYs for a randomly chosen person rises with age. The gain for a young adult aged 25–44 is 3.7 healthy *hours* (.00042 adjusted years); for a person aged 65 and above, the gain is ten times as large—38.1 healthy hours (.00435 years).

Application of the Cost-effectiveness Paradigm

The OTA pneumonia vaccine study employed age as the primary risk category. The cost-effectiveness of pneumococcal pneumonia vaccination, according to their results, improves with age from $77,200 per QALY for children aged 2–4 to $1,000 per QALY for persons aged 65 and over. The policy implication is clear. Vaccination should probably be encouraged for persons aged 65 and above, but probably not recommended for children. Under current FDA-approved indications, the vaccine is recommended for persons aged 50 and over (OTA 1979, p. 54).

Analyses derived from the OTA (1979), study show how policy-relevant risk factor classification can improve policy performance dramatically. If the pneumococcal pneumonia vaccine were offered to all persons aged 50 and above, and age-specific acceptance rates were similar to those observed for influenza vaccine in 1975, then a national program for the United States would cost $50 million and return a total of 27,200 QALYs. (Using linear interpolation, this calculation allocated three-fourths of the costs and benefits of the age category 45 through 64 to persons 50 and above). If age could not be used for allocating vaccinations, for example because it was considered an invidious basis for discrimination, and the vaccine were offered to all persons regardless of age, the cost would be $150 million (three times as high), while the number of QALYs would be increased by only 15%.

CE Ratios for Other Observable Risk Factors
for Pneumoccocal Pneumonia

In the absence of quantitative data relating chronic disease and risk of death due to pneumococcal pneumonia, the OTA (1979, p. 77) reported an illustrative hypothetical calculation. Persons with selected cardiovascular, bronchopulmonary, renal, and metabolic diseases were termed high-risk persons. It was assumed that their instantaneous mortality rate was five times as high as that for the general population, a factor derived from Fitzpatrick, Neutra, and Gilbert's (1977) study. The proportion of deaths due to pneumococcal pneumonia in high-risk persons was assumed to be 1.8 times as high as in the general population. The OTA illustration found, consistent with the FDA-approved indications for the varrine, that vaccination was more cost-effective in high-risk persons than in low-risk persons. Among persons aged 25 to 44, for example, the illustrative cost-effectiveness ratio was $7,300 per QALY in high-risk persons, compared to $33,000 per QALY in low-risk persons.

Latent Heterogeneity within Age Categories: Effect on Estimated Benefits

Even if the vaccine were offered to all persons of a given age regardless of risk status, stratification by risk group would be important when estimating the benefits. For a 50-year-old male, for example, we calculated that failure to stratify by other risk factors overestimates the gain in undiscounted life expectancy from the vaccine by about 20%. We interpolated this estimate from Table 4 in Shepard and Zeckhauser (1980a).[11] If mortality were the outcome measure, rather than life expectancy, the bias would be even more substantial, particularly at advanced ages. The bias in mortality at age 80, for example, is three times as large as the bias in life expectancy (Shepard 1977).

Latent Heterogeneity and the Bias in future Health Costs Estimates

Within each age group, high-risk person are those with other chronic conditions. A vaccination program increases the proportion of high-risk persons among survivors compared to what it would have been in the absence of intervention. Because of their chronic diseases, high-risk persons are likely to incur higher medical costs than the general population of the same age. Residents of chronic care facilities provide an extreme example. They are expected to reap large benefits from the vaccine (they were specifically mentioned in the FDA-approved indications for use), but their medical costs are probably five to ten times higher than others of the same age without the chronic condition.

In the OTA (1979) study, high-risk persons were estimated to comprise 17.3% of the population aged 25 to 44 (Bell 1980). Suppose the lifetime average prevalence of high-risk persons from a standardized assessment (weighted by the number of survivors and discounted) were 10% compared to 5% from a traditional assessment. Assume that the expected medical costs of the high-risk persons were five times that of low-risk persons. Expected medical costs for the mixed population would be 1.5 times that of low-risk persons under the standardized intervention compared to 1.25 times under the traditional assessment. Thus standardized cost-effectiveness estimates would be 20% (.25/1.25) more favorable than traditional estimates due to the bias in cost estimation alone. If the effectiveness bias were also overstated by 20% of the true value (as in the example above), the total bias would be approximately 44% too favorable.

Conclusion

Heterogeneity among members of the population in their responsiveness to interventions—both beneficial and detrimental—is a central issue for policy-making. Battery plants are forced to make themselves safe for female workers in childbearing years, and air pollution standards are set supposedly to protect the most susceptible members of the population. Flu innoculations are dispensed according to a priority schedule based primarily on medical need. Regulatory and reimbursement policies for health care may start by examining the consequences for health and resources of offering different procedures to different categories of individuals, and then try to channel patients and providers in cost-effective directions. Society is increasingly confronting the salient issue of crafting policies that recognize heterogeneity within the population. This analysis provides some lessons and principles that might make that confrontation more productive.

We hope to have demonstrated that: (1) population heterogeneity may be an important factor even when heterogeneity is latent; (2) traditional methods for predicting the benefits of interventions in populations with latent heterogeneity are biased; (3) the bias generally causes us to overstate the benefits and cost-effectiveness of helpful interventions; (4) attention to latent heterogeneity can improve inferences and extrapolations about the benefits alternative policies will provide to populations; (5) observed heterogeneity raises interesting efficiency and equity issues in setting priorities for receipt of interventions; and (6) calculations attending to heterogeneity are feasible as a guide when making policy choices.

Appendix A

A Comparison of Traditional and Appropriately Standardized Assessment Procedures

In this appendix we prove that under common assumptions, the traditional assessment underestimates mortality and overestimates life expectancy under beneficial intervention.

After three lemmas, Theorem 2 presents two important extensions of Theorem 1, which we proved earlier in the text. Under two very common models of mortality, the multiplicative and logistic models, the covariance is positive so that the traditional assessment overstates the reduction in mortality. Finally, it can easily be shown that life expectancy behaves inversely to mortality. We state as a corollary to Theorem 2 that these two models overstate life expectancy. Similarly, they overstate gains in life expectancy. This statement applies also to expected utility and to quality-adjusted life expectancy.[12] Thus, if the traditional assessment gives too low an estimate of mortality, it gives too high an estimate of life expectancy.

Lemma 1[13]

Let

$$| \ell_{jk} | = \begin{vmatrix} \ell_{1j} & \ell_{1k} \\ \ell_{2j} & \ell_{2k} \end{vmatrix} .$$

Then

$$\Delta m(x) = \frac{1}{\ell_1. \, \ell_2.} \sum_j \sum_{k>j} r_j r_k (\mu_{2k} - \mu_{2j}) | \ell_{jk} | .$$

Proof

By definition,

$$\Delta m(x) = \sum_j \mu_{2j} \frac{r_j \ell_{2j}}{\ell_2.} - \sum_j \mu_{2j} \frac{r_j \ell_{1j}}{\ell_1.} .$$

Now substitute the definition of $\ell_i.$ (from equation (2)) and write the result over a common denominator:

$$\Delta m(x) = \frac{1}{\ell_1. \, \ell_2.} [\sum_j \sum_k \mu_{2j} r_j r_k \ell_{2j} \ell_{1k}$$

$$- \sum_j \sum_k \mu_{2j} r_j r_k \ell_{1j} \ell_{2k}] .$$

Now the first double summation above can be rewritten with j and k reversed, since the indices of summation are symmetrical. The sum becomes

$$\sum_j \sum_k \mu_{2k} r_j r_k \ell_{1j} \ell_{2k}$$

Now the two double sums can be combined, yielding

$$\Delta m(x) = \frac{1}{\ell_1. \, \ell_2.} \sum_j \sum_k (\mu_{2k} - \mu_{2j}) r_j r_k \ell_{1j} \ell_{2k} .$$

For $j = k$ the summand vanishes. We can group the terms with each combination of different subscripts to obtain

$$\Delta m(x) = \frac{1}{\ell_1.\ell_2.} \sum_j \sum_{k>j} (\mu_{2k} - \mu_{2j}) r_j r_k (\ell_{1j}\ell_{2k} - \ell_{2j}\ell_{1k}).$$

Rewriting the last factor as a 2×2 determinant yields the required formula.

Q.E.D.

Lemma 2

Let risk groups j be numbered in order of increasing risk in the absence of treatment at the initial time $x_0, \mu_{1j}(x_0)$. Assume that this numbering ranks risk groups in order of increasing risk for all ages $x, x_0 < x < x_1$. Let treatment lower mortality according to a multiplicative model, i.e., for all x

(A.1) $\mu_{2j}(x) = a\mu_{1j}(x)$ where $0 < a < 1$.

Then for $k > j, |\ell_{jk}| > 0$.

Proof

Inserting (A.1) into the definition of the survival function (1) gives

$$\ell_{2j} = \exp\left[- \int_0^x a\mu_{1j}(t) dt\right] ,$$

so

$$\ell_{2j} = \ell_{1j}^{\,a} .$$

Thus

$$|\ell_{jk}| = \begin{vmatrix} \ell_{1j} & \ell_{1k} \\ \ell_{1j}^a & \ell_{1k}^a \end{vmatrix} = \ell_{1j}\ell_{1k}^a - \ell_{1j}^a\ell_{1k}$$

$$= (\ell_{1j}\ell_{1k})^a [\ell_{1j}^{(1-a)} - \ell_{1k}^{(1-a)}] .$$

The ordering of the risk classes implies that for $k > j, \mu_{1j}(x) < \mu_{1k}(x)$ so $\ell_{1j} > \ell_{1k}$ and $\ell_{1j}^{(1-a)} > \ell_{1k}^{(1-a)}$. Thus $|\ell_{jk}| > 0$.

Q.E.D.

Lemma 3

Assume the risk groups j can be ordered as in Lemma 2. Divide the interval (x_0, x) into n equal intervals. Let $\ell_{jk}^{(m)}$ be the survival matrix on the mth interval. Assume that on each interval m, treatment lowers mortality according to a logistic model, i.e., treatment lowers the odds of mortality by a constant fraction. For an interval of Δx starting at time x.

$$q_{2j} = 1/[1 + \exp(b_j + \alpha)] \; ,$$

where b_j is defined such that

$$q_{1j} = 1/[1 + \exp(b_j)]$$

and $\alpha > 0$. Let $\ell_{jk}^{(m)}$ be the survival matrix on the mth interval and let ℓ_{jk} be the composite survival matrix over the interval (x_0, x) with element ℓ_{ij} defined by

$$\ell_{ij} = \prod_{m=1}^{n} \ell_{ij}^{(m)} \; .$$

Then $|\ell_{jk}| > 0$.

Proof

We proceed by induction. Let $\ell_{jk}^{(M)}$ denote the composite survival matrix over the first M intervals, so $\ell_{ij}^{(M)} = \prod_{m=1}^{M} \ell_{ij}^{(m)}$.

1) First, we establish that if $M = 1, |\ell_{jk}^{(1)}| > 0$. To show this we substitute

$$|\ell_{jk}^{(1)}| \;\; = \frac{\exp(b_j)}{1 + \exp(b_j)} \times \frac{\exp(b_k + \alpha)}{1 + \exp(b_k + \alpha)}$$

$$- \frac{\exp(b_j + \alpha)}{1 + \exp(b_j + \alpha)} \times \frac{\exp(b_k)}{1 + \exp(b_k)} \; .$$

The above expression may be rewritten with a common denominator as

$$[\exp(b_j + b_k + \alpha)]\Big\{[1 + \exp(b_j + \alpha)][1 + \exp(b_k)]$$

$$- [1 + \exp(b_j)][1 + \exp(b_k + \alpha)]\Big\} \; ,$$

divided by the product of the four denominators above. Since the denominator and the first factor in the numerator are all positive, the sign of $|\ell_{jk}^{(1)}|$ is identical to the sign of the factor in braces, which simplifies to

(A.2) $\qquad$ $[\exp(b_k)][1 + \exp(b_j - b_k)\exp(\alpha)$

$\qquad\qquad - \exp(b_j - b_k) - \exp(\alpha)]$.

The steps below establish that the factor in braces is positive. Since for $k > j, g_{ij} < g_{1k}, b_j > b_k$. Thus

$$1 - \exp(b_j - b_k) > 0 .$$

Further, $\alpha > 0$ implies

$$1 - \exp(\alpha) < 0 .$$

The second factor in (A.2) is the product of the two inequalities above, not shown to be positive. This completes the proof for $M = 1$.

2) Next we establish that if $|\ell_{jk}^{(M)}| > 0$, then $|\ell_{jk}^{(M+1)}| > 0$. We define the matrices

$$A = \ell_{jk}^{(M)}$$
$$B = \ell_{jk}^{(m+1)}$$

and

$$C = \ell_{jk}^{(M+1)} .$$

Then $C_{ij} = A_{ij}B_{ij}$. Since $|A| > 0$ by hypothesis,

(A.3) $\qquad$ $A_{11}A_{22} - A_{12}A_{21} > 0$.

Since B represents the survival matrix for a single period under a logistic model, $B > 0$ by an argument identical to the one above for $|\ell_{jk}^{(1)}| > 0$. Thus

(A.4) $\qquad$ $B_{11}B_{22} - B_{12}B_{21} > 0$.

Since all the elements of logistic model survival matrices are positive, the factors $B_{11}B_{22}$ and $A_{12}A_{21}$ and both positive. The inequalities (A.3) and (A.4) may be multiplied by positive factors without changing their direction. Multiplying (A.3) by the first factor and (A.4) by the second and adding the resulting inequalities gives

$$A_{11}A_{22}B_{11}B_{22} - A_{12}A_{21}B_{12}B_{21} > 0$$

or

$$C_{11}C_{22} - C_{12}C_{21} > 0 .$$

Thus $|C| > 0$. This completes the proof of the inductive part of the lemma.

Q.E.D.

Theorem 2

Assume the risk groups can be ordered as in Lemma 2, and assume that treatment lowers mortality according to a multiplicative model (as defined in Lemma 2) or a logistic model (as defined in Lemma 3). Then

$$\Delta m(x) > 0 \ .$$

Proof

Under either the logistic or multiplicative models, Lemmas 2 and 3 establish that for $k > j, |\ell_{jk}| > 0$. The ordering of risk groups assumes that for $k > j, \mu_k - \mu_j > 0$. With $\Delta m(x)$ written as a summation in Lemma 1, each of the summands is the product of positive factors. Thus, $\Delta m(x) > 0$. Q.E.D.

Corollary

Let $\overset{\circ}{e}_{x_0}$ and $\overset{\circ}{e}'_{x_0}$ be the life expectancy at age x_0 using mortality forces $m_2(x)$ and $m'_2(x)$, respectively. Life expectancy is defined by

$$\overset{\circ}{e}_{x_0} = [\int_{x_0}^{\infty} \ell_2(x)\,dx]/\ell_2(x_0) \ .$$

Assume treatment lowers mortality according to a multiplicative or a logistic model. Then

$$\overset{\circ}{e}_{x_0} > \overset{\circ}{e}'_{x_0} \ .$$

Proof

From the definition of the survival function in equation (1), it is clear that lower mortality rates lead to higher survival rates. Life expectancy, as the integral of the survival function, changes in the same direction as the survival function.
Q.E.D.

Appendix B

Model for Changes in Age-Specific Mortality Over Time

We assume that the cohort of white males attaining age 30 at the beginning of each decade consists of a specified proportion of normal and weak persons. Within both the normal and weak groups there is an average annual mortality, $\mu_{ij}(30)$, for the decade of age centered at age 30 (i.e., between 25 and 34 inclusive). The risk category j denotes a normal ($j = 1$) or weak person ($j = 2$). Here the "treatment" i corresponds to the year in which mortality is observed (1930 through 1970); it is an index of the state of medical technology and environmental conditions.

We further assume that the base mortality force (i.e., the rate at age 30) for each group changes in a log-linear relation with calendar year, i,

$$\ell n\, \mu_{ij}(30) = \ell n\, \mu_{1930,j}(30)$$

$$+ \left[\ell n\, \frac{\mu_{1970,j}(30)}{\mu_{1930,j}(30)} \right] \left[\frac{i - 1930}{1970\text{-}1930} \right] \; .$$

Our model treats an individual's risk category as being fixed for life. It has mortality within a risk category in decade i increasing with age x (in years) according to the Gompertz curve, one of the simplest expressions for mortality,

$$\mu_{ij}(x) = [\mu_{ij}(30)]\, e^{b(x - 30)} \; .$$

Finally, we assume that the proportion of high-risk persons in the cohort at age 30 in year i, $r_{i2}(30)$ increases in a log-linear relationship with time. (The increase is postulated because reductions in infant and child mortality have presumably benefited weak persons most.)

$$\ell n\, r_{i2}(30) = \ell n\, r_{1930,2}(30)$$

$$+ \left(\ell n\, \frac{r_{1970,2}(30)}{r_{1930,2}(30)} \right) \left(\frac{i - 1930}{1970\text{-}1930} \right) \; .$$

Our model thus has seven free parameters: the parameter b; $\mu_{ij}(30)$ for $i = 1930$ and 1970, and for $j = 1$ (normal) and 2 (weak); and $r_{i2}(30)$ for $i = 1930$ and 1970. (The values for $r_{i1}(30)$ are not free since by definition they equal $1\text{-}r_{i2}(30)$.) Using this model, we computed age- and risk-specific mortality rates for cohorts attaining age 30 from 1890 to 1970, inclusive. Using those rates, the proportion of each risk cohort surviving each decade was estimated by

$$\ell_{i + 10,j}(x + 10) = \ell_{ij}\exp[-10\mu_{ij}(x)] \; ,$$

where

$$x = 30 \text{ is the starting age,}$$

and

$$\ell_{ij}(30) = 1 \quad \text{for all } i,j \; .$$

The overall survival for an age cohort is the weighted sum of the survival fractions for each risk group, weighted by the proportion of the cohort initially at each risk level,

$$\ell_{1.}(x) = (1 - c)\ell_{i,1}(x) + c\ell_{i,2}(x)$$

where

$$c = r_{i-(x-30),2}(30) \ .$$

From these age-specific survival rates, corresponding average annual mortality rates can be derived:

$$m_i(x) = -\frac{1}{10} \ell n \frac{\ell_{i+10,.}(x + 10)}{\ell_{i.}(x)} \ .$$

Since the risk factor j is not directly observable, only $m_i(x)$ and not $\mu_{ij}(x)$ could be observed.

The test of our model is how closely the calculated $m_i(x)$ replicate reported age-specific mortality rates. We selected as a goodness of fit criterion the weighted absolute percentage error. If $m_i^*(x)$ is the true mortality for age x in year i, the percentage error is $|m_i^*(x) - m_i(x)|/m_i^*(x)$. Reasoning that low rates were more subject to random variation, being based on fewer deaths, we wanted to give greater weight to errors on the higher mortality rates. We therefore chose as a weighting factor for each error $\sqrt{m_i^*(x)}$. Our final criterion was thus the weighted sum of percentage errors. Our sample consisted of mortality rates at the beginning of each decade from 1930 to 1970, inclusive, and for decades of age centered at 30 through 80, inclusive. They are shown in Table 9.A.1. The number of observations was thus $5 \times 6 = 30$. Using a nonlinear optimization routine[14] we found the following values for the parameters:

$$r_{1930,2}(30) = .1085, \ r_{1970,2}(30) = .3849,$$
$$\mu_{1930,1}(30) = 2.4023, \ \mu_{1930,2}(30) = 19.2184,$$
$$\mu_{1970,1}(30) = 1.8686, \ \mu_{1970,2}(30) = 1.6853, \ \text{and}$$
$$b = .0798$$

where mortality rates are in deaths per thousand per year.[15] The mortality rates calculated with our model are presented above the empirically observed rates in Table 9.A.1. The weighted average of the percentage errors was 6.23%.

Since reported mortality data are based on census rather than sample data, test of statistical significance are not appropriate to judge goodness of fit.[16] The weighted average error of 6.23% may be contrasted with the fit achieved by a naive model with the same number of parameters—a general quadratic function of i and x (with six free coefficients) multiplied

Table 9.A.1   Predicted and Actual Mortality Forces for White Males by Decade 1930 to 1970[a]

Ten Years Centering At Age		Annual Mortality Rates Per 1,000[b]					Percentage Reduction 1930–1970
		1930[c]	1940	1950	1960	1970	
30	model	4.1	3.4	2.8	2.3	1.8	56.1
	actual	4.1	2.8	1.9	1.6	1.8	56.2
40	model	7.2	6.6	5.8	4.9	4.0	43.7
	actual	6.7	5.1	3.9	3.3	3.4	49.3
50	model	12.8	12.5	11.7	10.5	9.0	29.0
	actual	12.6	11.4	10.0	9.3	8.8	29.8
60	model	26.4	25.1	24.1	22.6	20.2	23.3
	actual	25.8	25.1	23.5	22.3	22.1	14.3
70	model	58.5	55.0	51.8	48.9	45.2	22.7
	actual	57.2	54.4	49.5	48.9	49.1	14.2
80	model	130.0	120.0	114.6	107.7	101.0	22.3
	actual	130.0	127.8	111.2	106.4	105.3	19.0

[a]Actual rates are from National Office of Vital Statistics (1956), National Vital Statistics Division (1963), and National Center for Health Statistics (1974). Annual rates (q) per 1,000 per year were converted to instantaneous rates (μ) per 1,000 per year by the equation

$$\mu = -1000 \; \ell n (1 - q/1000).$$

[b]Except for 1970, the rate represents the average of three years centered at year indicated. For 1970, the rate was extrapolated at the average of 1968–70 plus the increase from 1967 to 1968.
[c]Death registration states only (Continental U.S. excluding Texas).

by an exponential function of x, giving a seventh parameter. Using the same nonlinear optimization procedure, the polynomial could achieve a fit with a weighted percentage error of 9.27%.[17]

Notes

1. For certain combinations of rates of increase for an individual's risk and heterogeneity among individuals' risk, there will be no change in observed loss rates over time. Shepard (1977) examined the special case of an exponential increase in the individual's loss rate (at rate k per year) and a gamma distribution for initial loss rates among individuals (with scaling parameter β). There is an infinite number of pairs (where k equals β) for which the two effects precisely balance.

2. To simplify notation, the age variable x in $\mu_{ij}(x)$, $r_{ij}(x)$, $g_{ij}(x)$, and $\ell_{ij}(x)$ will sometimes be omitted.

3. A factor extraneous to our analysis—the eligibility of patients and classification of deaths (Kolata 1980)—has created a further complication in assessing the validity of this

particular experiment; we shall leave this problem aside and assume all classifications are correct.

4. It is not automatic that our model would be able to fit the observed data. It is true that we have six parameters (four loss rates which are constant over time, μ_{ij}, and two initial prevalences, $r_j(0)$, for i and j equal to 1 and 2), with which to fit only four pieces of data, the four rates in Table 9.1. However, the equality constraint

$$r_1(0) + r_2(0) = 1$$

effectively gives another piece of data, and all six parameters are also subject to nonnegativity constraints. Nevertheless, since our solution is not a corner solution, an infinite number of parameter combinations (of one dimension) within a narrow range of the foregoing values are consistent with the data and restrictions. Here, as in other examples, limited population data are not sufficient to identify a structure of risks exactly, but can suggest possibilities that merit further investigation.

5. Strictly speaking, straight addition is only appropriate in a society that organizes itself so that public expenditures are fungible among these three categories, and so that public and private expenditures are equally productive of welfare at the margin. Moreover, prices would have to reflect resource costs. The world is not perfectly efficient in this way. However, we are not prepared to discuss here what nonequal weights should be established for these different classes of resources.

6. In a subsequent analysis we hope to look at issues of discounting. For an individual who has time preference for QALYs, to discount seems unambiguous. However, this seems to us to provide no guidance on how to weight QALYs to different generations.

7. We do sidestep one point here, the role of income distribution. Our line of argument, for the most part, assumes that individuals have relatively equal incomes, or that for other reasons income distribution is not a primary issue in relation to these decisions. How to deal with income-distributional concerns is a matter for another day.

8. We might wish to judge the taxing of smoking from an original position. Then, if elasticities of response are low, the taxes primarily represent a random financial imposition. Given risk aversion, a population some of whose members might smoke might choose not to have smoking taxes if such taxes had little effect on behavior. (We have asked a number of academic audiences their attitudes on smoking taxes. Over 90% of their members favor such taxes. This is less surprising when we observe that only a small fraction of such audiences smokes.)

9. As a means of raising the overall price of cigarettes, the strategy of denying beneficial medical interventions to smokers as opposed to raising per pack taxes would be reinforced if, as seems likely, the marginal damage of a cigarette is greater for smokers who manifest signs of illness or increased risk, as opposed to those who appear healthy.

In practice, some interventions targeted along grounds of cost-effectiveness, such as the large scale Multiple Risk Factor Intervention Trial, will favor smokers. If that is the predominant pattern, cigarette taxes should be correspondingly higher.

10. Various studies have shown that practically all (96%) of lobar pneumonia is pneumococcal (Heffron 1979, pp. 1–2). Moreover, the other major type of pneumonia, bronchopneumonia, is believed to have a similar case fatality rate (Heffron 1979, p. 304).

11. In computing the entries for the table, the odds ratio (approximately equal to the risk ratio) for the risk indicator "other chronic disease" for all causes of death was taken to be 5. This is the ratio Shepard (1977) found applied to survivors of heart attacks compared to the general population of the same age and sex, and the ratio Fitzpatrick, Neutra, and Gilbert (1977) used for high-risk candidates for gall bladder surgery. The risk ratio for the "treatment," vaccination, was taken to be 1.012. This ratio is calculated as 1 plus the product of the share of deaths due to pneumococcal pneumonia (39,600/2,000,000) times the percentage of pneumococcal pneumonias due to valences in the vaccine (75%) times the efficacy of the vaccine against included valences (80%) in the OTA (1979) study.

12. See, for example, Pliskin, Shepard, and Weinstein (1980).

13. Emmett Keeler helped us generalize this lemma to a risk factor with more than two categories.

14. The procedure was steepest descent with synthetic derivatives under the IBM scientific subroutines package.

15. Our fitting procedure did not prevent the mortality rates in the two risk groups from crossing. It so happened with the best-fitting parameters that the mortality of the weak risk group actually fell below that of the normal risk group in the last decade (between 1960 and 1970). The mortality of the weak group could have been constrained not to fall below that of the normal group with little degradation of the fit.

16. It is worthwhile to note that our model can also reproduce the backwards J-shaped decline in mortality rates as a function of age. (That is, the decline is greatest at low ages, but greater at the highest ages than for some in the middle.) To get a significant rise for the older ages, the percentages of high-risk individuals, the r_{i2}s, would have to be much greater than those estimated here.

17. The equation is

$$m(x,y) = (.1335x^2 + .1259xy + .0197y^2$$
$$- 1.4771x - .9543y + 9.4501)e^{.6848x} ,$$

where $m(x,y)$ is mortality force per thousand per year, $x = \frac{1}{10}$ (age–30) is age decade, and $y = \frac{1}{10}$ (year–1870) is calendar decade.

There is no unequivocal methodology by which one should compare two quite dissimilar models. That ours, with its logical underpinnings, outperformed the polynomial formulation is reassuring. The triumph is perhaps enhanced because this was the only functional form that was tried for our model.

References

Anturane Reinfarction Trial Research Group. 1980. Sulfinpyrazone in the prevention of sudden death after myocardial infarction. *New England Journal of Medicine* 302:250–56.

Austrian, R., and Gold, J. 1964. Pneumococcal bacteremia with especial reference to bacteremic pneumococcal pneumonia. *Annals of Internal Medicine* 60:759–76.

Bell, J.C. 1980. Personal communication to the authors.

Fitzpatrick, G.; Neutra, R.; and Gilbert J.P. 1977. Cost-effectiveness of cholecystectomy for silent gallstones. In J.P. Bunker, B.A. Barnes, F. Mosteller, eds., *Costs, risks, and benefits of surgery*. New York: Oxford University Press.

Fuchs, V.R. 1974. *Who shall live?* New York: Basic Books.

Heffron, R. 1979 (reprint of 1939 edition). *Pneumonia, with special reference to pneumococcus lobar pneumonia*. Cambridge: Commonwealth Fund, Harvard University Press.

Kolata, G.B. 1980. FDA says no to Anturane. *Science* 208:1130–32.

McNamara, J.J.; Molot, M.A.; Stremple, J.F.; et al. 1961. Coronary artery disease in combat casualties in Vietnam. *Journal of the American Medical Association* 216:1185–87.

Mufson, M.A.; Kruss, D.M.; Wasil, R.E.; and Metzger, W.I. 1974. Capsular types and outcome of bacteremic pneumococcal disease in the antibiotic era. *Archives of Internal Medicine* 134:505–510.

National Center for Health Statistics. 1974. *Vital statistics of the United States 1972.* Vol. 2, sec. 5, life tables. DHEW Publ. No. (HRA) 75–1147. Washington: U.S. Government Printing Office.

National Office of Vital Statistics. 1956. Death rates by age, race and sex, United States 1900–1953: selected causes. *Vital statistics–special reports* 43(1). Washington: U.S. Government Printing Office.

National Vital Statistics Division, 1963. *Vital statistics of the United States 1960.* Vol. 2, part A. Washington: U.S. Government Printing Office.

Neuhauser, D. 1977. Elective inguinal herniorrhaphy versus truss in the elderly. In J.P. Bunker, B.A. Barnes, F. Mosteller, eds., *Costs, risks, and benefits of surgery.* New York: Oxford University Press.

Office of Technology Assessment, U.S. Congress, 1979. *A review of selected federal vaccine and immunization policies.* Washington.

Oseasohn, R., et al. 1978. Pneumonia in a Navajo community. *American Review of Respiratory Diseases* 117:1003.

Pliskin, J.S.; Shepard, D.S.; and Weinstein, M.C. 1980. Utility functions for life years and health status. *Operations Research* 28:206–24.

Schelling, T.C. 1968. The life you save may be your own. In S.B. Chase, Jr., ed., *Problems in Public Expenditure Analysis.* Washington: Brookings Institution.

Shepard, D.S. 1977. Prediction and incentives in health care policy. Ann Arbor: Xerox University Microfilms (#77–11744).

Shepard, D.S., and Thompson, M.S. 1979. First principles of cost-effectiveness analysis in health. *Public Health Reports* 94:535–43.

Shepard, D.S., and Zeckhauser, R.J. 1977. Heterogeneity as a factor in surgical decision making. In J.P. Bunker, B.A. Barnes, F. Mosteller, eds., *Costs, risks, and benefits of surgery.* New York: Oxford University Press.

Shepard, D.S., and Zeckhauser, R.J. 1980a. Long-term effects of intervention to improve survival in mixed populations. *Journal of Chronic Diseases* 33:413–33.

Shepard, D.S., and Zeckhauser, R.J. 1980b. The anturane reinfarction trial (letter). *New England Journal of Medicine* 303:49.

Sullivan, R.J.; Dowdle, W.R.; Marine, W.M., et al. 1972. Adult pneumonia in a general hospital. *Archives of Internal Medicine* 129:935–42.

Willems, J.S.; Sanders, C.R.; Riddiough, M.R.; and Bell, J.C. 1980. Cost-effectiveness of vaccination against pneumococcal pneumonia. *New England Journal of Medicine* 303:553-59.

Zeckhauser, R.J., and Shepard, D.S. 1976. Where now for saving lives? *Law and Contemporary Problems* 40(Fall):5–45.

Zook, C.J., and Moore, F.D. 1980. The high cost users of medical care. *New England Journal of Medicine* 302:996–1002.

Zook, C.J.; Moore, F.D.; and Zeckhauser, R.J. 1981. "Catastrophic" health insurance—a misguided prescription? *The Public Interest* 62(Winter):66–81.

10 Medical Care, Medical Insurance, and Survival Probability: The True Cost of Living

Theodore C. Bergstrom

In this paper we construct a much simplified model of private and public social decision-making related to health care and health insurance. The model is designed to clarify the logical relationships among health insurance plans, life insurance and annuities, consumption, medical care and nursing care. The paper characterizes an efficient allocation of health care and describes decentralized insurance markets that would sustain an efficient allocation. The analysis is similar in spirit to papers by Arrow (1976) and Nordquist and Wu (1976) presented at an earlier NBER conference on health economics.

Individual Preferences and Plans

Imagine an economy with a large number of consumers, all with identical tastes. There are two commodities, bread and medical care. Tomorrow each consumer will receive a free medical check-up. There are n possible diagnoses, $d_1, \ldots, d_n$. Suppose that today the individuals' probability distributions over diagnoses are independent and identically distributed. Let π_i be the probability that any particular consumer will be diagnosed as being in condition i. We assume a simple medical technology. Regardless of the diagnosis, there are at most two things that can happen. The patient can painlessly be restored to perfect health or he can die. Let the conditional probability that someone with diagnosis i who receives m_i units of medical care will survive be $\theta_i(m_i)$.

Suppose that the amount of medical care that a person receives can be made to depend on the diagnosis of his condition. Suppose further that the amount of bread that he (or his heirs) receive can depend both on his

Theodore C. Bergstrom is at the University of Michigan.

diagnosis at the check-up and on whether he survives after being given the chosen medical care. As we shall later see, provision of these contingent commodities could be arranged either through a centrally imposed national plan or in a decentralized way through health insurance and life insurance contracts. Possible medical histories can be denoted d_i^0 and d_i^1, where d_i^0 denotes the event that one receives diagnosis i and proceeds to die and d_i^1 denotes the event that one survives after having diagnosis i. A *consumption strategy* is a vector (M, B) where $M = (m_1, \ldots, m_n)$ specifies the amount m_i of medical care that the consumer will receive if his diagnosis is i and where $B = (b_1^0, \ldots, b_n^0, b_1^1, \ldots, b_n^1)$ specifies the amounts b_i^0 and b_i^1 of bread that the consumer will consume if he has diagnosis i and dies or lives, respectively. We will sometimes speak of M as the consumer's "medical strategy" and B as his "bread-consumption strategy."

In the model discussed, the probability that the consumer has a particular medical history is determined by the medical strategy M. The probability of medical history d_i^x given strategy M will be denoted $\pi(d_i^x | M)$. In particular, our assumptions imply that

$$(1) \qquad \pi(d_i^1 | M) = \pi_i \theta_i(m_i)$$

and

$$(2) \qquad \pi(d_i^0 | M) = \pi_i(1 - \theta_i(m_i)).$$

The von Neuman-Morgenstern expected utility of a consumer with medical strategy M and consumption strategy B will take the form:

$$(3) \qquad V(M, B) = \sum_{x=0,1} \sum_{i=1}^{n} \pi(d_i^x | m_i) u(d_i^x, m_i, b_i^x).$$

Recall that we have assumed that medical care does not affect utility directly, and that after medical treatment one is either restored to perfect health or one is dead. Thus the utility function takes the special form

$$(4) \qquad u(d_i^x, m, b_i^x) \equiv u_x(b_i^x)$$

where $u_1(b)$ can be viewed as the utility of the prospect of surviving and consuming b units of bread and $u_0(b)$ as the utility of the prospect of dying and leaving b units of bread to one's heirs. From equations (1) – (4) we see that (3) could be written equivalently as:

$$(5) \qquad V(M, B) = \sum_{i=1}^{n} \pi_i \theta_i(m_i) u_1(b_i^1)$$
$$+ \sum_{i=1}^{n} \pi_i(1 - \theta_i(m_i)) u_0(b_i^0)$$

In most of the remaining discussion we will assume that the functions $u_0(\cdot)$, $u_1(\cdot)$ and $\theta_i(\cdot)$ are nondecreasing and concave. Assuming concavity of $u_1(\cdot)$ and $u_0(\cdot)$ is equivalent to assuming that the consumer is either risk-averse or risk-neutral with respect to bets that leave his survival probability unchanged. Concavity of the θ_i's means diminishing marginal returns to medical care.

An Optimal Centrally Imposed Health Plan

Having examined individual preferences for medical care and bread, we now consider the options available to the economy as a whole. We begin by considering a hypothetical central authority that seeks to impose a national health care plan. We define an "allocation of consumption strategies" to be a list, $(M^1, B^1, \ldots, M^K, B^K)$, of the consumption strategies, (M^k, B^k), of each consumer k. Since all consumers have identical preferences and the same prospects before their medical check-ups, it is of special interest to consider those allocations that offer all consumers the same consumption strategy. Such an allocation plan will be called a "uniform national plan."

Let $[M, B]$ be a uniform national plan that offers each consumer the consumption plan, (M, B). If the number of consumers is K, then the total number of persons with diagnosis i will be $K\pi_i$ and total consumption of medical care by these persons will be $K\pi_i m_i$.[1] Therefore average per capita consumption of medical care in the economy is certain to be

$$(6) \qquad \bar{M}(M) \equiv \sum_{i=1}^{n} \pi_i m_i$$

if the national plan is (M, B).

If the national health plan is $[M, B]$, then the proportions of the population with medical histories d_i^1 and d_i^0 are $\pi_i \theta_i(m_i)$ and $\pi_i(1 - \theta_i(m_i))$ respectively. Therefore average per capita bread consumption in the economy will be

$$(7) \qquad \bar{B}(M, B) \equiv \left[\sum_{i=1}^{n} \pi_i \theta_i(m_i) b_i^1 + \sum_{i=1}^{n} \pi_i(1 - \theta_i(m_i)) b_i^0 \right]$$

The feasibility of a national plan depends on whether the economy can supply the total outputs $K\bar{M}$ and $K\bar{B}$. We develop here a very simple model of the productive capacity of the economy which is sufficient to illustrate the relevant issues. Suppose that it is technically possible to convert one unit of bread into $\frac{1}{p}$ units of medical care (regardless of how many units are produced). Suppose also that there is an initial endowment of b units of bread per consumer and that each consumer who survives produces h units of bread (or equivalently $\frac{h}{p}$ units of medical care). Consumers who do not survive produce nothing.

The proportion of the population that survives is determined by M and can be written as:

$$(8) \qquad \Pi_1(M) \equiv \sum_{i=1}^{n} \pi_i \theta_i(m_i).$$

Therefore the total output of the economy measured in terms of bread must be $K[\tilde{b} + \Pi_1(M)h]$ and the constraint on the feasibility of a national plan, (M, B) is:

$$(9) \qquad K[\bar{B}(M,B) + p\bar{M}(M)] = K[\tilde{b} + \Pi_1(M)h].$$

Since consumers are assumed to have identical preferences, we don't need a deep welfare economic analysis to arrive at a criterion for an optimal national plan. We simply seek a national plan that maximizes the utility of a representative consumer on the set of feasible plans. We define an "optimal uniform national plan" to be a uniform national plan (M, B) that maximizes $V(M, B)$, as defined in equation (5) subject to the feasibility constraint expressed in equation (9). Although an optimal uniform national plan is, by definition, not dominated by any feasible allocation that treats all consumers in exactly the same way, there might conceivably be feasible allocations that are Pareto superior to an optimal uniform national plan but treat some consumers differently from others. The following proposition, which is proved in the Appendix to this paper establishes conditions under which there are no such allocations.

Proposition 1

For an economy, let the set of feasible allocations of consumption strategies be those such that:

$$\sum_{k=1}^{K} [\bar{B}(M^k, B^k) + p\bar{M}(M^k, B^k)]$$

$$= K\tilde{b} + \sum_{k=1}^{K} \Pi_1(M^k)h.$$

If $u_0(\cdot)$ and $u_1(\cdot)$ are concave functions, then an optimal uniform national plan is Pareto optimal.

Proposition 1 enables us to restrict our search for an equalitarian Pareto optimal allocation strategy to the set of uniform national plans. Proposition 2 allows us to further limit the domain of search.

Proposition 2

Let $V(M, B)$ be the expected utility function defined in equation (5). If $u_0(\cdot)$ and $u_1(\cdot)$ are concave functions, and if (M, B) satisfies the feasibility constraint (9), then there exists a consumption plan, $(M, \bar{B})$ such that $V(M, \bar{B}) \geqq V(M, B)$, $(M, \bar{B})$ satisfies the budget equation (24), and $\bar{B} = (\bar{b}^1, \ldots, \bar{b}^1, \bar{b}^0, \ldots, \bar{b}^0)$ gives the consumer or his heirs a bread consumption that depends only on whether he lives or dies and not on the diagnosis he receives.

Proof:

If (M, B) satisfies (24), then so does $(M, \bar{B})$ where $\bar{B} = (\bar{b}^0, \ldots, \bar{b}^0, \bar{b}^1, \ldots, \bar{b}^1)$

where $\qquad \bar{b}_1 = \left(\dfrac{1}{\Pi_1(M)}\right) \sum\limits_{i=1}^{n} \pi_i \theta_i(m_i)$ and $\bar{b}_0$

$$= \left(\dfrac{1}{1 - \Pi_1(M)}\right) \sum\limits_{i=1}^{n} \pi_i(1 - \theta_i(m_i)).$$

Furthermore, since $u^1(\cdot)$ and $u^0(\cdot)$ are concave functions, it must be that

$$u_1(\bar{b}^1) \geq \left(\dfrac{1}{\Pi_1(M)}\right) \sum\limits_{i=1}^{n} \pi_i \theta_i(m_i) u_1(b_i^1) \text{ and } u_0(\bar{b}^0)$$

$$\geq \left(\dfrac{1}{1 - \Pi_1(M)}\right) \sum\limits_{i=1}^{n} \pi_i(1 - \theta_i(m_i)) u_0(b_i^0).$$

It follows that $V(M, \bar{B}) \geq V(M, B)$.
Q.E.D.

Proposition 2 enables us to confine our search for an optimal uniform national plan to those plans in which consumption strategies, (M, B), have the property that

(10) $\qquad b_1^1 = b_2^1 = \ldots = b_n^1 \equiv b^1$

and

(11) $\qquad b_1^0 = b_2^0 = \ldots = b_n^0 \equiv b^0.$

We will frequently denote such strategies by (M, b^0, b^1) and their expected utilities by

(12) $\qquad V(M, b^0, b^1) \equiv \Pi_1(M) u_1(b^1) + (1 - \Pi_1(M)) u_0(b^0).$

The definition (7) of $\bar{B}(M, B)$ reduces to

(13) $\qquad \bar{B}(M, b^0, b^1) = [\Pi_1(M) b^1 + (1 - \Pi_1(M)) b^0]$

Thus the constraint in (9) can be written

(14) $\qquad K[\Pi_1(M) b^1 + (1 - \Pi_1(M)) b^0$

$\qquad \qquad + p\bar{M}(M)] = K[\bar{b} + \Pi_1(M) h].$

or equivalently:

(15) $\qquad \Pi_1(M)(b^1 - h) + (1 - \Pi_1(M)) b^0 + p\bar{M}(M) = \bar{b}.$

Assuming that the derivatives, $u_0'(\cdot), u_1'(\cdot)$, and $\theta_i'(\cdot)$, exist everywhere, the first-order necessary conditions for an interior solution to the maximization of (12) subject to (15) can be written:

(16) $$u_1'(b^1) = u_0'(b^0)$$

and for $i = 1, \ldots, n$:

(17)
$$\frac{\partial \Pi_1(M)}{\partial m_i} \left[\frac{u_1(b^1) - u_0(b^0)}{u_1'(b^1)} \right] = p \frac{\partial \bar{M}(M)}{\partial m_i}$$
$$+ \ [b^1 - h - b^0] \ \frac{\partial \Pi_1(M)}{\partial m_i}$$

From the definitions of $\Pi_1(M)$ and $\bar{M}(M)$, it follows that (17) is equivalent to

(18)
$$\theta_i'(m_i) \left[\frac{u_1(b^1) - u_0(b^0)}{u_1'(b^1)} + h + b^0 - b^1 \right] = p.$$

Equations (16) and (17) have simple and rather interesting interpretations. Equation (16) require that the marginal rate of substitution between bread contingent on being alive and bread in one's estate should be unity. Notice that this is true regardless of the probability distribution of medical histories. Typically one would expect the functions $u_1(\cdot)$ and $u_0(\cdot)$ to have the property that if $u_1'(b^1) = u_0'(b^0)$ then $u_1(b^1) > u_0(b^0)$. Operationally this means that at an optimal solution, consumers would prefer a higher survival probability to a lower one.

On the left side of (17) the rate of change of survival probability due to an increment in m_i is multiplied by an individual's marginal rate of substitution between survival probability and bread. This expresses the rate at which an individual would be willing to make a small exchange of bread for an increase in the amount of medical care he would receive if he had diagnosis i. On the right side of (17) the term $p\frac{\partial \bar{M}}{\partial m_i}$ is the direct resource cost of increasing m_i while the term $[b^1 - h - b^0]$ $\frac{\partial \Pi_1(M)}{\partial m_i}$ represents the per capita effect on net bread requirements due to the fact that increasing m_i also increases the proportion of the population that is consuming b^1 and producing h units of bread, and reduces the proportion of the population whose heirs must be given b^0 units of bread.

From equation (18) it follows that:

(19)
$$\theta_1'(m_i) = \ldots = \theta_n'(m_n)$$

$$= p \div \left[\frac{u_1(b^1) - u_0(b^0)}{u_1'(b^1)} + h + b^0 - b^1 \right].$$

Thus we see that an optimal health plan has the property that the marginal contribution of medical care to the conditional probability that one survives contingent on a diagnosis is equalized for all diagnoses.

Equation (19) emphasizes a fact that, on reflection, should have been obvious from the start. An optimal health plan will exclude some technically possible medical treatments on the grounds that they are too expensive. Equalizing θ_i' across diagnoses certainly need not imply equalizing θ_i across diagnoses. In fact, in an optimal medical plan there may be diagnoses for which only a small amount of medical care is given and from which recovery is then unlikely even though there exists a medical cure which, though very expensive, would ensure that persons with this diagnosis survive.

A Decentralized Economy with Actuarially Fair Insurance

We now consider provision of medical services and bread by means of private markets. We will show that an optimal national plan could also be reached as a competitive equilibrium with appropriate insurance markets. Let each consumer own an initial endowment of $\bar{b}$ units of bread. If and only if he survives, he will produce an additional h units of bread. As before we assume that one unit of bread can always be costlessly converted into one unit of medical care.

In this paper, a "health insurance plan" is a contract that specifies a vector $\mu = (\mu_1, \ldots, \mu_n)$ where a positive μ_i is the net amount, measured in units of bread, that the insurance company will pay a consumer enrolled in the plan if the consumer has diagnosis i. If μ_i is a negative number, then the consumer will pay the insurance company a net amount μ_i if the consumer's diagnosis is i. The expected value of payments to the consumer under health insurance plan μ is then $\sum_{i=1}^{n} \pi_i \mu_i$.

If transactions costs for the insurance company can be ignored and if the number of identical consumers is large enough so that the variance in the proportion of the population with a given diagnosis is negligible, then, to a close approximation, in competitive equilibrium, insurance companies must be willing to offer any actuarially fair health insurance plan. Thus an equilibrium health insurance plan must satisfy

(20)
$$\sum_{i=1}^{n} \pi_i \mu_i = 0$$

Here we will treat insurance plans that are commonly called "life insurance" and "annuities" as two different kinds of bets that could be made between a consumer and a life insurance company. For us, a life insurance-annuity plan is a contract that states payments (measured in units of bread) to be made from the insurance company to the consumer (or vice versa) where the direction of net payments depends on whether the consumer lives or dies. Any life insurance-annuity plan is described by a vector (α^0, α^1). If α^0 is positive and α^1 is negative, the plan is called "life insurance". If the signs are reversed, the plan is called an "annuity". If (α^0, α^1) is life insurance, then the consumer's estate receives a net payment (measured in units of bread) of α^0 if he dies, while the consumer pays the insurance company α^1 if he survives. If (α^0, α^1) is an annuity, then the consumer pays the insurance company a net amount α^0 if he dies and receives a net amount α^1 if he survives.

As we did with health insurance, we assume away transactions costs and asymmetries of information, and assume that statistical variation in the proportion of the population having any particular life history is negligible. Therefore the supply side conditions for competitive equilibrium require that life insurance-annuity plans be actuarially fair. In this case, the condition for actuarially fair insurance is a bit more complicated than in the case of health insurance. One's survival probability depends on how much medical care he would obtain in the event of each possible diagnosis. Therefore actuarially fair life insurance-annuity plans must in general have rates that depend on the amount of medical care one will purchase in each contingency. On the face of it, it would seem unreasonably difficult to enforce a contract, signed between the insurance company and the consumer before the physical check-ups are made, requiring the consumer to purchase no less or more medical care in the event of each contingency than is specified in the life insurance or annuity contract.

As it turns out, a consumer who has chosen an insurance plan that gives him the best ex ante prospects possible with an actuarially fair plan will not in the event of any realized diagnosis be able to afford a combination of bread and medical care that he prefers ex post to that provided by the consumption strategy chosen ex ante. This is true even if medical insurance takes the form of lump sum payments contingent on one's diagnosis and not tied to any particular level of purchases of medical care. Therefore an insurance company can offer actuarially fair rates simply by setting its rates as a function of one's health insurance plan.

A "consumer's consumption strategy" is a vector (M, B) where $M = (m_1, \ldots, m_n)$ states the amount, m_i, of medical care that the individual plans to consume if he has diagnosis i and where $B = (b_1^0, \ldots, b_n^0, b_1^1, \ldots, b_n^1)$ states the amount b_i^0 of bread that he plans to consume if he has diagnosis i and dies and the amount b_n^1 that he plans to consume if he has diagnosis i and lives. We call M his medical care strategy and B his bread consumption strategy. A consumer's "insurance plan" consists of a health insurance plan and a life insurance-annuity plan. A "health insurance" plan is a vector $\mu = (\mu_1, \ldots, \mu_n)$ where μ_i represents net payments (possibly negative) measured in units of bread from a health insurance company to a consumer in the event that he has diagnosis i. A "life insurance-annuity" is a vector (α^0, α^1) where α^0 and α^1 represent net payments (possibly negative) from a life insurance company to a consumer respectively if he dies or lives. A health insurance plan, μ, is "actuarially fair" if it satisfies equation (20). A life insurance-annuity plan is actuarially fair *contingent on M* if

$$(21) \qquad \Pi_1(M)\alpha^1 + (1 - \Pi_1(M))\alpha^0 = 0$$

The insurance plan $(\mu, \alpha^0, \alpha^1)$ is said to be actuarially fair *with respect to M* if it is actuarially fair, and (α^0, α^1) is actuarially fair with respect to M.

Suppose a consumer chooses the insurance plan $(\mu, \alpha^0, \alpha^1)$. If he then has diagnosis i and survives, his net receipts from the insurance companies will be $\mu_i + \alpha^1$. He has an initial allotment of $\bar{b}$ units of bread and he produces an additional h units. Thus he has a total number of $\mu_i + \alpha^1 + \bar{b} + h$ units of bread to be spent on medical care and bread. His purchases in this event must therefore satisfy

$$(22) \qquad pm_i + b_i^1 = \mu_i + \alpha^1 + \bar{b} + h$$

If a consumer has diagnosis i and dies, he and his estate receive $\mu_i + \alpha^0$ from the insurance companies. He has an initial endowment of $\bar{b}$ and produces no additional bread. Therefore his purchases in the event of this medical history must satisfy

$$(23) \qquad pm_i + b_i^0 = \mu_i + \alpha^0 + \bar{b} \ .$$

An insurance plan μ, (α^0, α^1) is said to "sustain" the consumption plan (M, B) if equations (22) and (23) are satisfied for $i = 1, \ldots, n$.

All of the propositions to be developed here assume implicitly the special structure of our model. However, each of them can be extended in a fairly transparent way to much more general models.

Proposition 3

If the consumption plan (M, B) can be sustained by an insurance plan, $(\mu, \alpha^0, \alpha^1)$ that is actuarially fair with respect to M, then (M, B) must satisfy the following budget constraint:

$$(24) \qquad \sum_{i=1}^{n} \pi_i [pm_i + \theta_i(m_i)(b_i^1 - h) \\ + (1 - \theta_i(m_i))b_i^0] = \bar{b}$$

Proof:

For each i, multiply both sides of equation (22) by $\pi_i \theta_i(m_i)$ and both sides of equation (23) by $\pi_i(1 - \theta_i(m_i))$ and add the resulting $2n$ equations. This yields:

$$(25) \quad \sum_{i=1}^{n} \pi_i[pm_i + \theta_i(m_i)b_i^1 + (1 - \theta_i(m_i))b_i^0]$$

$$= \sum_{i=1}^{n} \pi_i[\mu_i + \theta_i(m_i)\alpha^1 + (1 - \theta_i(m_i))\alpha^0 + \theta_i(m_i)h] + \bar{b}$$

Since the insurance plans are assumed to be actuarially fair, equations (20) and (21) apply. Using (20) and (21) and slightly rearranging terms one obtains (24) from (25).
Q.E.D.
From Propositions 2 and 3, we arrive at the following result.

Proposition 4

Let (M, b^0, b^1) be a consumption plan that maximizes

$$(26) \quad V(M, b^0, b^1) \equiv \Pi_1(M)u_1(b^1) + (1 - \Pi_1(M))u_0(b^0)$$

over all $(M, b^0, b^1) \geq 0$ such that:

$$(27) \quad \bar{M}(M) + \Pi_1(M)(b^1 - h) + (1 - \Pi_1(M))b^0 = b.$$

Then $V(M, B) \geq V(M', B')$ if (M', B') can be sustained by an insurance plan that is actuarially fair with respect to M'.

Proposition 5

If (M, b^0, b^1) satisfies equation (27), then there exists an insurance plan, $(\mu, \alpha^0, \alpha^1)$ that sustains (M, b^0, b^1) and is actuarially fair with respect to M.

Proof:

We prove Proposition 5 by exhibiting the claimed insurance plan. Given M and (b^0, b^1), let:

$$(28) \quad \mu_i = p[m_i - \sum_{i=1}^{n} \pi_i m_i] \quad \text{for } i = 1, \ldots, n$$

$$(29) \quad \alpha_1 = p \sum_{i=1}^{n} \pi_i m_i + b^1 - h - \bar{b}$$

$$(30) \quad \alpha_0 = p \sum_{i=1}^{n} \pi_i m_i + b^0 - \bar{b}$$

It is easily verified that the insurance plans defined in (28), (29), and (30) satisfy equations (20), (22), and (23). Furthermore, if equation (27) is satisfied, it is a matter of straightforward verification to show that equation (21) is satisfied. Therefore (M, B) is sustained by the insurance plan $(\mu, \alpha^0, \alpha^1)$, the health insurance plan, μ, is actuarially fair, and the life insurance-annuity plan, (α^0, α^1), is actuarially fair contingent on M. Q.E.D.

From Propositions 4 and 5 we deduce:

Proposition 6

If (M^*, b^{0*}, b^{1*}) solves the constrained maximization problem posed in Proposition 5, then (M^*, b^{0*}, b^{1*}) maximizes $V(M, B)$ on the set of consumption strategies (M, B) that can be sustained by an insurance plan that is actuarially fair contingent on M.

Supply considerations require that a competitive equilibrium insurance plan be actuarially fair. Demand conditions require that an equilibrium insurance plan sustain a consumption strategy that consumers like at least as well as any consumption plan sustainable by another insurance plan. These considerations, together with Proposition 1, suggest the appropriateness of the following definitions.

We define a "competitive consumption strategy" for a consumer to be a strategy (M^*, b^{0*}, b^{1*}) that solves the constrained maximization problem posed in Proposition 4. A "competitive equilibrium insurance plan" is defined to be an insurance plan, $(\mu^*, \alpha^{0*}, \alpha^{1*})$ that sustains the competitive consumption strategy (M^*, B^*) and is actuarially fair with respect to M^*.

Proposition 7

If preferences are continuous and if $\Pi_1(M)$ is bounded away from 0 and from 1 for all M, then there exists a competitive equilibrium insurance plan.

Proof:

If $\Pi_1(M)$ is bounded away from 0 and 1, it is easy to see that the set of consumption plans $(M, b^0, b^1) \geq 0$ satisfying (27) is closed and bounded. Continuity of preferences implies continuity of the function, $V(M, B)$. Since continuous functions take maxima on compact sets, there exists a competitive consumption strategy, (M^*, B^*). According to Proposition 5, there exists an actuarially fair insurance plan, $(\mu^*, \alpha^{0*}, \alpha^{1*})$ that sustains (M^*, B^*). Q.E.D.

Observe that the constrained maximization problem that defines a competitive consumption strategy is formally the same as the maximization problem that defines an optimal uniform national plan. As a consequence of Proposition 7, we therefore have the following result.

Proposition 8

An allocation of consumption strategies in which each consumer has a competitive consumption strategy is Pareto optimal.

Propositions 7 and 8 show that an allocation of competitive consumption strategies exists and is Pareto optimal. Proposition 6 gives us reason to think that competitive consumption strategies deserve the title "competitive" since they are, in a sense, the best strategies a consumer can accomplish by means of a competitive insurance plan.

There remains some room for doubt. Even if an insurance plan leads to the best achievable strategy, ex ante, can we be sure that in the event of an announced diagnosis, the consumer might not wish to and have the ability to purchase a different amount of medical care than the optimal plan specifies? Thus we might wonder whether a consumer who has a positive initial endowment of bread and who receives an additional amount of bread μ_i after diagnosis i is announced would indeed choose the amount of medical care that was anticipated in the competitive plan. If, say, the diagnosis were that he is almost certain to die if he does not buy a very large amount of medical care and if the competitive plan does not provide a very large amount, might he not then try to spend more on medical care than the competitive plan provides? (Even if he can not raise a large enough amount of bread to pay for a cure, he could possibly bet whatever bread he has in a lottery, such that if he wins the lottery he could afford a cure.) If this were the case, then in order for a competitive life insurance-annuity contract to be workable, not only would it have to include a provision specifying the exact amount of medical care the consumer is to purchase in the event of each diagnosis, but that contract would sometimes have to be enforced, after the medical check-ups, against consumers who may be able to and wish to spend more (or less) than the contracted amount on medical care. Proposition 9, however, establishes that this is not a problem. In fact, from Proposition 9, we see that a competitive equilibrium health insurance plan could take the form of a lump sum payment (positive or negative) the size of which is contingent on the diagnosis. Even if all of the consumer's assets, including expected earnings if he survives and the expected value of his life insurance or annuity plans, could be converted freely at market value after the diagnosis to buy alternative bundles of medical care and bread, the consumer will be best off holding to the competitive consumption strategy that was sustained by the original competitive health insurance plan. A formalization of this result follows.

Proposition 9

Let (M^*, b^{0*}, b^{1*}) be a competitive consumption strategy that is sustained by the insurance plan, (μ^*, b^{*0}, b^{*1}). Then for every event i, a consumer's ex post utility function:

(31) $\qquad \theta_i(m_i) u_l(b^1) + (1 - \theta_i(m_i)) u_0(b^0)$

is maximized at (m_i^*, b^{1*}, b^{0*}) subject to the constraint:

(32) $\qquad \theta_i(m_i)(b^1 - h) + (1 - \theta_i(m_i)) b^0 + p m_i$

$\qquad \leq \mu_i + \bar{b} + \theta_i(m_i) \alpha^1 + (1 - \theta_i(m_i)) \alpha^0.$

Proof:

A competitive consumption strategy (M^*, B^*) maximizes

$$\sum_{i=1}^{n} \pi_i \left[\theta_i(m_i) u_1(b_i^1) + (1 - \theta_i(m_i)) u_0(b_i^0) \right]$$

over all (M, B) such that:

$$\sum_{i=1}^{n} \pi_i [p m_i + \theta_i(m_i)(b_i^1 - h) + (1 - \theta_i(m_i)) b_i^0] \leq \bar{b}.$$

Therefore, if

$$\theta_i(m_i) u_1(b_i^1) + (1 - \theta_i(m_i)) u_0(b_i^0)$$

$$> \theta_i(m_i^*) u_1(b^{1*}) + (1 - \theta_i(m_i^*)) u_0(b_0^*),$$

it must be that

$$p m_i + \theta_i(m_i)(b_i^1 - h) + (1 - \theta_i(m_i)) b_i^0$$

$$> p m_i^* - \theta_i(m_i)(b^{1*} - h) + (1 - \theta_i(m_i)) b^{0*}.$$

Equations (22) and (23) imply that

$$p m_i^* + \theta_i(m_i)(b^{1*} - h) + (1 - \theta_i(m_i)) b^{0*}$$

$$= \mu_i + \theta_i(m_i) \alpha^{1*} + (1 - \theta_i(m_i)) \alpha^{0*}.$$

Substituting from this equation into the last inequality yields the conclusion of Proposition 9.
Q.E.D.

Expression (31) is the expected utility function for a consumer who knows he has diagnosis i. Equation (32) describes the budget that would be available to him if he could make any actuarially fair revision of his bets. One might argue that it is not realistic to suppose all such bets to be available to him. But if this is the case, our interpretation of the result remains intact. If the consumer can not improve on his existing contracts when all actuarially fair rearrangements are possible, then certainly he can not improve his prospects if only some of them are available.

Applications of the Analysis

A health insurance plan, as modelled in this paper, consists of a payment between the insurance company and the consumer, the size of which depends only on the consumer's diagnosed condition. In fact, as we showed in the proof of Proposition 5, if $M^* = (m_1^*, \ldots, m_n^*)$ is an optimal medical care plan, then M^* is sustained by an insurance plan in which the net payment between the insurance company and the consumer in the event of diagnosis i is $m_i^* - \bar{m}^*$ where $\bar{m}^* \equiv \sum_{i=1}^{n} \pi_i m_i^*$ is the expected cost of medical care in an optimal medical strategy. Such a plan amounts to having the consumer pay an insurance premium equal to $\bar{m}^*$ regardless of his health state. In return the consumer receives, contingent on diagnosis i, the amount m_i^* which is the full cost of the efficient level of medical care for someone with diagnosis i.

In most existing medical plans the payment to a consumer is made contingent, not on the diagnosis of his health, but rather on the amount he actually spends on medical care.[2] If consumers were to be reimbursed for the entire cost of any level of medical care they chose to purchase, one would expect that they would want to purchase more than the amount that is efficient. Thus some health insurance plans reimburse essentially all medical costs up to a predetermined maximum amount that depends on the nature of the ailment that is treated. If that maximum were approximately equal to the optimal m_i^* for each diagnosis, then a plan of this type would be equivalent to the efficient diagnosis-specific insurance we have modelled. Even where an insurance plan does not specifically limit the amount to be spent on particular illnesses, it seems likely that restraints are placed on the amount of care by current practice of physicians and hospitals. Thus if doctors were to prescribe the efficient amount, m_i^*, to patients with illness i and not offer them any other alternatives, then a health insurance plan offering full coverage would be efficient.

Many existing health care plans are characterized by coinsurance, where the insurance company pays some fixed fraction of actual medical expenditures. Since the consumer shares in the cost of medical care, he has some incentive to economize on its use. On the other hand, if the consumer does not have full coverage then he is left to bear some residual risk. Coinsurance is analyzed formally by Arrow (1976), who displays necessary conditions for an optimal rate of coinsurance.

For a model of the type we have studied, however, an optimal level of coinsurance is only second best. In Arrow's model, payments from the insurance company to the consumer are required to depend only on the amount of medical care purchased and not on the patient's diagnosis. The second best optimal rate of coinsurance results in too much medical care being purchased and too little risk-pooling relative to the optimum for the model studied here. To see this we notice that with coinsurance, the consumer is able to choose his quantity of medical care while paying less than its full marginal cost. Furthermore, because the full cost is not paid, his consumption level is not fully insured.

In the model presented above, health insurance in which payments are conditional on diagnoses does better than coinsurance. As we showed, not only are consumers left with an incentive to purchase efficient amounts of medical care, they also are able to achieve full risk-pooling.

Before we attribute practical significance to this result, it is appropriate to ask whether the case is prejudiced by the very special structure of our model. Conspicuously missing from this model are costs of information, moral hazard, adverse selection, deception, and fraud. It is reasonable to ask whether, in a model with imperfect information, coinsurance offers advantages that are not apparent in our special model. In a world where information is costly, it might be that medical expenditures are more readily observed and measured than diagnoses. Still, before a physician decides what medical treatment to perform, he has to make a diagnosis. Thus diagnosis-specific insurance should not require the acquisition of knowledge that wasn't all ready available to the doctor. There also may be greater opportunities for fraud in the case of diagnosis-specific insurance, although fraudulent reporting of diagnosis would appear to require cooperation of the patient and physician. However, particularly if second opinions are required, it is not clear that the possibilities for fraudulent reporting of diagnoses are greater than the possibilities for fraudulent reporting of expenditures.

The model we have discussed treats only a single time period. If we were to extend the model to realistically treat the passage of time, the list of possible diagnoses becomes extremely long and complicated, since each time path of medical and diagnostic history would have to be treated as a distinct event. An insurance plan that determines what happens in each case would have to be extremely elaborate. Consumers may find decision-making about such complicated alternatives too difficult to handle intelligently. Coinsurance presents a very easily stated rule determining the payments in each possibility. However, even if an insurance policy that pays different amounts for each possible diagnosis were too complicated to deal with, it should be possible to find simplified approximations to such plans that would not be unreasonably difficult to understand or administer.

A remaining question is whether diagnostic-specific health insurance is better than coinsurance in a world where there is moral hazard and adverse selection. This is an issue that deserves much more careful attention than we have time or space to deal with in this paper.

A separate issue from the question of coinsurance versus diagnostic-specific insurance is whether private competitive health plans would perform as well as governmentally imposed plans. If, for example, it is thought that private consumers typically do not think intelligently and objectively about health-related matters then a case exists for imposed solutions. Where there is moral hazard and adverse selection, little is known about the existence and welfare economic properties of competitive insurance market equilibrium. Thus it might be that in more realistic models, the case for private insurance is less good than in the model presented above.

There is a widespread view that existing private medical insurance plans, as well as medicare and medicaid, are deficient in their provision of "catastrophic health insurance". Private insurance plans typically place a ceiling on the total amount of payments they will make in a year. Private plans, medicare, and medicaid also typically limit the number of days of hospitalization for which they will pay. It seems intuitively appealing to think that health insurance plans that will not pay for the very expensive medical care that would accompany a catastrophic illness are not fulfilling the main function of insurance, namely pooling the risks of big losses for risk-averse consumers. Perhaps the main selling point of the national health insurance bills that have in recent times appeared in Congress, such as the Long-Ribicoff bill and the Kennedy-Mills bill, is the fact that both provide essentially unlimited coverage in the event of catastrophic illness.

The model presented here suggests that a case can be made that an efficient national health insurance plan should put some limits on the amount of medical care offered, even in the event of catastrophic illness. In fact, it is hard to resist making some wild guesses about how high such a ceiling might be. In particular, imagine an illness that one might get with some very small probability, π_i. Suppose that there are two feasible treatments of this illness. One treatment costs a negligible amount and leaves only a small probability that the patient will survive. A second treatment costs $\$c$ and is sure to cure the patient. How large can c be if the optimal medical strategy is to choose the second treatment? The per capita cost of providing all consumers with the second treatment rather than the first will be approximately $\$\pi_i c$. The gain in ex ante survival probability to each consumer from using the second plan rather than the first is just π_i. Thus the per capita cost per unit of survival probability added by choosing the second treatment is just $\$\pi_i c \div \pi_i = \$c$. An efficient medical strategy would choose the more expensive treatment if and only if c is less than the marginal cost at which survival probability can be increased by other means, such as improving the construction of highways, or reducing occupational hazard. These numbers should, in turn, be equal to individual willingness to pay for increased survival probability. Rosen and Thaler (1975) have estimated, from the wage premiums paid for occupational risk of death, a marginal rate of substitution between survival probability and wealth that amounted to between twenty and forty times the annual wage of the population studied. Thus according to their estimates, someone with an annual income of $20,000 should be willing to buy actuarially fair insurance against a relatively unlikely illness that costs $400,000 or possibly up to $800,000 to cure. The benefit ceilings on the existing medical plans that I have heard described are much lower than that. Of course, most medical treatments are not nearly as effective as the one we have just modelled. Typically the treatment will make only a small change in the conditional probability that one survives, and furthermore it may restore one not to full health but to some relatively unpleasant form of invalidism.

One feature of catastrophic illness that is not well described by the analysis so far is the fact that medical care not only takes the form of reducing the probability of death, but may take the form of easing the discomfort of prolonged convalescence or permanent disability. Treatment in such cases may be extremely expensive, and the absence of treatment may be extremely unpleasant. For illnesses of this kind, one might reasonably wonder whether, say, the feature of the current medicare plan that limits the number of days of hospitalization that will be paid for to 150 days is appropriate. The next section deals with this issue in the context of a more general model which allows other states of health besides "healthy" and "dead."

Invalidism and Nursing Care

In this section we consider a model with several different possible conditions of physical well-being. These include various conditions of survival with impaired health as well as death and full health. Again, we suppose that before medical treatments there are several possible medical diagnoses. The probability that someone with a particular diagnosis will reach a given condition of health depends on how much medical treatment he purchases. Formally, we let the possible states of health be denoted by $j = 0, 1, \ldots, \ell$, where states 0 and 1 are death and full health respectively. We let possible diagnoses be denoted by $i = 1, \ldots, n$. The probability that someone receives diagnosis i is π_i and the conditional probability that someone with diagnosis i and the amount, m_i, of medical care will arrive in health state j is $\theta_i^j(m_i)$. Therefore if someone adopts a medical strategy $M = (m_1, \ldots, m_n)$, the probability that he will arrive in health state j is

(33)
$$\Pi^j(M) \equiv \sum_{i=1}^{n} \pi_i \theta_i^j(m_i).$$

Suppose that one's utility depends on the state of his health and the amount of bread that he consumes. Let a bread consumption strategy consist of a vector $b = (b^0, b^1, \ldots, b^n)$ specifying the amount b^j of bread that an individual will consume if he arrives in each health condition j. The expected utility of a consumer with the consumption strategy (M, b) is then:

(34)
$$V(M, b) \equiv \sum_{j=0}^{\ell} \Pi_j(M) u_j(b^j).$$

As in our earlier discussion we can find necessary conditions for an optimal uniform national plan. Suppose that there is an initial endowment of $\bar{b}$ units of bread per capita and that an individual in health state j can produce h^j units of bread. Then the feasibility constraint for a uniform national plan is

(35)
$$\sum_j \Pi^j(M)(b^j - h^j) + p(\bar{M}(M)) = \bar{b}$$

(where $\bar{M}(M)$ is defined in (6).) Maximizing (34) subject to the constraint, (35), yields the following conditions:

(36)
$$u_j'(b^j) = u_1'(b^1) \text{ for } j = 1, \ldots, n$$

and

(37)
$$\sum_{j=0}^{\ell} \left[\left(\frac{u_j(b^j)}{u_1'(b^1)} \right) + h^j - b^j \right] \frac{d\theta_i^j}{dm_i} = p.$$

Since the conditional probabilities of the various outcomes must sum to one, it follow that:

(38)
$$\sum_{j=0}^{\ell} \frac{d\theta_i^j}{dm_i} = 0$$

for each i.

Therefore (37) can be written equivalently as:

(39)
$$\sum_{j=1}^{\ell} \left[\frac{u_j(b^j) - u_0(b^0)}{u_1'(b^1)} (b^j - h^j - b^0 + h^0) \right] \frac{d\theta_i^j}{dm_i} = p.$$

for all i.

Where h^0 is assumed to be zero, it is clear that (39) generalizes (18).

Equations (36) and (39) can be given reasonable economic interpretations without a great deal of difficulty. Furthermore, results analogous to those in the previous sections on the sustainability of an optimum by actuarially fair insurance plans can be found. I think, however, that more insight can be gained by looking carefully at a very special case. In particular, suppose that we let the expected utility representation take the following form:

(40) $\qquad u^0(b^0) = f(\beta_0 + b^0)$: where $\beta_0 > 0$.

(41) $\qquad u^1(b^1) = \alpha^1 + f(b^1)$: where $\alpha_1 > 0$

(42) $\qquad u^2(b^2) = \alpha^2 + f(b^2 - \beta_2)$ if $b^2 > \beta_2$ and

$\qquad\qquad u^2(b^2) = f(0)$ if $b^2 \leq \beta_2$: where $\beta_2 > 0$ and $\alpha^2 < \alpha^1$.

These functional forms were chosen to crudely depict the following features of preferences. The α's represent a pure preference over health states, independent of consumption. The presence of the parameter β_0 in $u^0(\cdot)$ represents the notion that the needs of one's family for consumption goods are reduced if one dies. The particular representation chosen here is entirely for analytic convenience. The parameter β_2 in $u^2(\cdot)$ represents a cost of nursing care that is not needed by healthy people, but without which invalids would be extremely miserable. Once the amount of nursing care, β_2, is provided, the individual enjoys the same *marginal* (but not *total*) utility schedule for consumption as he would if he were healthy.

Assuming that $f''(b) < 0$ for all $b \geq 0$, the first-order conditions in (36) together with the functional specifications in (40)–(42) imply that for the optimal consumption plan:

(43) $\qquad\qquad b^0 = b^1 - \beta_0$ and

(44) $\qquad\qquad b^2 = b^1 + \beta^2$.

Then in an optimal plan it follows that

(45) $\qquad\qquad u(b^0) = u(b^1) - \alpha_1 = u(b^2) - \alpha_2$.

Thus the optimal plan provides the most consumption goods (including nursing care) in the event that the consumer becomes an invalid and the least in the event that he dies.

In the previous section, we offered the suggestion that it may be socially efficient to provide no health insurance for people who have ailments that are extremely expensive to cure. In such cases an efficient plan might allow those who contract such diseases to expire without expensive treatment. The critical level of costs in this case is the amount that the society is willing to spend on saving a life by other means.

The analysis of nursing care is rather different in character. In our model, nursing care has no effect on the probability distribution of health states; it simply makes the state of invalidism less unpleasant. So long as an individual can not choose immediate and painless death as an alternative to invalidism, the amount, β_2, which is efficient for him to spend on nursing care could quite possibly exceed the maximum amount that an efficient plan would spend on curing an illness. Thus the size of efficient "catastrophe insurance" benefits for nursing care might possibly be larger than is appropriate for medical care devoted to "curing".

Returning to our formal analysis, we find another, perhaps surprising, effect. Let us also suppose that the individual will have earnings, h, if he is healthy and zero otherwise. Let there be only one diagnosis and let $\theta^i(m)$ be the probability that one reaches health state i if he spends m on medical treatment. The condition in (39) then reduces to

$$(46) \quad \left[\frac{\alpha_1}{u_1'(b^1)} + (h - \beta_0) \right] \frac{d\theta^1}{dm}$$

$$+ \left[\frac{\alpha_2}{u_1'(b^1)} - (\beta_0 + \beta_2) \right] \frac{d\theta^2}{dm} = p$$

The left side of (46) is the marginal contribution of a unit of medical treatment to utility. This contribution comes in part from its effect on the probability of being healthy and in part from its effect on the probability of being an invalid. Each of these effects in turn consists of two components, a direct effect on utility and a "budget effect". The budget effects register the influence of a change in the probability distribution of health state on the expected value of consumption net of earnings. Typically one would expect the sign of the first term in brackets to be positive, indicating that when both direct and budget effects are accounted for one would prefer to have a higher probability of being healthy and a lower probability of being dead. The sign of the second bracketed term could reasonably be either positive or negative, depending on how unpleasant and how costly it is to be an invalid. It is interesting to notice that even where $\alpha_2 > 0$ so that one prefers the prospect of being an invalid (with the consumption assigned by an optimal plan) to the prospect of being dead, the second bracketed term in (46) could be negative. If this were the case, a medical treatment that increased the probability of being an invalid and lowered the probability of dying, without changing the probability of being healthy, would be socially undesirable even if it were free. The reason, of course, is that in this model being an invalid and being cared for at the efficient level is much more expensive than being dead. Thus if the extra pleasure from the prospect of being a well-cared-for invalid rather than being dead is not large, an investment in achieving this status may not be worthwhile.

Appendix

Proof of Proposition 1

We will prove Proposition 1 with the aid of two lemmas which are in themselves of some general interest. We will need just a bit of additional definitional structure. A "convex symmetric economy" is defined as follows. Let there be m consumers and a set F of feasible allocations. Where $(x_1, \ldots, x_m) \varepsilon F$ is an allocation, x_i is the consumption bundle consumed by consumer i. All consumers, i, have identical concave utility functions $u(x_i)$. The set F is convex and symmetric, where by symmetric we mean that if $(x_1, \ldots, x_n) \varepsilon F$, then $(x_1', \ldots, x_n') \varepsilon F$ if $(x_1', \ldots, x_n')$ can be obtained from $(x_1, \ldots, x_n)$ by reassigning the same commodity bundles to different individuals. (More formally, if $(x_1, \ldots, x_n) \varepsilon F$ and $x_i' = x_{\pi(i)}$ for all i where $\pi(\cdot)$ is a permutation on the set of consumers, then $(x_1', \ldots, x_n') \varepsilon F$.)

An "optimal uniform allocation" is an allocation $(\bar{x}, \bar{x}, \ldots, \bar{x}) \varepsilon F$ that maximizes $u(x)$ subject to the constraint $(x, x, \ldots, x) \varepsilon F$. A "Pareto optimal allocation" is an allocation $(x_1, \ldots, x_n)$ such that there exists no $(x_1', \ldots, x_n') \varepsilon F$ such that $u(x_i') \geqq u(x_i)$ for all i with strict inequality for some i.

Lemma 1

In a convex, symmetric economy, an optimal uniform allocation is Pareto optimal.

Proof:

Let $(\bar{x}, \ldots, \bar{x})$ be an optimal uniform allocation and suppose that for $(x_1^*, \ldots, x_n^*) \varepsilon F$, $u(x_i^*) \geqq u(x_i)$ for all i with strict inequality for some i. Define $\bar{x}^* \equiv \dfrac{1}{m} \sum_{i=1}^{n} x_i^*$. Since F is symmetric and convex, it follows that $(\bar{x}^*, \ldots, \bar{x}^*) \varepsilon F$. But since $u(\cdot)$ is a concave function, $u(\bar{x}^*) \geqq \dfrac{1}{n} \sum_{i=1}^{n} u(x_i^*) > u(\bar{x})$. But this contradicts the hypothesis that $(\bar{x}, \ldots, \bar{x})$ is an optimal uniform allocation. It follows that $(\bar{x}, \ldots, \bar{x})$ is Pareto optimal.
Q.E.D.

If the utility function $V(M, B)$ in the text of our paper were concave and the set of feasible allocations were symmetric and convex, then Proposition 1 would be immediate from Lemma 1. Fortunately (for those who like tricky proofs) matters are not quite this simple. The function $V(M,B)$ is generally not concave under reasonable assumptions, nor is the set of feasible allocations as described in Proposition 1 a convex set. However, by a judicious transformation of variables one can demonstrate the equivalence of the economy of Proposition 1 to a convex, symmetric economy. Using this equivalence, we show that Proposition 1 follows from Lemma 1. In order to accomplish this program we will also need the following result.

Lemma 2

Let $u(x)$ be a concave function with domain the nonnegative orthant in Euclidean n space. For any positive scalar y and any vector x in the domain of $u(\cdot)$, define $V(y,x) \equiv yu(\frac{x}{y})$. Then $V(y,x)$ is a concave function on its domain.

Proof:

For λ between zero and one,

$$V(\lambda y + (1-\lambda)y', \lambda x + (1-\lambda)x')$$

$$= (\lambda y + (1-\lambda)y')u\left(\frac{\lambda x + (1-\lambda)x'}{\lambda y + (1-\lambda)y'}\right)$$

$$= (\lambda y + (1-\lambda)y')u\left(\frac{\lambda y\left(\frac{x}{y}\right) + (1-\lambda)\, y'\, \left(\frac{x'}{y'}\right)}{\lambda y + (1-\lambda)y'}\right)$$

$$\geqq (\lambda y + (1-\lambda)y')\left[\left(\frac{\lambda y}{\lambda y + (1-\lambda)y'}\right)u\left(\frac{x}{y}\right)\right.$$

$$\left. + \frac{(1-\lambda)y'}{\lambda y + (1-\lambda)y'}\, u\left(\frac{x'}{y'}\right)\right]$$

$$= \lambda yu\left(\frac{x}{y}\right) + (1-\lambda)y'u\left(\frac{x'}{y'}\right)$$

$$= \lambda V(y,x) + (1-\lambda)V(y',x').$$

The resulting inequality proves the lemma.
Q.E.D.

Proof of Proposition 1

We make a change of variables by defining a one-to-one transformation T that maps the set of feasible consumption strategies for each individual into its image as follows:

$$T(M,B) = (Y,Z)$$

where

$$(Y,Z) \equiv (y_1, \ldots, y_n, z_1^0, \ldots, z_n^0, z_1^1, \ldots, z_n^1)$$

with:

(A.1) $y_i \equiv \pi_i \theta_i(m_i)$

(A.2) $z_i^0 \equiv \pi_i(1 - \theta_i(m_i))b_i^0$

and

(A.3) $z_i^1 \equiv \pi_i \theta_i(m_i)(b_i^1 - h).$

To see that T is one-to-one we notice that (for predetermined $(\pi_1, \ldots, \pi_n)$ and h) the equations A.1–A.3 can be inverted to solve uniquely for the m's and b's in terms of the y's and z's. In particular, we have:

(A.4) $m_i = \theta_i^{-1}\left(\dfrac{y_i}{\pi_i}\right)$

(A.5) $b_i^0 = \dfrac{z_i^{\,0}}{\pi_i - y_i}$

(A.6) $b_i^1 = \dfrac{z_i}{y_i} + h$

Our objective is now to show that where we describe the economy constructed in the text of the paper in terms of the transformed variables, we have a convex, symmetric economy. Using equations (5) of the text and A.4, A.5 and A.6, we can write:

(A.7) $V^*(Y,Z) \equiv V(T^{-1}(Y,Z)) = \displaystyle\sum_{i=1}^{n} y_i u_1\left(\dfrac{z_i^1}{y_i} + h\right)$

$+ \displaystyle\sum_{i=1}^{n} (\pi_i - y_i) u_0\left(\dfrac{z_i^{\,0}}{\pi_i - y_i}\right).$

From the assumption that u_1 and u_0 are concave functions, from Lemma 2, and from the fact that the sum of concave functions is concave, it follows that $V^*(Y, Z)$ is a concave function.

We next rewrite the feasibility constraint of Proposition 1 in terms of the variables (Y, Z). Using (A.4)–(A.6) and slightly rearranging terms we can describe the feasible set as follows. A typical allocation is denoted $(Y^1, Z^1, \ldots Y^m, Z^m)$ where consumer k's utility is $V^*(Y^k, Z^k)$. The set of feasible allocations is:

$$(A.8) \qquad F^* = \{(Y^1, Z^1, \ldots, Y^m, Z^m)$$

$$\mid \sum_{k=1}^{m} \sum_{i=1}^{n} \left(z_i^1 + z_i^0 + p\,\pi_i\,\theta_i^{-1}\left(\frac{y_i}{\pi_i} \right) \right) \le m\bar{b}\}.$$

Clearly F^* is a symmetric set. Since $\theta_i(\cdot)$ is assumed a concave function for each i, $\theta_i^{-1}(\cdot)$ must be a convex function. It is then easy to show that F^* is a convex set.

The economy in which consumers have utility functions $V^*(Y, Z)$ and in which the set of feasible allocations is described by A.8 must therefore be a convex, symmetric economy which we will call the "derived economy." If $(\bar{M}, \bar{B})$ is an optimal uniform national plan, then $V(\bar{M}, \bar{B}) \ge V(M', B')$ if the allocation in which all consumers have M', B' is feasible. Where $(\bar{Y}, \bar{Z}) = T(\bar{M}, \bar{B})$ it follows from our definitions that $(\bar{Y}, \bar{Z})$ is an optimal uniform allocation in the derived economy. From Lemma 1 it follows that $(\bar{Y}, \bar{Z})$ is also Pareto optimal for the derived economy. But it is then easy to show that $(\bar{M}, \bar{B}) = T^{-1}(\bar{Y}, \bar{Z})$ must be Pareto optimal for the original economy.
Q.E.D.

Notes

1. Here and subsequently we proceed as if the proportion of the population having each diagnosis takes on exactly its expected value. Of course the "law of large numbers" tells us only that this proportion comes arbitrarily close to its expected value with arbitrarily high probability for a large enough population. If we were to pursue this more accurate representation carefully, we would find that for large populations, the residual social risk can be shared, so as to have negligible effects on individual utilities. Thus our shortcut has a negligible effect on the results, but much eases exposition.

2. Useful discussions of a variety of existing and proposed private and public health plans can be found in Davis (1975) and Reed and Cass (1970).

References

Arrow, K.J. 1976. Welfare analysis of changes in health coinsurance rates. in R.N. Rosett, ed., *The role of health insurance in the health services sector.* NBER Conference Series, No. 27. New York: National Bureau of Economic Research.

Davis, K. 1975. *National health insurance.* Washington: The Brookings Institution.

Nordquist G., and Wu S. 1976. The joint demand for health insurance and preventative medicine in Rosett, op. cit.

Reed L.S., and Carr, W. 1970. The benefit structure of private health insurance, 1968. Research Report No. 32, Social Security Administration. Washington: U.S. Government Printing Office.

Rosen, S., and Thaler, R. 1975. The value of saving a life: evidence from the labor market. In Nestor E. Terleckyi, ed., *Household Production and Consumption.* NBER Studies in Income and Wealth, Volume 40. New York: Columbia University Press.

List of Contributors

Drs. Lee and Alexandra Benham
Division of Health Care Research
Washington University School of
    Medicine
4566 Scott Avenue, Box 8113
St. Louis, MO 63110

Professor Theodore Bergstrom
Department of Economics
University of Michigan
Ann Arbor, MI 48104

Professor Victor R. Fuchs
National Bureau of Economic
    Research
204 Junipero Serra Boulevard
Stanford, CA 94305

Dr. Michael Grossman
National Bureau of Economic
    Research
269 Mercer Street
New York, NY 10003

Jeffrey Harris, M.D.
7 Spruce Court
Boston, MA 02108

Dr. Will Manning
RAND Corporation
1700 Main Street
Santa Monica, CA 90406

Dr. Joseph Newhouse
RAND Corporation
1700 Main Street
Santa Monica, CA 90406

Professor Sherwin Rosen
Department of Economics
University of Chicago
1126 East 59th Street
Chicago, IL 60637

Dr. Mark Rosenzweig
Department of Economics
University of Minnesota
Minneapolis, MN 55455

Professor David Salkever
School of Hygiene and Public Health
Johns Hopkins University
615 North Wolfe
Baltimore, MD 21205

Professor T. Paul Schultz
Economic Growth Center
Box 1987 Yale Station
New Haven, CT 06520

Dr. Robert A. Shakotko
Department of Economics
Columbia University
810 International Affairs
New York, NY 10027

Professor Donald Shepard
Center for Analysis of Health
   Practices
Harvard School of Public Health
677 Huntington Avenue
Boston, MA 02115

Professor Paul Taubman
Department of Economics
3718 Locust Walk CR
University of Pennsylvania
Philadelphia, PA 19104

Dr. John E. Ware, Jr.
Senior Social Psychologist
RAND Corporation
1700 Main Street
Santa Monica, CA 90406

Professor Richard Zeckhauser
Kennedy School of Government
Harvard University
Cambridge, MA 02138

Author Index

Subject Index

Age: and health, 125, 126; and maternal education, 26, regressions of health status on, 114

Age-specific mortality: changes in, 290–93; rates for white males, 267

American College of Obstetricians and Gynecologists, 17

American Psychiatric Association, 206, 207

Annuities, 306

Bayesian sufficiency, 189

Becker-Lewis-Tomes interactive model, 55

Birth characteristics: and estimates of marginal products of inputs at sample means, 76; and socioeconomic variables and health programs, 78–81; production function estimates, 70–78; white population, 89–89

Birth order and child health, 80

Birthweight: adjusted for neonatal mortality rate, 40; and gestational age, 35; and health-related behavior of mothers, 81; and neonatal mortality, 38; and relation to neonatal mortality, 39; by gestation, 64; in relation to neonatal care and month of initiation, 42; normalized for gestation, 65; production function estimates for white population, 90–91; production function estimates normalized for gestation, 74–75; specific mortality and relation to prenatal care, 41

Black mothers, 15; and gestation period, 78; and live births, 18; and termination of pregnancy, 26; sample characteristics of pregnancies, 24

Catastrophic health insurance, 314

CAT scanners, 279

Center for Health Administration Studies, 144

Central Limit Theorem, 156

Certificate of Need, 275

Child health: and birth order, 80; and delay in seeking prenatal care, 80; and parental behavior factors, 60; and smoking during pregnancy, 80

Child health endowments and family consumption decisions, 224

Child health input, demand equation estimates, 68–70

Child health variables: effects on maternal labor supply and earnings, 234–35; effects on paternal labor supply and earnings, 237–39

Children and chronic health conditions, 222

Children's disabilities: and maternal labor, 223; and parental labor supply, 223

Chronic health conditions and children, 220

Cigarette smoking and socioeconomic variables, 112

Cobb-Douglas case, 67, 68

Coinsurance, 166, 312

Commission on the Cost of Medical Care, 275

Cost-effectiveness paradigm and health intervention, 271